# 101
# Clinical Cases in Emergency Room

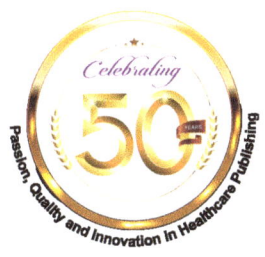

# 101
# Clinical Cases in Emergency Room

## Second Edition

*Editor*

**Badar M Zaheer** MD

Board Certified in Emergency Medicine and Family Medicine
Associate Professor
UIC College of Medicine
Chicago, Illinois, USA

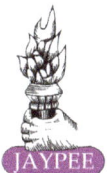

**JAYPEE BROTHERS MEDICAL PUBLISHERS**
*The Health Sciences Publisher*
New Delhi | London

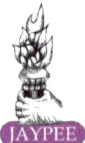 **Jaypee Brothers Medical Publishers (P) Ltd.**

**Headquarters**
Jaypee Brothers Medical Publishers (P) Ltd
4838/24, Ansari Road, Daryaganj
New Delhi 110 002, India
Phone: +91-11-43574357
Fax: +91-11-43574314
E-mail: jaypee@jaypeebrothers.com

**Overseas Office**
JP Medical Ltd
83 Victoria Street, London
SW1H 0HW (UK)
Phone: +44 20 3170 8910
Fax: +44 (0)20 3008 6180
E-mail: info@jpmedpub.com

Website: www.jaypeebrothers.com
Website: www.jaypeedigital.com

© 2020, Jaypee Brothers Medical Publishers

The views and opinions expressed in this book are solely those of the original contributor(s)/author(s) and do not necessarily represent those of editor(s) of the book.

All rights reserved. No part of this publication may be reproduced, stored or transmitted in any form or by any means, electronic, mechanical, photocopying, recording or otherwise, without the prior permission in writing of the publishers.

All brand names and product names used in this book are trade names, service marks, trademarks or registered trademarks of their respective owners. The publisher is not associated with any product or vendor mentioned in this book.

Medical knowledge and practice change constantly. This book is designed to provide accurate, authoritative information about the subject matter in question. However, readers are advised to check the most current information available on procedures included and check information from the manufacturer of each product to be administered, to verify the recommended dose, formula, method and duration of administration, adverse effects and contraindications. It is the responsibility of the practitioner to take all appropriate safety precautions. Neither the publisher nor the author(s)/editor(s) assume any liability for any injury and/or damage to persons or property arising from or related to use of material in this book.

This book is sold on the understanding that the publisher is not engaged in providing professional medical services. If such advice or services are required, the services of a competent medical professional should be sought.

Every effort has been made where necessary to contact holders of copyright to obtain permission to reproduce copyright material. If any have been inadvertently overlooked, the publisher will be pleased to make the necessary arrangements at the first opportunity. The **CD/DVD-ROM** (if any) provided in the sealed envelope with this book is complimentary and free of cost. **Not meant for sale.**

**Inquiries for bulk sales may be solicited at:** jaypee@jaypeebrothers.com

*101 Clinical Cases in Emergency Room*

*First Edition:* 2014
*Second Edition:* 2020

ISBN: 978-93-5270-333-3

**Dedicated to**

*The memory of my father Dr Abdul Hafeez who used to say, "be an asset to your community, society, and nation at large and make a difference in somebody's life." I'll consider myself fortunate to follow in your footsteps.*

# Preface to the Second Edition

Just as the field of emergency medicine has evolved over the last several years, we have sought to evolve and enhance our understanding of this exciting field with the second edition of this book. We have worked hard to update you with the most common emergencies and the most up-to-date methods to deal with those emergencies.

In this edition, we have laid out the management of critical emergencies such as STEMI, non-STEMI, and "unstable angina". With the rapid growth of STEMI centers, the protocols and guidelines are very precise allowing emergency providers to save more lives. We have also included the new classification guidelines of "myocardial infarction" with an explanation of the different types of MI. Additionally, stroke guidelines are clearer than ever before, and similarly have allowed improved patient outcomes. Finally, we know that sepsis is the leading cause of mortality in the developing world. Thus, we have sought in this book to increase understanding of sepsis management and the rule of 1-1-1. Our hope with this second edition is that you learn to manage these complex emergencies that we have worked to simplify.

We know that students learn best with visual aids, thus we have gone to great lengths to add visual diagrams, tables, and organizers to present the information in a manner that will reinforce learning. In simplifying the complexities of medical emergencies with visual aids, this book serves as a practical manual/handbook for the successful clinical management of emergencies we come across in daily life.

**Badar M Zaheer**

# Preface to the First Edition

Emergency care, a staple of Western medicine, remains severely inadequate in many areas of the developing world. Every minute, thousands of people die from a lack of basic emergency services. Even in these resource-limited settings, many causes of injury and death can be prevented or treated with simple procedural skills and a knowledge of core priorities in critical care. The assessment and treatment of patients in many acute medical and trauma situations should be based on the ABCD (airway, breathing, circulation, and deformity) protocol. With 25 years of personal ER experience and updated guidelines in emergency care, I have written *101 Clinical Cases in Emergency Room* for training the reader to efficiently address immediate life-threatening concerns so as not to waste valuable time in trying to reach a final diagnosis. This book can be easily understood by all healthcare providers and first-responders in an emergency setting, including physicians, nurses, technicians, assistants, and students.

This book includes 101 real-world emergency cases grouped into 21 chapters based on body systems and other relevant scenarios. Each case is accompanied by tables, charts, and simple illustrations to clarify the content and facilitate the learning process. "Clinical pearls and pitfalls" are provided to emphasize the importance of "cannot-miss" diagnoses and the legal consequences of failing to identify these conditions. I also mention a few relevant historical cases that make the subject interesting and more memorable. Standard guidelines of treatment are stressed, and fundamental concepts in emergency medicine (e.g. the golden hour of opportunity in stroke and MI management) are discussed to optimize patient care and quality-of-life. I have included a chapter on preventable injuries like drownings and burns from fires, chemicals, and electrical sources. The last chapter deals with disaster management, triaging techniques, and the training of healthcare workers for efficient management of mass casualties. I also stress the importance of coordination between law enforcement and local communities for primary prevention of these disasters.

Each case study is designed to train readers to identify the acute issue and quickly formulate an appropriate treatment plan, especially in the setting of limited resources seen in developing nations. I hope this book is an enjoyable read compared to the average textbook, but at the same time a valuable resource for up-to-date information on the care of critically ill patients.

If I can save a single life with my educational points, the purpose of this book will be fulfilled.

**Badar M Zaheer**

# Acknowledgments

Saving a life is like saving a nation, as commanded by our faith, and I am thankful to our Creator for giving me this opportunity to serve his creations.

First of all, I would like to thank my family for their support and encouragement throughout the process. My wife, Qudsia Zaheer MD and our children Fatima Zaheer MD, Zubair Zaheer DO, Naima Zaheer MS, and Zaki Zaheer MS (for his surprising help in preparing for board questions) as well as my mother Nurjehan for her prayers and blessings. Special note to Lisan Zahirsha as well.

To my professional mentors Judith E Tintinalli MD, author of Emergency Medicine Manual from University of North Carolina and Beatrice Hoffman from Johns Hopkins for their encouraging remarks.

*To my teachers who have inspired me:* First of all my elder brother Khutub M Uddin MD, my professional mentor Khaja Ahmed Shamsi MD, my primary school teacher Syed Sirajuddin, and my teachers from medical school, Late TP Gopinath MD and the late Prasad Rao MS who influenced me through their dedication and love for teaching medicine.

Special thanks to Amer Aldeen MD and Sh Zakaria Khudeira.

This book was only possible due to the continuous support of Jaypee Brothers Medical Publishers, New Delhi, India.

# Contents

1. Head and Neck — 1
2. Chest — 31
3. Abdomen — 119
4. Pelvic and Urogenital — 138
5. Musculoskeletal — 143
6. Neurology — 164
7. Endocrine — 201
8. Psychiatric Emergencies — 215
9. Environmental Injuries, Toxicology, and Animal Bites — 220
10. Sexually Transmitted Infections — 270
11. Pediatrics — 275
12. Obstetrics and Gynecology — 302
13. Ear, Nose and Throat Emergencies — 310
14. Hematology/Oncology — 323
15. Trauma in Extremes of Age — 330
16. Infectious Diseases — 341
17. Renal Emergencies — 346
18. Medical Errors — 352
19. Water and Electrolyte Imbalance — 356
20. Ocular Emergencies — 374
21. Disaster Management — 380

Index — 387

# CHAPTER 1

# Head and Neck

## CASE STUDY 1: SUBDURAL HEMATOMA (SDH)

*I would especially like to commend the physician who, in acute diseases, by which the bulk of mankind are cutoff, conducts the treatment better than others.*

—Hipporcrates

### CASE HISTORY

A 55-year-old male presents to a small rural emergency department (ED) after a fall. The patient was attempting to fish during a beer festival event by standing on a rock. The patient slipped on the rock and subsequently fell and struck his head. On his arrival to the ED, his Glasgow coma scale (GCS) is 13. His alcohol level is 200 mg/dL. His complete blood count (CBC) is within normal limits, and urine toxicology screen is negative. The patient's vitals are unremarkable, so it is deemed safe to obtain computed tomography (CT) scan of the head. A noncontrast CT scan reveals a subdural hematoma. A neurosurgeon at a nearby hospital is contacted, and the patient is immediately airlifted to the awaiting operating room for surgery.

Figures 1 and 2 represent the subdural hematoma and its treatment.

### DISCUSSION

Subdural hematoma is the most common cause of intracranial mass lesion.[1,2] It is defined as a collection of blood on the surface of the brain which may be acute, subacute, or chronic. The acute type is usually caused by a high-speed impact to the skull. It is caused by ruptured bridging veins, which occurs during the impact of high acceleration injuries, which, in turn, is caused by high strained falls and assaults.[3] Risk factors include chronic alcoholism, epilepsy, coagulopathy, arachnoid cysts, anticoagulant therapy, cardiovascular disease, thrombocytopenia, and diabetes. The cause is secondary to the shearing forces of small surface or bridging blood vessels. Subdural hematoma has

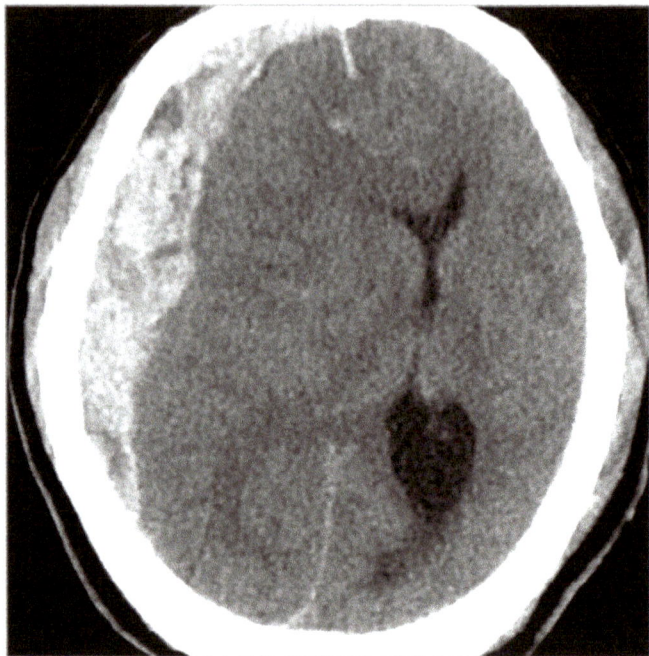

**Fig. 1:** Subdural hematoma.
*Source:* http://www.ncbi.nlm.nih.gov/pmc/articles.

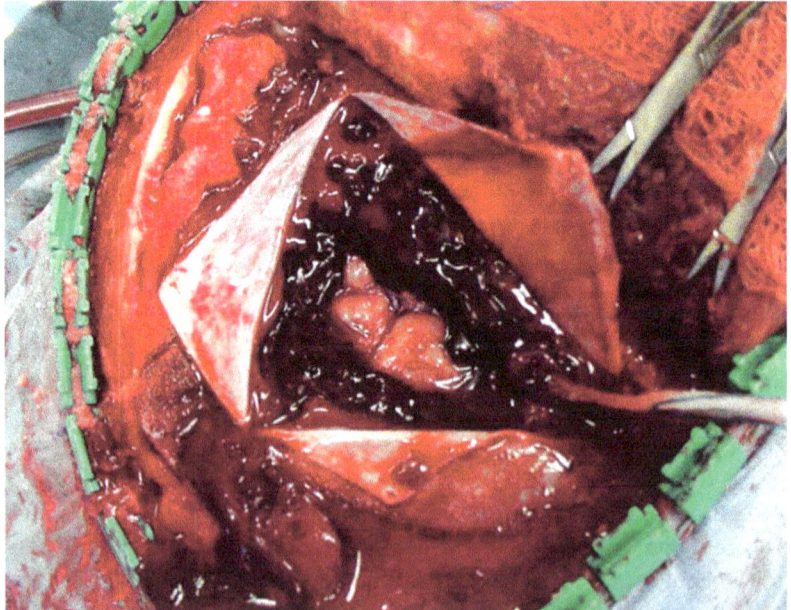

**Fig. 2:** Chronic subdural hematoma treatment.
*Source:* Available online from http://www.health-reply.com/chronic-subdural-hematoma-treatment/.

**Table 1:** Comparison between different intracranial hemorrhages.

| | Epidural hematoma | Subdural hematoma | Subarachnoid hemorrhage |
|---|---|---|---|
| Vessel involved | Arterial bleeding | Venous bleeding | Arterial–venous |
| Presentation | Lucid interval | Progressively worsening headache | Thunderclap headache, "worst headache of my life" |
| CT | Elliptical/lens shaped | Crescent | Star shaped, "The Lone Star Flag of Texas" |
| Prognosis | Immediately fatal, if not evacuated | Slower progression than epidural fatal | Fatal if not treated |
| Risk factors | None | Elder persons, alcoholics, Alzheimer patients | Family history of Berry aneurysms |
| CT images (Figs. 3 to 5) | Fig. 3: Epidural hematoma. | Fig. 4: Subdural hematoma. | Fig. 5: Subarachnoid hemorrhage. |

a distinctive appearance on CT compared to epidural hematoma as it may appear as a crescent-shaped mass (Table 1). The risk of severe brain damage is much higher than with epidural hematoma, and increased intracranial pressure (ICP) is correlated with a worse prognosis (Fig. 1).

Presentation, which is usually gradual in onset, may include decreased level of consciousness, headache, difficulty in walking, cognitive dysfunction, personality changes, motor deficit, and aphasia. It is essential to consult a neurosurgeon as soon as a subdural hematoma is suspected because the definitive treatment will require craniotomy.

Initial management should include the monitoring of airway, breathing, and circulation (ABC), obtaining CT head, monitoring GCS, and obtaining laboratory tests values, such as that of CBC, coagulation profile, basal metabolic profile (BMP), type and screen, and drug and alcohol screening, to correlate clinical findings. Management should be done as discussed previously for decreasing ICP: start normal saline; elevate head of bed; optimized hyperventilation should be there, and mannitol should be administered. Consider the procedure of creating burr holes in the cases of rapid deterioration. Always maintain hemostasis when patients have been taking anticoagulants. Intubate if GCS is <12.

Modern term for trepanation is craniotomy which is used for epidural and subdural hematoma (Figs. 6 and 7).

There is a 30% reduction in mortality if surgery is done within the first hour. Prognosis depends on initial neurological examination, sex, postoperative ICP and multimodality-evoked potentials.[4]

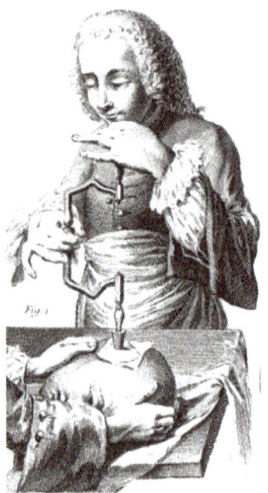

**Fig. 6:** 18th century French illustration of trepanation.
*Source:* http://en.wikipedia.org/wiki/Trepanning.

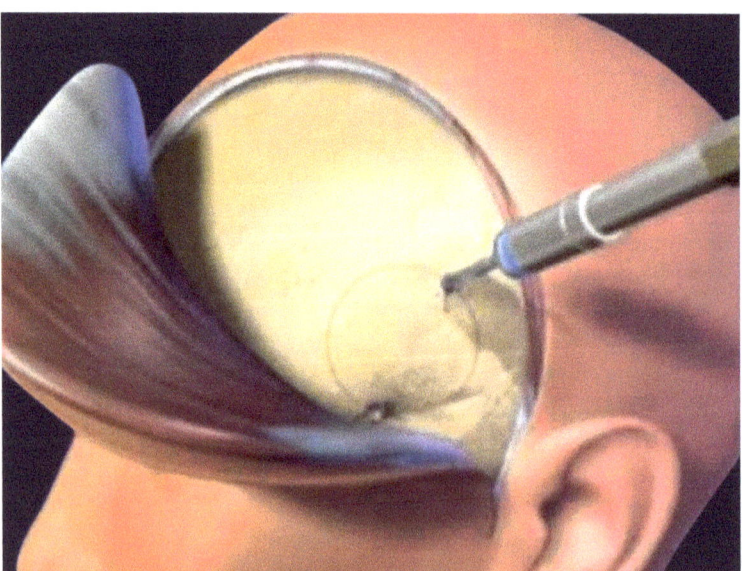

**Fig. 7:** Modern term for trepanation is craniotomy which is used for epidural and subdural hematoma.
*Source:* Watch this video for a demonstration on traditional pterional craniotomy by Hrayr Shahinian, MD: California, USA. http://www.youtube.com/watch?v=qfRelImEEfU.

Head and Neck

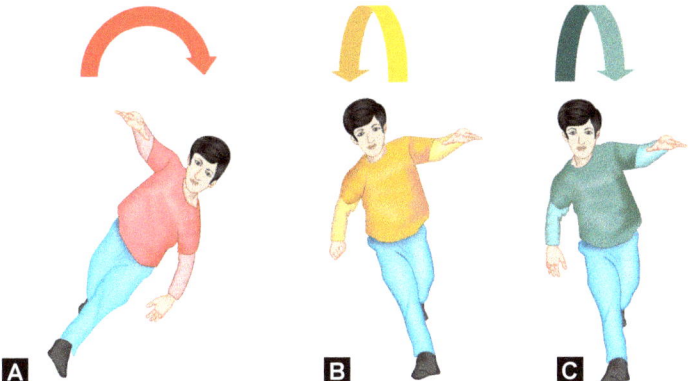

**Figs. 8A to C:** Mechanism of fall in children: (A) Fall sideways highest risk; (B) Fall backwards moderate risk; (C) Fall forward lowest risk.

## Learning Points for Reading CT of the Head

Remember the mnemonic: ABBBC, when reading the CT head.
- *Air sacs*: Sinuses; mastoid air cells fractures, and infections
- *Bones*
- *Blood*: Different types of hemorrhages
- *Brain*: Infarction, edema, masses, and mid-line shift
- *CSF spaces*: Ventricles, atrophy, hydrocephalus, edema.

## PRACTICE POINT

If our paramedics and the emergency staff refer the cases with subdural hemorrhage to a nearest facility which has the capacity to diagnose and drain the hematoma by a neurosurgeon, the mortality can be significantly reduced.

In children, if the child falls forward, there is less risk of hemorrhage. However, if the child falls backwards, it is moderate risk. Moreover, if the child falls on the side, it is considered severe risk (Figs. 8A to C).

- Maintain inline immobilization to protect the cervical spine to avoid immediate quadriplegia and establish a definitive airway. Paramedics should know how important it is to avoid legal ramifications for improper care and transport of head injury patients.
- With severe head injuries it is important to avoid hypotension.
- For ALL injured Rh-neg pregnant women Rh-immunoglobulin should be given.
- With ALL head injuries it is important to be aware of the signs and symptoms of increased intracranial pressure (ICP). These symptoms include irregular respiration, decreased pulse, but increased blood pressure, known as Cushing's Triad. Additional symptoms include severe headache, vomiting without nausea and altered mental status (AMS).
- Nobody should miss unequal pupils on exam because it requires immediate neurosurgical intervention.

## REFERENCES

1. Yadav YR, Parihar V, Namdev H, Bajaj J. Chronic subdural hematoma. Asian J Neurosurg. 2016;11(4):330-342. doi:10.4103/1793-5482.145102.
2. Advanced trauma life support (ATLS®). J Trauma and Acute Care Surgery. 2013;74(5):1363-1366. doi:10.1097/ta.0b013e31828b82f5.
3. Gennarelli TA, Thibault LE. Biomechanics of acute subdural hematoma [Abstract]. J Trauma—Inj Infect Crit Care. 1982;22. Retrieved December 14, 2016.
4. Seelig JM, Becker DP, Miller JD, et al. Traumatic acute subdural hematoma. New Eng J Med. 1981;304(25):1511-1518. doi:10.1056/nejm198106183042503

## FURTHER READING

1. http://www.youtube.com/watch?v=qfRellmEEfU.

## CASE STUDY 2: EPIDURAL HEMATOMA (EDH)

*It is common to overlook what is nearby keeping the eye fixed on something remote.*

—Samuel Johnson

## CASE HISTORY

A 10-year-old school boy presents to the emergency department (ED) after being attacked by a gang. The boy reports that five individuals gathered around the boy and beat him with baseball bats. Upon initial presentation to the ED, the boy is neurologically intact with normal mentation and Glasgow coma scale (GCS) is 15. Initial evaluation includes unremarkable vital signs and some bruising throughout on examination. While finishing the remainder of the examination, the patient becomes stuporous and comatose. Repeat GCS has decreased to 7 and pupils are now sluggish to react. Vitals are reassessed as temperature 37°C (98.6°F) blood pressure 180/90 mm Hg, pulse rate 50 bpm, respiratory rate 12 breaths/min, and $O_2$ saturation level 93%. The patient is intubated and taken immediately for computed tomography (CT) which reveals an epidural hematoma in the right temporal region. A neurosurgeon is called, and the patient is taken immediately to the operation room for surgical evacuation of the bleed. What type of bleeding is this patient likely to have?

## FEATURES

Epidural hematoma is represented in Figures 1 and 2.

Epidural hematoma is defined as a collection of blood between the dura mater and the skull. It is most commonly caused by blow to the head. Generally, the underlying brain tissue is spared which makes the overall prognosis extremely good if an immediate action is taken.

Head and Neck

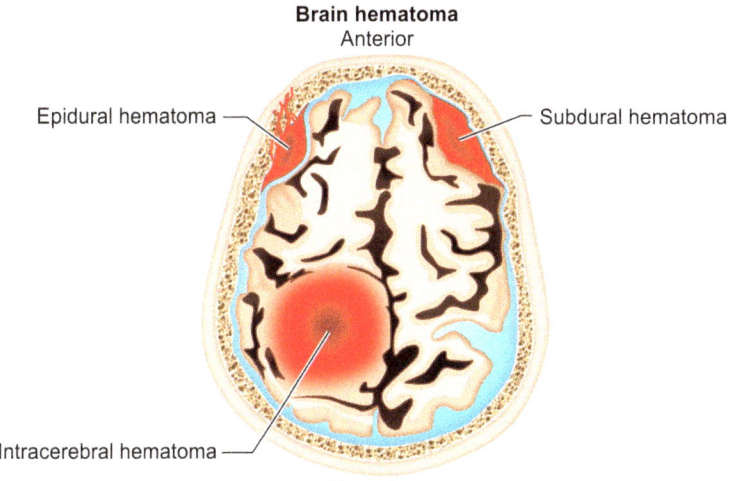

**Fig. 1:** Epidural hematoma.
*Source:* Available online from http://www.images.emedicinehealth.com/images eMedicine Health/illustrations/brain-hematoma.jpg; Copyright: 2009, MedicineNet, Inc.

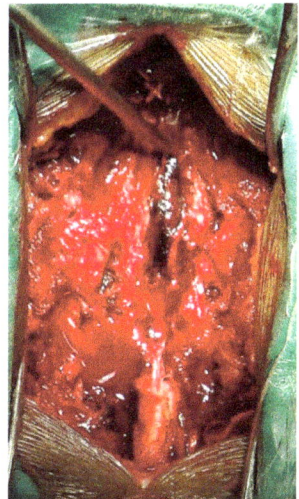

**Fig. 2:** Neurosurgical exposure of the epidural hematoma.
*Source:* Singh P, Joseph B. Paraplegia in a patient with dengue. Neurol India. 2010;58:962-3. Available from: http://www.neurologyindia.com/text.asp? [serial online].

## PRESENTATION

Only 20% of patients have the classic lucid interval. Patients may have severe headache, vomiting, or seizures. Signs of increased intracranial pressure include hypertension, bradycardia, and bradypnea. The medical professional should look for signs of herniation which would include a triad of coma, fixed pupils, and decerebrate posturing in conjunction with contralateral hemiplegia.

It occurs most commonly in the temporoparietal region due to location of the meningeal artery.

## MANAGEMENT

Protect the airway by intubating, maintain blood pressure, elevate head of bed, consider optimized hyperventilation, mannitol to reduce cerebral edema, and phenytoin should be given for seizure prophylaxis. Early neurosurgical consult is an absolute requirement.

### Conservative Method

A study of nonoperative management of epidural hematomas (EDH) and subdural hematomas (SDH) is done to investigate whether it is safe in lesions measuring ≤1 cm, (http://www.ncbi.nlm.nih.gov/pubmed/17693838) shows that EDH or SDH <1 cm thick can be safely managed nonoperatively unless there is concomitant cerebral edema.

### Surgical Approach

Early involvement of a neurosurgeon is the most important duty of the emergency room physician. Surgical intervention is necessary for larger to intermediate epidural hematoma. It needs continuous careful individualized clinical approach based on radiological parameters: like thickness, midline shift, mass effect, and EDH location. For example, one of the studies, where a thickness of EDH >18 mm, a midline shift >4 mm, and a moderate to severe mass effect, and the location fairly predicted the outcome of epidural hematoma.

The surgical approach depends on the age, sex, GC score (Glasgow coma scale) mechanism of injury, interval between injury, and the CT scan findings.

### PRACTICE POINT

A recent high-profile case of epidural hemorrhage occurred in 2009 when actress Natasha Richardson (Fig. 3) suffered a head injury while skiing.

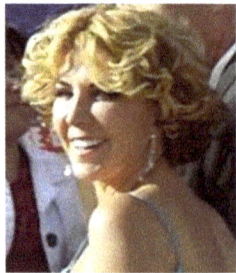

**Fig. 3:** Natasha Richardson: English actress of stage and screen who unfortunately died of epidural hemorrhage.
*Source:* Wikipedia.

After the injury, Natasha experienced a lucid interval and dismissed the paramedics and ambulance assistance. She refused the medical care twice, but 3 h later, she developed a headache and was taken to a local hospital. Despite the best efforts of physicians and transfer to two other hospitals, she died the following day. Autopsy revealed that she had suffered an epidural hematoma due to blunt impact to the head. This case has helped raise the public awareness of the dangers of head trauma and has provided a needed reminder that headache can be the first sign of a major pathology. During the lucid interval, patients may be reluctant to agree to testing or hospitalization, emphasizing the importance of education on the dangers of epidural hematoma.

## FURTHER READING

1. http://www.ncbi.nlm.nih.gov/pubmed/17693838.
2. http://www.ncbi.nlm.nih.gov/pubmed/9348150.
3. Natasha Richardson. Wikipedia. http://en.wikipedia.org/wiki/Natasha_Richardson. Published July 13, 2018. Accessed July 17, 2018

## CASE STUDY 3: SUBARACHNOID HEMORRHAGE

*If you cannot make a judgment or a decision in 30 seconds, do not become an ER doctor.*

—Badar M Zaheer

## CASE HISTORY

A 30-year-old male presents to the emergency room (ER) and mentions to have experienced the worst headache of his life. The patient was sitting down for dinner after work, when all of a sudden he had severe pain in his head. The pain has been persistent for the last hour despite taking over-the-counter pain medications at home. The patient does not have any history of headaches in the past. He has faced no other medical problems in the past. He recalls that one of his relatives died suddenly at a young age from a bleed in his brain. The patient has smoked about a pack of cigarettes a day for the last 15 years. Vitals are as follows: temperature 38.5°C, blood pressure 190/100 mm Hg, pulse rate 120 bpm, respiratory rate 25 breaths/min, and $O_2$ saturation level 93% on room air. On physical examination, patient's alertness is waxing and waning. Emergency computed tomography (CT) has revealed subarachnoid hemorrhage (SAH). Nimodipine is started to control blood pressure. The head of bed is elevated to decrease intracranial pressure (ICP). Emergent neurosurgical consultation is obtained for evacuation of the bleed.

## DISCUSSION

By definition, SAH is bleeding into the subarachnoid space which is the space between the brain and the tissues that cover it. Causes include arteriovenous malformation, bleeding disorders, cerebral aneurysms, head injuries, idiopathic, and use of blood thinners. SAH from injuries is more common in the elderly population. In younger individuals, the most common cause is motor vehicle accidents. Bleeding from aneurysmal rupture happens in about 40–50/100,000 people over the age of 30 years. Risk factors include aneurysm in other blood vessels, fibromuscular dysplasia and other connective tissue disorders, high blood pressure, history of polycystic kidney disease, and smoking. Family history of aneurysms also increases your risk.[1]

Clinically, the main symptom is a severe, sudden onset of headache near the back of the head. The pain may have started with a "popping" or "snapping" feeling also described as "thunderclap headache." Other symptoms include altered mental status, photophobia, mood and personality changes, myalgia, especially in the neck and shoulders, nausea and vomiting, loss of sensation, seizures, neck stiffness, vision problems including double vision, blind spots, vision loss, eyelid drooping, and pupil size difference. Physical findings may include a stiff neck, focal neurologic deficits, and/or decreased eye movements. Testing may include lumbar puncture, cerebral angiography, CT head, transcranial Doppler ultrasounds, magnetic resonance imaging (MRI), and magnetic resonance angiogram (MRA).

Goals of treatment are to repair the cause of bleeding, relieve symptoms, and prevent complications, such as brain damage and seizures. Consultation from neurosurgeon should be done. Interventions may include a craniotomy and aneurysm clipping to remove pressure on the brain and close the aneurysm. Endovascular coiling may be used to reduce the risk of the aneurysm bleeding any further. In the absence of aneurysm, treat the increased ICP and monitor airway, breathing, and circulation. Blood pressure should be controlled. Maintain systolic blood pressure to <160 mm Hg or maintain mean arterial pressure (MAP) of 110 mm Hg. Use nimodipine to prevent vasospasm in all patients.

Prognosis depends on the location and severity of the bleeding. The more complications, the worse the prognosis. Older age is also a poor indicator of outcome. Complications include repeated bleeding, coma, or death. Other complications may occur as a result of the surgery, medication, seizures, or stroke. New guidelines have been developed by the University of Ottawa for managing patients with suspected SAH.

The study applies to patients with nontraumatic headache and suggests them that they need further workup. The patient groups consist of
- Age over 40 years, neck pain or stiffness, witnessed loss of consciousness, and onset occurs on exertion
- Arrival by emergency medical services, age over 45 years, vomiting at least once, diastolic blood pressure higher than 100 mm Hg

- Arrival by emergency medical services, age from 45 years to 55 years, neck pain or stiffness, systolic blood pressure higher than 160 mm Hg.

Although these guidelines are promising in identifying patients at the highest risk for SAH, results must be validated in other setting before being put into widespread use.

To understand the surgical procedure, please watch the YouTube video: https://www.youtube.com/watch?v=Ji7fohBEPnM.

## LESSONS TO LEARN FROM A LEGAL POINT

A patient may present to the emergency department with a headache and may be treated as sinusitis, especially where there are residency-teaching programs. Unless we have a high index of suspicion for headaches, we may miss a SAH, central nervous system tumors, etc. Diagnosis should not be done hastily, especially when you suspect a subarachnoid bleed or a tumor, and you treat them with antibiotics for sinusitis or NSAIDs for headaches, the results may turn fatal. If a physician is not thorough in testing for SAH and the outcome results in death, there will be hefty medicolegal and ethical consequences!

Figures 1 to 6 represent the subarachnoid hemorrhage.

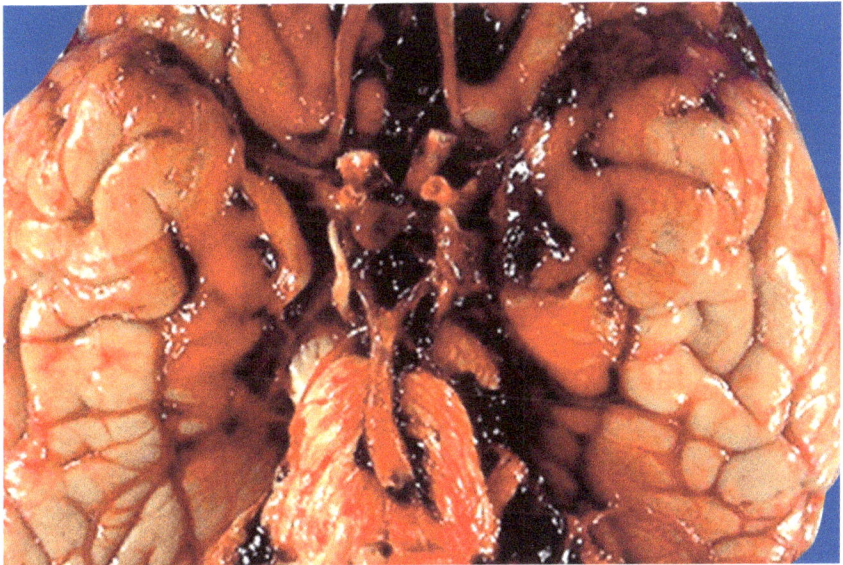

**Fig. 1:** Subarachnoid hemorrhage.
*Source:* http://emedicine.medscape.com/article/252142-overview.

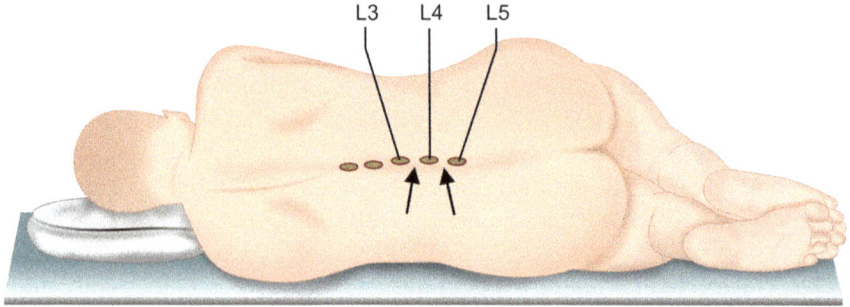

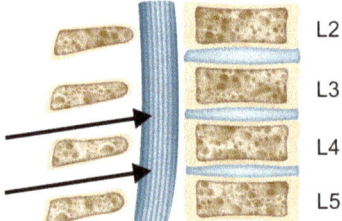

**Fig. 2:** Lumbar puncture locations.
*Source:* http://www.cdc.gov/meningococcal/about/diagnosis-treatment.html.

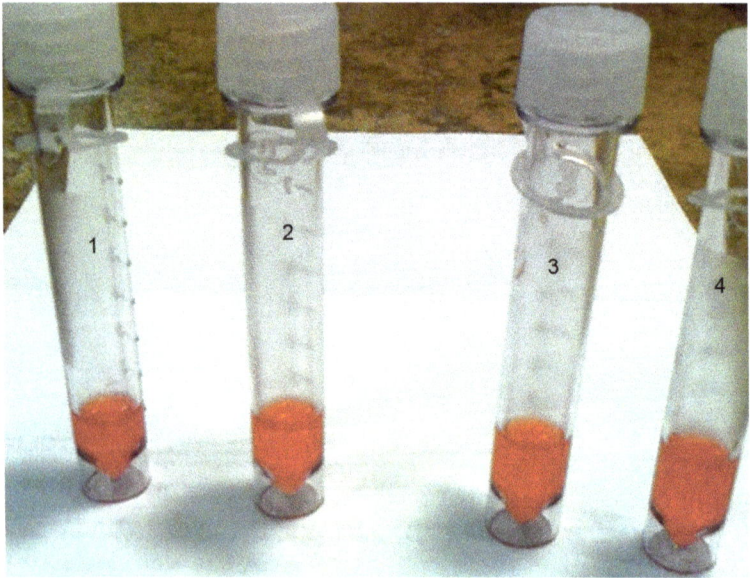

**Fig. 3:** Draw test tubes with CSF to evaluate for xanthochromia. (CSF: cerebrospinal fluid)
*Source:* From Medscape, New York, USA.

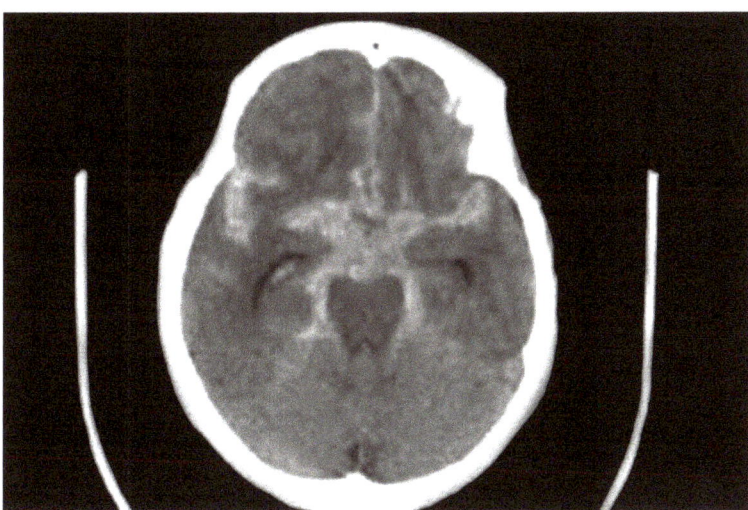

**Fig. 4:** Star shaped, "The Lone Star Flag of Texas" blood (bright white) is seen in the subarachnoid space on noncontract CT. (CT: computed tomography)
*Courtesy:* Badar M Zaheer, Chicago, USA.

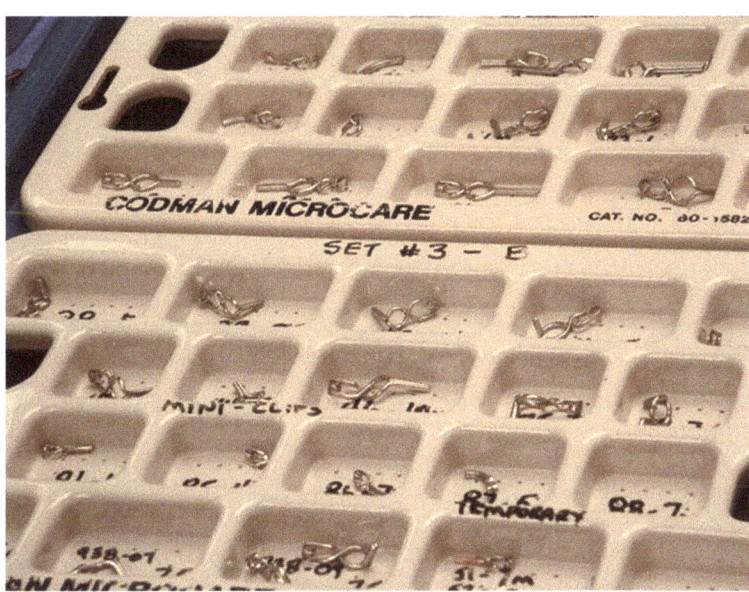

**Fig. 5:** A selection of Mayfield and Drake aneurysm clips ready for implantation.
*Source:* Wikipedia.

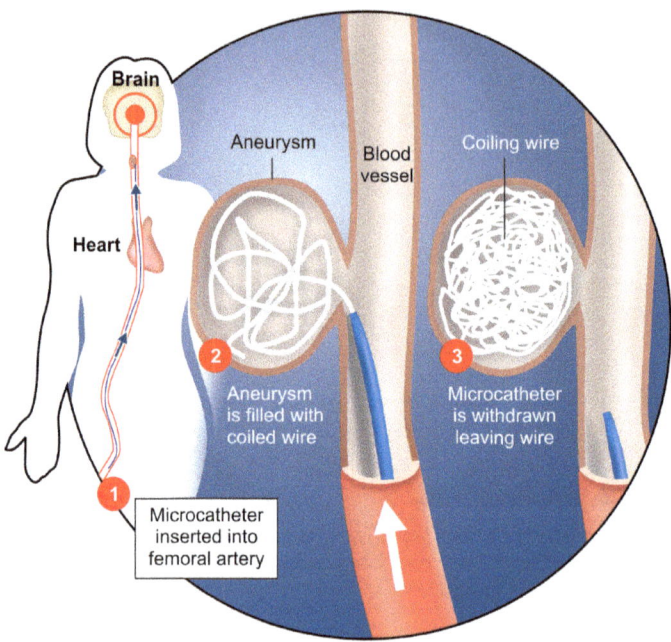

**Fig. 6:** Coils are inserted as a prevention of aneurysm ruptures.
*Source:* http://www.dailymail.co.uk/health/article-2054726/The-tiny-coil-wire-inserted-body-saves-thousands-stroke.html.

## REFERENCE

1. Perry JJ, Stiel IG, Sivilotti ML, et al. High risk clinical characteristics for subarachnoid haemorrhage in patients with acute headache: prospective cohort study. BMJ. 2010;341:c5204. http://www.medscape.com/viewarticle/761589_2.

## CASE STUDY 4: TRAUMATIC BRAIN INJURY

*The wind does not always blow in the direction you desire.*

—Arab Proverb

## CASE HISTORY

A 40-year-old female presents to the trauma bay after a motor vehicle accident (MVA). She was an unrestrained passenger in an accident in which a driver ran a red light and struck the driver side of her car. The driver also lost consciousness but was taken to another hospital. Initial assessment includes an intact airway with cervical collar in place. Patient is breathing spontaneously with adequate saturations. No signs of obvious bleeding are present. Distal pulses are all palpable and within the normal limits. Ecchymosis is found to be present periorbitally and on the abdomen. Glasgow coma scale

(GCS) is 7. Due to GCS score, the patient is intubated before being assessed further. The patient is unresponsive, and no family member is present. Vital signs are as follows: temperature 36°C, blood pressure 90/60 mm Hg, and pulse rate 125 bpm. The patient is now on the ventilator. Normal saline bolus is given. Intracranial and intra-abdominal bleeding is suspected. Patient is sent for further imaging of head, cervical spine, chest, and abdomen. Basilar skull fracture, subarachnoid hemorrhage (SAH), and intra-abdominal hemorrhage due to liver laceration are revealed. Surgical and neurosurgical consultations are obtained. Careful monitoring of vitals is continued before the patient is sent to the operation room (OR) for definitive management.

## DISCUSSION

Traumatic brain injury (TBI)[1] is a dynamic injury process due to cerebral edema, an increase in intracranial pressure (ICP), and anoxia (Fig. 1). It is usually related to rapid deceleration as seen in an MVA, diving accident, or blunt trauma. Initially, bleeding may be present followed by secondary injury due to cerebral edema. These injuries may have permanent consequences. There are 1.4 million cases in the United States per year with 50,000 deaths. A total of 235,000 hospitalizations and 1.1 million treated in the emergency department (ED). Of those, that present to the ED, 80% are discharged, 10% are mild, and 10% are serious.

Causes include falls (28%), automobile accidents (20%), being struck by car (19%), and assaults (11%). Mild injuries are usually associated with a

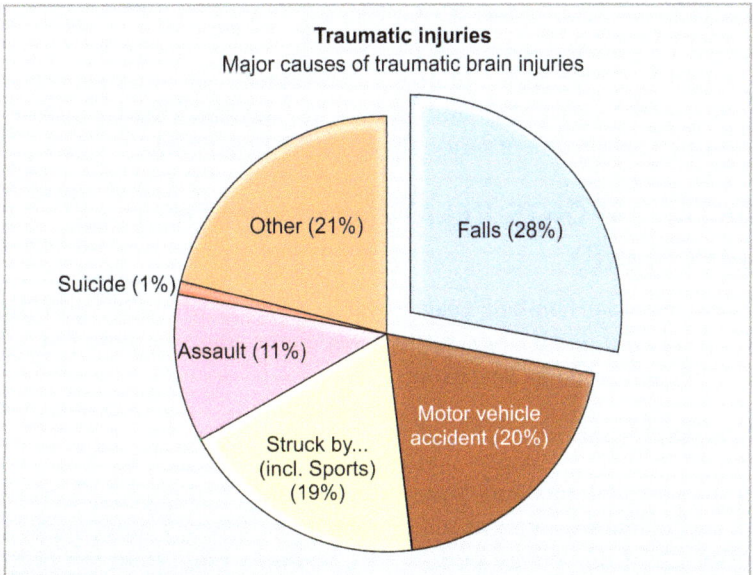

**Fig. 1:** Major causes of traumatic brain injuries.
*Source:* National Center for Injury Prevention and Control, CDC, Atlanta, USA.

concussion because the effects are not generally life-threatening. (Please see concussions case for further discussion).

Severe TBI may lead to death or severe disability. There are two types of these injuries: closed and penetrating. Closed injuries are due to movement of the brain within the skull. These injuries result from falls, MVAs, or blunt trauma. Penetrating injuries are caused by the entry of a foreign object into the skull. Initially, assessment should include the GCS. Scores of 3–8 are consistent with severe TBI; scores of 9–12 are associated with moderate TBI; and finally scores of 13–15 are considered mild TBI.

Potential outcomes of severe TBI include coma, amnesia, decreased attention and memory, extreme weakness, impaired coordination and balance, loss of sensation including hearing, vision and perception loss, depression, anxiety, aggression, impulse control, and personality changes. The effects of these symptoms impact both the patient's family and the society.

Immediate treatment should be focused on maintaining airway, breathing and circulation (ABC) and assessment using trauma protocols to assess for other injuries. All patients should receive 100% oxygen and two large bore intravenous (IV) lines. In severe cases, appropriate neurosurgery or neurology consultations should be obtained. Severely injured patients should be intubated and admitted to the appropriate intensive care unit for further management. Goals should include controlling blood pressure, decreasing ICP, and seizure prophylaxis. Cervical spine X-rays should be obtained due to the High risk of associated cervical spine fracture. Emergent head computed tomography (CT) should be obtained for all patients with GCS <14.[2] If SAH is present, nimodipine should be administered to prevent vasospasm. [Please see SAH for further discussion]. A recent study suggests that measurement of plasma S100-B on admission of patients who have a minor head injury can be helpful to the physician to prevent ordering an unnecessary CT scan in certain low-risk cases.[3] The study shows that elevated S100-B proteins in the blood can be indicative of serious brain injury in patients.

## CONTACT SPORTS-RELATED TRAUMATIC BRAIN INJURY

Famous National Football League (NFL) athletes who suffered disability, depression, and death from this horrible sports injury include Junior Seau, Dave Duerson, and Ray Easterling.

## PREVENTION

Educate your patients and community at large by supporting government laws and policies to prevent motor vehicle crashes and other sport-related injuries. Educational handouts like a take-home point from the doctor are always helpful. Always wear your seat belt when traveling in the car and wear your helmet when traveling by motorcycle! Wear protective gear while playing contact sports.

## PRACTICE POINT

It is very important to note that patients with severe traumatic brain injury, profound hypocapnia (hypocarbia) should be prevented, as this can lead to cerebral vasoconstriction with diminished perfusion. Therefore, avoid hyperventilation.

## REFERENCES

1. Traumatic Brain Injury & Concussion. Centers for Disease Control and Prevention. https://www.cdc.gov/traumaticbraininjury/. Published July 6, 2017. Accessed July 17, 2018
2. Ma OJ, Cline D. Emergency Medicine Manual. New York: McGraw-Hill, Medical Pub. Division; 2004
3. Zongo D, Ribéreau-Gayon R, Masson F, et al. S100-B protein as a screening tool for the early assessment of minor head injury. Ann Emerg Med. 2012;59(3):209-18.

## CASE STUDY 5: CERVICAL SPINE INJURY

*Things cannot always go your way.*

—Sir William Osler

## CASE HISTORY

A 45-year-old African–American male lost control of his vehicle during a snowstorm. The vehicle flipped three times in a row before coming to rest in the ditch at the side of the road. The patient was extricated from his vehicle and transported to a nearby hospital. On arrival, the patient is immobilized and has a large scalp hematoma. All imaging findings, including cervical-spine (C-spine) X-ray, are interpreted as normal despite having a poorly visualized cervicothoracic junction (Figs. 1 and 2). Based on negative studies and absence of pain, the nurse has removed the C-spine collar. After walking just down the hallway, the patient collapses. It is now found that the patient has experienced an anterior subluxation of the C-spine. Is this case approached correctly? How can we prevent spinal cord injury? What imaging is required to rule out C-spine injury during trauma?

|                  | *Radiography* | *CT* |
| --- | --- | --- |
| Cost             | +      | +++  |
| Radiation        | +      | ++   |
| Time             | +++    | +    |
| Sensitivity      | 94%    | 99%  |
| Specificity      | 78–89% | 93%  |
| Technical issues | +++    | +    |

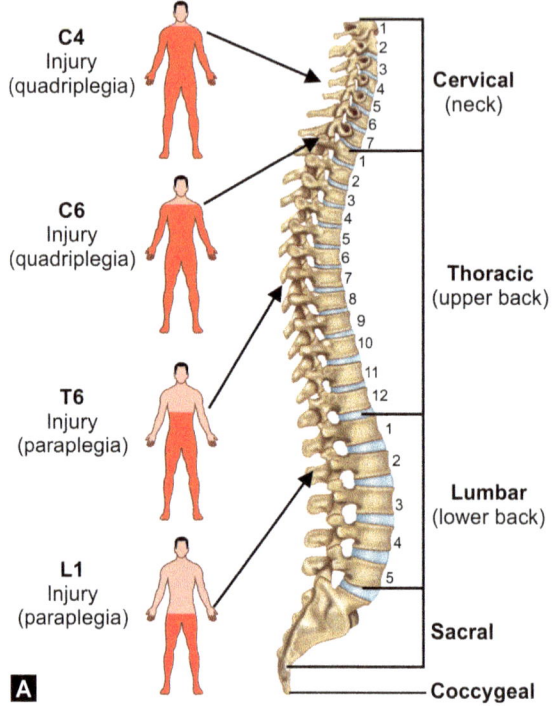
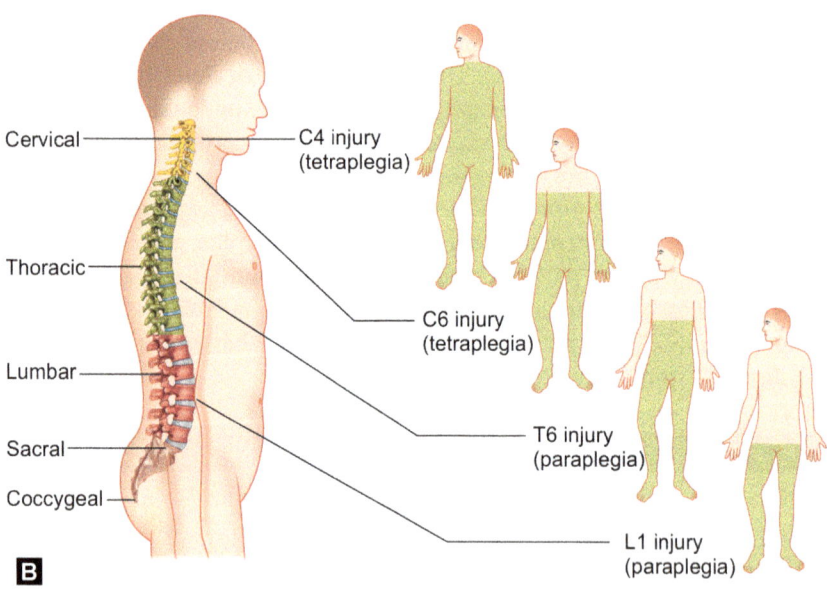

**Figs. 1A and B:** Levels of injury and extent of paralysis.
*Source:* Healthwise, incorporated.

Head and Neck

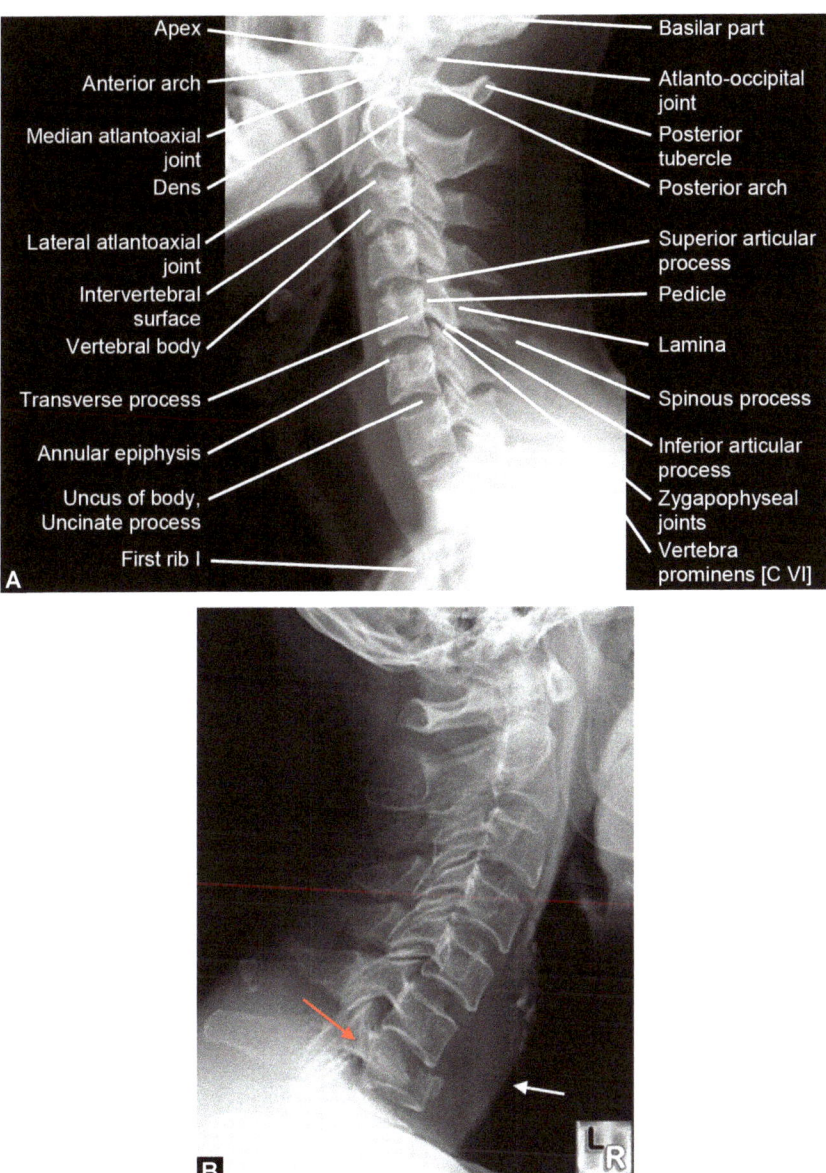

**Figs. 2A and B:** (A) Anatomy of cervical spine; (B) C7 fracture from (http://www.learning radiology.com/archives06/cow%20194-Brust%20fx/burstfxcorrect.htm).
*Source:* IMAIOS for Figure 2A.

## DISCUSSION

Cervical spine is the most vulnerable to injury because of its high mobility and exposure. The cervical canal is wider in the upper part from the foramen

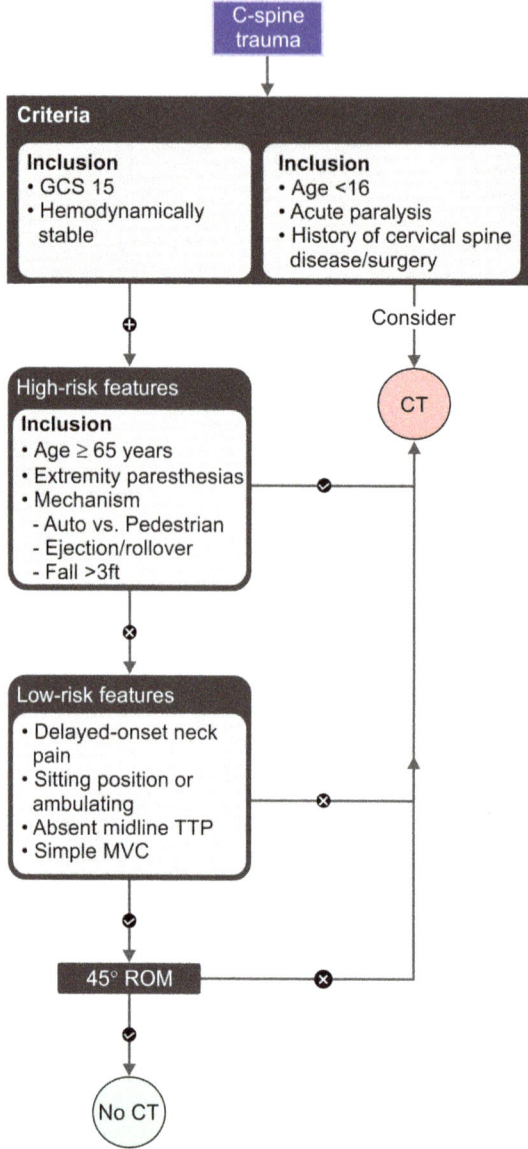

**Fig. 3:** Algorithm for evaluation of cervical spine injuries (Canadian C-spine rule). *Source:* Wikipedia.

magnum to the lowest part of C2. The majority of patients with injuries around C2 vertebra who survive are neurologically intact when they arrive to the hospital. One third of patients who have upper cervical injuries die at the scene of the injury secondary to apnea caused by an injury at C1 vertebra which denervates the phrenic nerves.

It is important to have a systematic approach for cervical spine assessment as not to miss any abnormalities. First, inspect for signs of blunt and penetrating injury, tracheal deviation, and use of accessory respiratory muscles. Always palpate for tenderness, deformity, swelling, subcutaneous emphysema, tracheal deviation, and symmetry of pulses. Obtain a computed tomography (CT) of the cervical spine or lateral, cross-table cervical spine X-ray. Throughout all evaluations and testing, always maintain adequate in-line immobilization and protection of the cervical spine (Fig. 3).[1]

Certain guidelines are in place for when a C-spine collar may be removed. If a patient is awake, alert, sober neurologically intact, and without neck pain or midline tenderness, he is unlikely to have a C-spine fracture. Movement is generally safe when performed by the patient. However, if pain or midline tenderness is present, one must exclude a C-spine injury.[2]

As always, use a systematic approach when assessing bony films. Look for signs of bone deformity. Assess for fracture of the vertebral body or process. Look for loss of alignment of the posterior aspect of the vertebral bodies. Check for increased distance between the spinous process at one level. Assess for narrowing of the vertebral canal and increased prevertebral soft tissue space.

Recent developments in treatment of cervical spine injuries include the use of stem cells to help regrow nervous tissue in the cervical spine.

Ten percent of patients with cervical spine injury will have a second noncontiguous vertebral fracture. If the spine is protected, further examination can be deferred until Airway, breathing, circulation, deformity (ABCD) are addressed. Look for the presence of hypotension, especially bleeding in other organs. Also, look for the causes of respiratory inadequacy.

## PRACTICE PEARL

- CT is cost effective, if fracture risk >4%
- CT saves money, if fracture risk >10%.

Always remember the cost of lawsuit by missing one fracture which changes the life of the person. Our job is not to hurt the patient but at the same time you do not want to get hurt yourself by getting involved in a lawsuit.

## PITFALL

Do not leave the patient on a hard surface, such as a backboard, for a long period of time. This may lead to formation of serious decubitus ulcers in patients with spinal cord injuries. The patient should be evaluated by the appropriate specialist and removed from the spine board as quickly as possible. Nobody should be left on the spine board for >2 h. If a patient has to be immobilized for >2 h, he must be logrolled every 2 h, maintaining the integrity of the skin and spine.

## REFERENCES

1. American College of Surgeons Committee on Trauma. Advanced Trauma Life Support Program for Doctors, Student Course Manual (ATLS). 8th ed. Chicago, IL: American College of Surgeons; 2002
2. http://www.youtube.com/watch?v=s7gULAPLY8U.

## CASE STUDY 6: ATYPICAL HEADACHE

*Gathering the appropriate studies in advance saves a lot of headaches.*
—Badar M Zaheer

### CASE HISTORY

A 40-year-old female presents to the emergency department (ED) with a headache persisting over the past several weeks. The patient has never had headaches like this before. The headache is unilateral on the right side. The patient is thought to have migraine headaches and is discharged home with oral analgesics for pain and antiemetics to control her nausea. One week later, emergency medical service (EMS) is called again because the patient is found to be unresponsive. Narcan is given which results in some mild improvement. The patient is thought to have been overusing hydrocodone and is sent home with further instructions for treating her migraine headache. The patient is dissatisfied with this diagnosis because she has never had migraine headaches before in her life. Subsequently, she decides to go to a different hospital. This time, computed tomography (CT) head is ordered, and the patient is found to have a large right frontal tumor. Before surgery can be scheduled, the patient passes away.

### DISCUSSION

This sad case can be taken as a lesson to look for red flag signs in headaches. Causes of headaches can range from simple tension headache to subarachnoid hemorrhage to malignancy and therefore must be taken seriously. In this case, the patient warranted a CT scan due to the new onset of the headaches. It would also be important to assess her neurologic status, because a tumor of this size may have caused neurologic abnormalities. Neurologic assessment may have been missed because the patient was incorrectly assessed as having abused her narcotic medication. This case also stresses the need for close monitoring and follow-up to ensure that patients do improve once they leave the ED.

Glioblastomas (malignant glioma) are the most common primary adult malignant brain tumors (Fig. 1), and 20% of all primary brain neoplasms are glioblastoma multiforme (GBM) tumors.[1] GBM is the highest grade form of astrocytoma and makes up about two thirds of all brain astrocytomas (Fig. 2).

Head and Neck

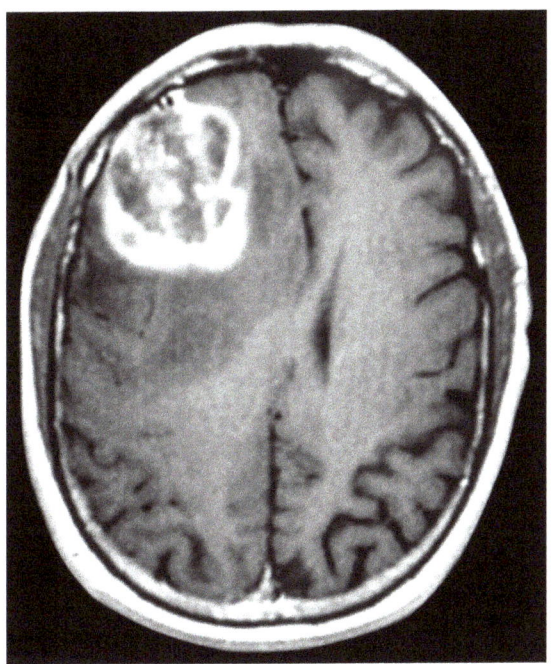

**Fig. 1:** Most common brain tumor, glioblastoma (stage IV astrocytoma).
*Source:* http://emedicine.medscape.com/article/340870-overview.

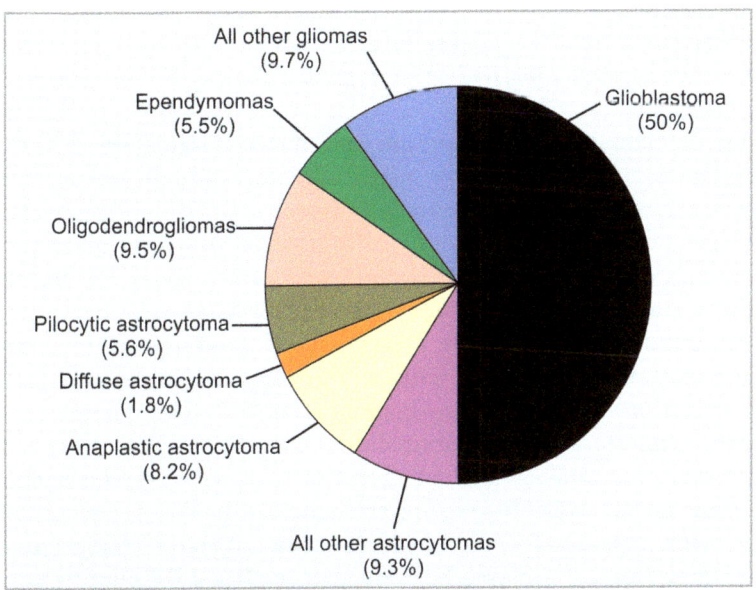

**Fig. 2:** Frequency of brain astrocytomas.
*Source:* Neurosurg focus 2006 American Association of Neurological surgeons.

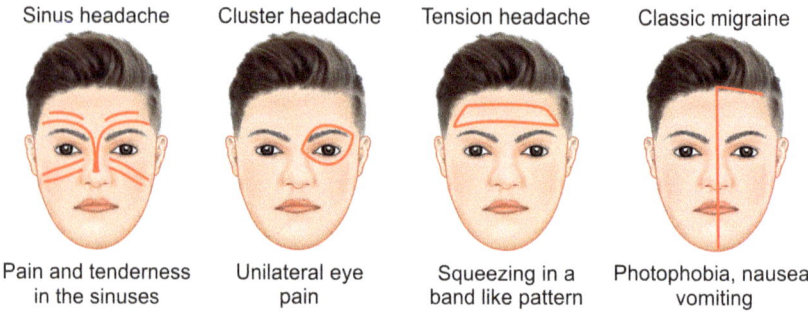

**Fig. 3:** Pain patterns in different types of headaches.
*Courtesy:* Badar M Zaheer, Chicago, USA.

**Flowchart 1:** Types of headache.

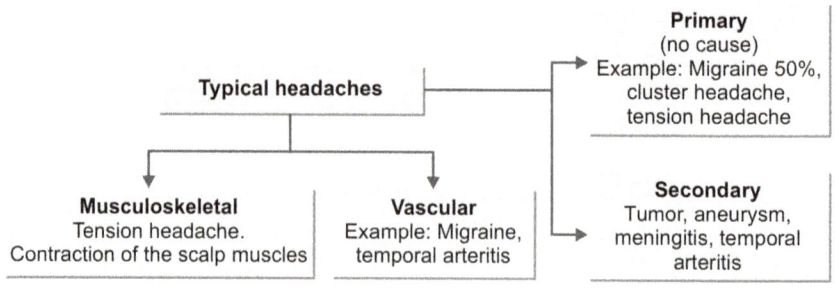

*Courtesy:* Badar M Zaheer, Chicago, USA.

The prognosis for this tumor is at the extreme worst end because of its high-grade status. Overall, metastatic tumors are the most common cause of brain neoplasms (Fig. 3).

Most of the metastatic tumors are caused by cell mutations. A history of irradiation to the head may also increase the risk of brain tumor development. In some, inherited diseases may be the cause and should be checked for with a patient and familial history. In HIV patients, primary central nervous system (CNS) lymphoma is a frequent cause of neoplasm. For metastatic neoplasms, lung is the most common cause of metastasis.

Presentation may include symptoms of headache (Flowchart 1), altered mental status, ataxia, nausea, vomiting, weakness, and gait disturbance. More focal symptoms include seizures, visual changes, speech deficits, or/and focal sensory normalities. Symptoms usually have a gradual onset. Complaints of headaches, one of the least-tolerated symptoms, occur later on and usually do not present alone. The headaches usually seem like tension-type nonspecific headaches. Mental status changes may be seen depending on the area of brain that is affected. Contrary to headaches, seizures may be an early sign, and are usually focal or generalized.

In general, ED management is not dependent on the type of tumor. The main concerns in the ED is managing intracranial pressure (ICP) that may result from the edema caused by the tumor. As a result of increased ICP, cerebral circulation may be impaired as well as shifting and herniation.

Physical examination should include a complete neurologic assessment. Look for localized deficits, papilledema, diplopia, impaired upward gaze, visual field deficits, anosmia, cranial nerve palsies, ataxia, nystagmus, or sensory deficits. When a neoplasm is suspected, patients should be screened with basic laboratory tests because they are at higher risk for medical complications, bleeding, and metabolic and endocrine disorders. CT is usually the first type of imaging done in the ED due to the ease of obtaining this test. Intravenous contrast CT can be used. Magnetic resonance imaging (MRI) is the preferred choice of imaging and should be done initially, if possible, but will be required either way for further management. Airway, breathing and circulation (ABC) should always be addressed. Cerebral edema may be treated with corticosteroids. Dexamethasone 4–24 mg daily may be used. Patients are generally admitted for further workup, and appropriate consultations should be obtained including neurosurgery.

## LESSONS FROM THE COURT

Keep in mind, every headache can be a big headache.

*Key pitfalls to avoid malpractice lawsuits:*
- Failure to diagnose by taking proper history and appropriate physical examination (42%)
- Failure to refer to a proper specialist
- Failure to follow-up
- Failure to order a proper diagnostic test (55%).

## REFERENCE

1. http://www.youtube.com/watch?v=PbMV0q2Hmyo.

## CASE STUDY 7: CONCUSSION

*Always wear your seat belt and remove tripping hazards in the home. Prevention and appropriate response to TBI can help save lives—CDC.*

—Badar M Zaheer

## CASE HISTORY

A 12-year-old male presents to the emergency department (ED) after being knocked out during a football game (Figs. 1A and B). The patient was running with the football when he was tackled, the opposing player put his helmet into the patient's helmet causing his head to fly back violently, and he lost consciousness for a few seconds. The patient is experiencing some nausea and has had several episodes of vomiting. He has never had a concussion before, other than the brief episode of loss of consciousness, he denies amnesia of the event. On examination, vitals are temperature 36.8°C, blood pressure 108/70 mm Hg, pulse rate 65 bpm, respiratory rate 15 breaths/min, and $O_2$ saturation level 100% on room air. The patient is found to be neurologically intact on cranial nerve, strength, sensation, and reflex examination. He is given Zofran and Tylenol and is then observed in the ED. Because the patient begins to experience worsening nausea, a computed tomography (CT) head is done which is found to be unremarkable. What is the next best step in management? What needs to be done before the patient can return to play?

## DISCUSSION

A concussion is a complex process affecting brain function induced by a traumatic biochemical force. Concussions predominantly occur between the ages of 12 years and 24 years, and more commonly in males. Risk factors include contact sports (especially football) and recent concussion (Figs. 2A to C). Prevention should include educating coaches and athletes, rule enforcement, and possibly rule changes. Current protective headgear has not been shown to prevent concussions; however, they are still mandatory. Improvement of such devices are being researched and developed.

Symptoms include confusion, post-traumatic amnesia, retrograde amnesia, loss of consciousness, disorientation, a "foggy feeling", inability to focus, delayed verbal and motor responses, slurred/incoherent speech, excessive drowsiness, headache, fatigue, disequilibrium, dizziness, visual disturbances, phonophobia, emotional liability, irritability, and sleep disturbance. Severity can only be assessed retroactively.

## PHYSICAL EXAMINATION

The physician should assess for airway, breathing and circulation (ABC), evidence of trauma, neurologic examination, and cervical spine injury.

Cafeteria list of symptoms.

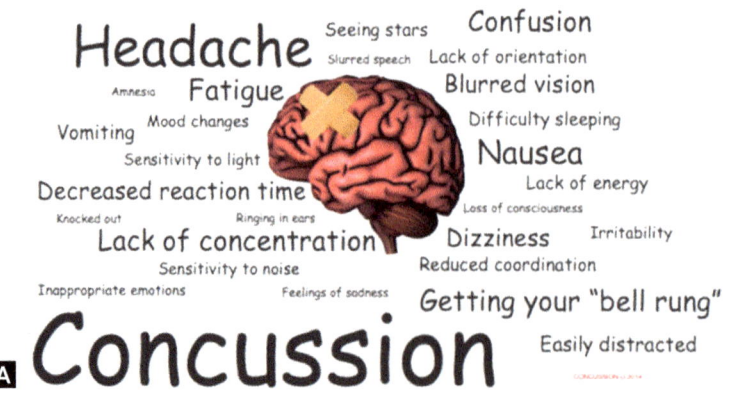

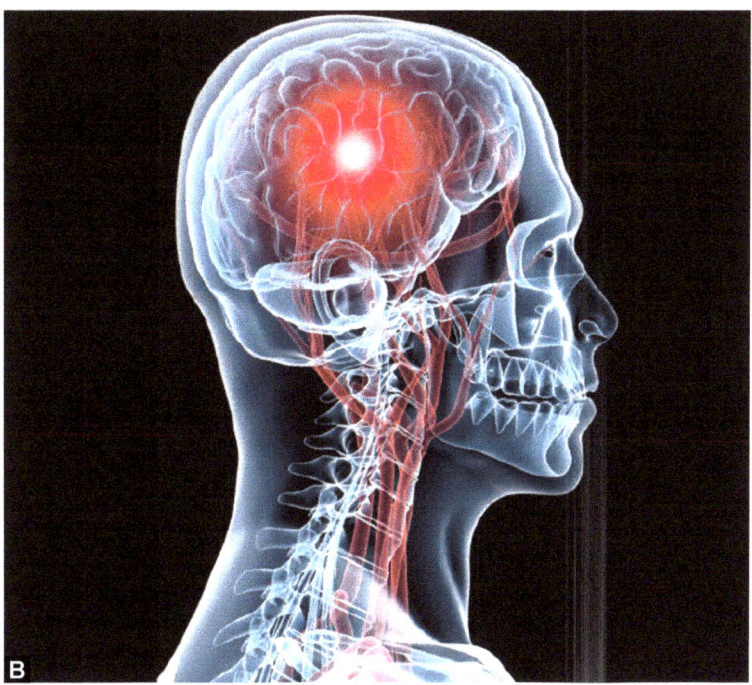

**Figs. 1A and B:** (A) Concussion; (B) Traumatic brain injury.
*Source:* (A) ConcussionU.wordpress.com; (B) Available online from http://www.cdc.gov/traumaticbraininjury/pdf/blue_book.pdf.

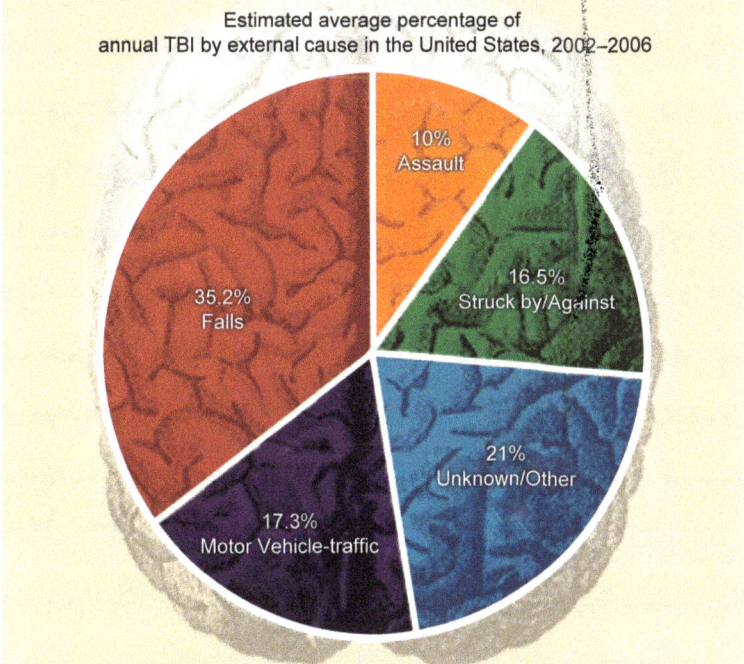

**Fig. 2A:** Estimated average percentage of annual TBI.

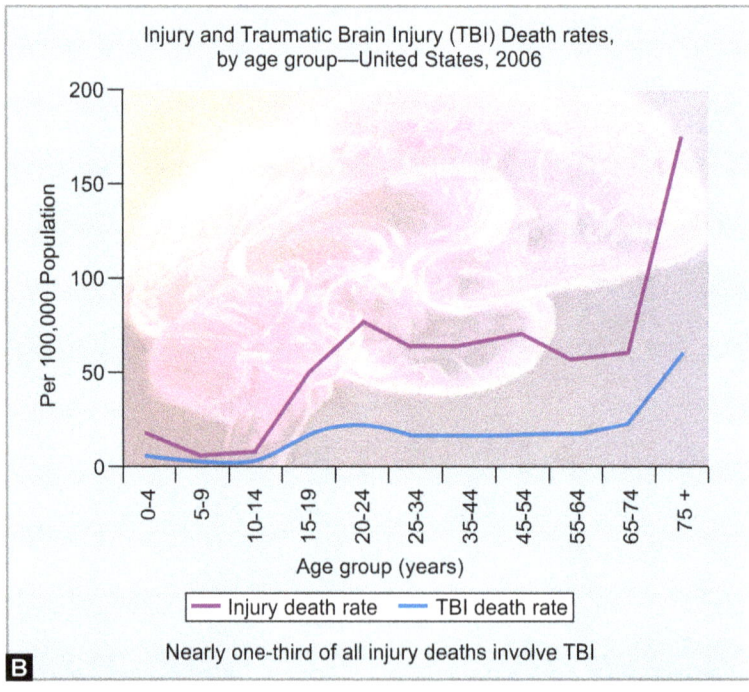

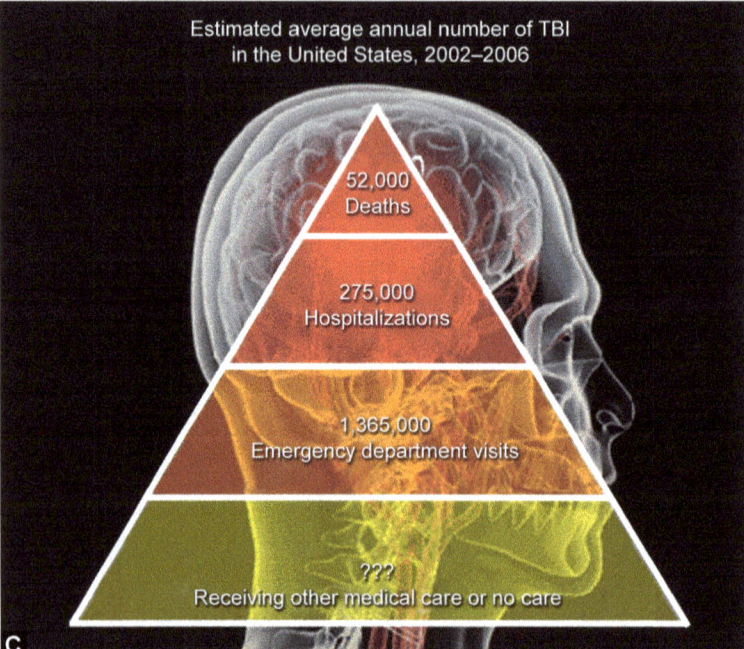

**Figs. 2B and C:** (B) TBI death rates; (C) Estimated average annual number of TBI.
*Source:* Available online from http://www.cdc.gov/features/dstbi_braininjury/.

Sideline assessment of concussion and serial cognitive evaluations may be used to determine if patient has returned to baseline. Patient must be assessed by a primary care doctor, not an emergency medicine physician in order to return to play.

Imaging is typically normal and should be considered if there is prolonged loss of consciousness, focal neurologic deficits, or worsening of symptoms. Cervical spine films should be ordered as indicated. Differential diagnosis includes concussion, subdural hematoma, epidural hematoma, cerebral contusion, and facial or skull fracture.

## TREATMENT

Treatment includes rest from physical and mental activities because both may worsen symptoms. That is, the patients should remain in place until they are symptom-free. Patients should reinitiate activity in a stepwise fashion with light activity first. Delay activity by 24 h if concussive symptoms return and then repeat. Ibuprofen or acetaminophen may be used for pain management. Treatment can usually be done by a primary care physician. More complicated cases should be referred to a sports medicine specialist or neurologist. Education regarding postconcussion symptoms and their treatment is very important. Complications to look for include delayed hematomas and recurrent concussion syndrome. Chronic traumatic brain injury can lead to cognitive decline and parkinsonian type syndromes.

With more knowledge being gained about concussion management, physicians, coaches, and players often disagree about playing time.[1] Coaches and players often want themselves to get right back into the game despite recommendations from the physician. More precautions regarding concussion management are being taken now more than ever.

Basic sideline management for concussions has been generally accepted, although randomized control data has been limited. If a patient shows any signs of a concussion, the player should be medically evaluated on the sideline and assessed for cervical spine injury. If no healthcare professional is present, then the player should be sent for further evaluation. The player should be initially treated with first aid guidelines and then assessed for signs and symptoms, such as loss of consciousness, headache, amnesia, nausea, or dizziness. Player should be accompanied by at least one friend or family member for the next 5 h. Players should not be allowed to return to play on the same day of injury with the exception of some adult athletes.[2]

## VIENNA CONCUSSION CONFERENCE: RETURN TO PLAY RECOMMENDATIONS

*Athletes should complete the following stepwise process before returning to play following their concussion:*
- Removal from contest following any signs/symptoms of concussion
- No return to play in the current game

- Medical evaluation following injury
  - Rule out more serious intracranial pathology
  - Neuropsychologic testing (considered a cornerstone of proper postinjury assessment).
- *Stepwise return to play*
  - No activity and rest until asymptomatic
  - Light aerobic exercise
  - Sport-specific training
  - Noncontact drills
  - Full-contact drills
  - Game play.

## REFERENCES

1. O'Reilly KB. "Put me in, Doc." American Medical News: Professional Issues. 2010.
2. Stevenson JH. Concussion. In: Domino FJ, editor. The 5-minute Clinical Consult: 2012. 20th edn.

## FURTHER READING

1. http://www.cdc.gov/features/dstbi_braininjury/.
2. Concussion Symptoms. Concussion-U. https://concussionu.wordpress.com/what-is-a-concussion-signs-and-symptoms/. Published June 6, 2015. Accessed July 17, 2018.

# CHAPTER 2

# Chest

## PULMONARY SYSTEM

### CASE STUDY 8: PULMONARY HYPERTENSION

### CASE HISTORY

#### Chief Complaints: Syncope and Dizziness History of Past Illness

Mrs. A is a 36-year-old female who is presented to the emergency department (ED) after an episode of syncope and continued dizziness. She was singing in church and suddenly felt dizzy and fell. She has been an avid church goer for much of her life and recently experienced the sudden passing of her aunt whom she considered a mother figure; she was 48 years of age and experienced a long battle with heart problems. The patient has been struggling with obesity for much of her life and has been taking "weight loss pills" in addition to starting multiple diet and exercise regimens.

On the way to the ED, the patient developed dyspnea and tachypnea. At the ED, she complains of chest pain, palpitation, and an on-and-off dry cough.

She denies any previous fainting episodes. She denies any history of seizure.

### PHYSICAL EXAMINATION

- *Cardiovascular*: Jugular venous pressure (JVP) is raised; loud P2, S3, and S4 are heard.
- *Respiration*: Tachypnea, no wheezing is heard.
- *Abdomen*: On palpation, slight hepatomegaly is found.
- *Extremities*: Pedal edema +1
- *Central nervous system (CNS)*: Intact.

## DIAGNOSTIC TESTS

- *Electrocardiogram (ECG)*: Right ventricular hypertrophy and right axis deviation
- *Pulmonary function test (PFT)*: Arterial hypoxemia, reduced diffusion capacity, and hypocapnia
- *Ventilation/Perfusion lung scan (V/Q scan)*: No proximal pulmonary artery emboli.

### Laboratory Tests

- Antinuclear antibody (ANA) is positive.
- D-dimer is negative.

### Imaging

- *Chest X-ray (CXR)*: It shows enlarged central pulmonary arteries and right ventricular enlargement (Fig. 1).
- *Echocardiography*: It shows right ventricular enlargement and overload. No atrial septal defect (ASD) is present and low mitral stenosis is found.
- *Enhanced computed tomography (CT) image* (Fig. 2).

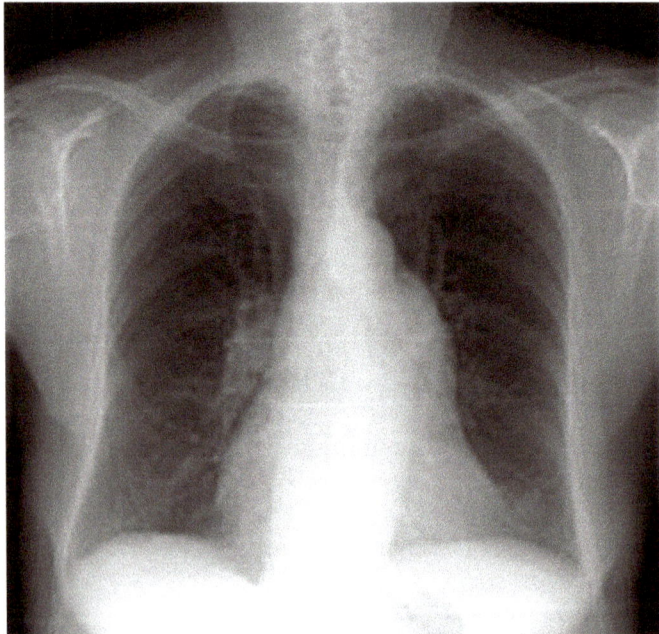

**Fig. 1:** Chest X-ray shows enlarged central pulmonary arteries and right ventricular enlargement.

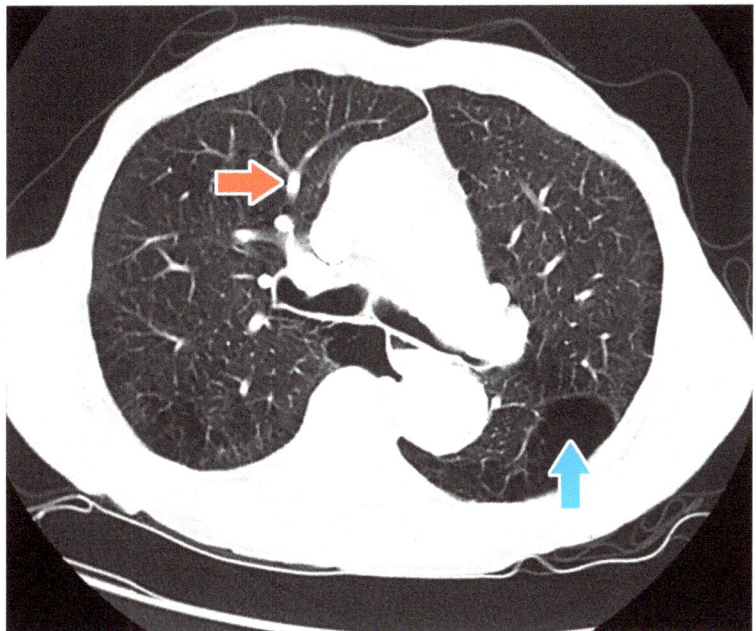

Fig. 2: Enhanced computed tomography (CT) image.

## DIAGNOSIS: PULMONARY/ARTERIAL HYPERTENSION

## Differential Diagnosis: For Patients with Syncope and Dizziness

- *Cardiovascular*: Aortic stenosis, asymmetric septal hypertrophy, ventricular tachycardia, supraventricular tachycardia, sinus node disorders (bradycardia), atrioventricular block (AVB)
- *Hemodynamic*: Decreased total peripheral resistance (TPR), subclavian steal, stroke, orthostatic hypotension
- *Respiratory*: Pulmonary embolism, pneumothorax, chronic obstructive pulmonary disease (COPD) exacerbation, asthma exacerbation
- *Endocrine*: Hypoglycemia, Addison disease (decreased TPR)
- *Neurologic*: Vasovagal reflex, complex seizure
- *Neoplasm*: Rare, but needs to be considered
- *Drugs*: Beta-blockers, vasodilators, nitrates, tricyclic antidepressant, phenothiazines, barbiturates, benzodiazepines, psychotropic drugs, alcohol.

## WORKUP: PULMONARY HYPERTENSION

### Rule out Secondary Causes

Pulmonary hypertension can often be secondary to other conditions. Left heart failure, for example, increases the resistance of blood flow away from the lungs. Conditions like COPD or sleep apnea can increase pulmonary blood pressure by causing vasoconstriction in areas of the lung where there is inadequate ventilation. Secondary causes of pulmonary hypertension need to be excluded first (Box 1).

| **Box 1:** World Health Organization's diagnostic classification of pulmonary hypertension. ||
|---|---|
| *Pulmonary arterial hypertension*<br>Primary pulmonary hypertension<br>  Sporadic disorder<br>  Familial disorder<br>Related conditions<br>  Collagen vascular disease<br>  Congenital systemic-to-pulmonary shunt<br>  Portal hypertension<br>  Human immunodeficiency virus infection<br>  Drug and toxins<br>    Anorectic agents (appetite suppressants)<br>  Others<br>    Persistent pulmonary hypertension of<br>    the newborn<br>  Others | *Pulmonary hypertension associated with<br>disorders of the respiratory system and/or<br>hypoxemia*<br>Chronic obstructive pulmonary disease<br>Interstitial lung disease<br>Sleep-disordered breathing<br>Alveolar hypoventilation disorders<br>Chronic exposure to high altitudes<br>Neonatal lung disease<br>Alveolar–capillary dysplasia<br>Others<br>*Pulmonary hypertension resulting from<br>chronic thrombotic and/or embolic disease*<br>Thromboembolic obstruction of proximal<br>pulmonary arteries |
| *Pulmonary venous hypertension*<br>Left-sided atrial or ventricular heart disease<br>Left-sided valvular heart disease<br>Extrinsic compression of central pulmonary veins<br>  Fibrosing mediastinitis<br>  Adenopathy and/or tumors<br>Pulmonary veno-occlusive disease<br>Others | Obstruction of distal pulmonary arteries<br>  Pulmonary embolism (thrombus, tumor,<br>ova, and/or parasites; foreign material)<br>In situ thrombosis<br>Sickle cell disease<br>*Pulmonary hypertension resulting from<br>disorders directly affecting the pulmonary<br>vasculature*<br>Inflammatory conditions<br>  Schistosomiasis<br>  Sarcoidosis<br>  Others<br>Pulmonary capillary hemangiomatosis |

*Source:* WHO.[1]

## Diagnostic Studies

### Chest X-ray and High-resolution CT Scan

In pulmonary hypertension, these studies show dilation and pruning of pulmonary arteries, and enlargement of right atrium and right ventricle. These studies can help to rule out other more obvious lung pathology (Fig. 1).

Prominence of both hila due to enlargement of pulmonary vessels is also a characteristic of pulmonary hypertension. There is blunting of both costophrenic angles which could represent small pleural effusion/pleural reaction. There is pruning of peripheral pulmonary vessels; findings are consistent with pulmonary hypertension. Figure 3 depicts ultrasound findings in pulmonary hypertension.

## Electrocardiography

This can show right atrial dilation, right bundle branch block (RBBB), right atrial enlargement, and right ventricular hypertrophy (Fig. 4).

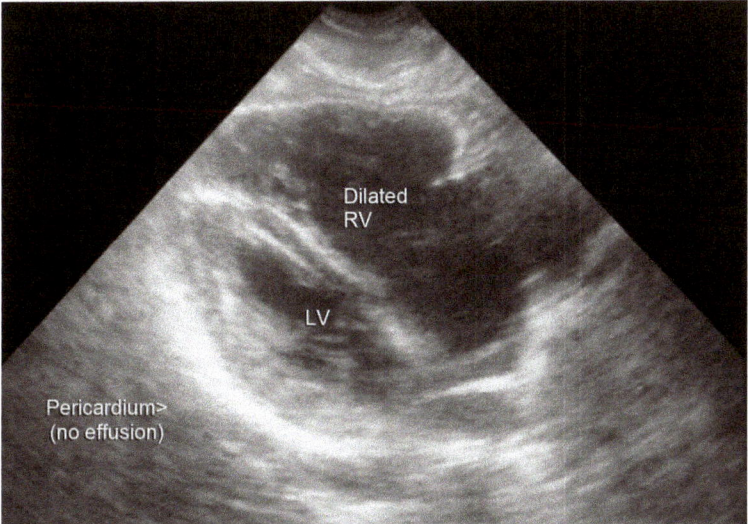

**Fig. 3:** Ultrasound shows dilated RV. (LV: left ventricle; RV: right ventricle).
*Courtesy:* Badar M Zaheer MD.

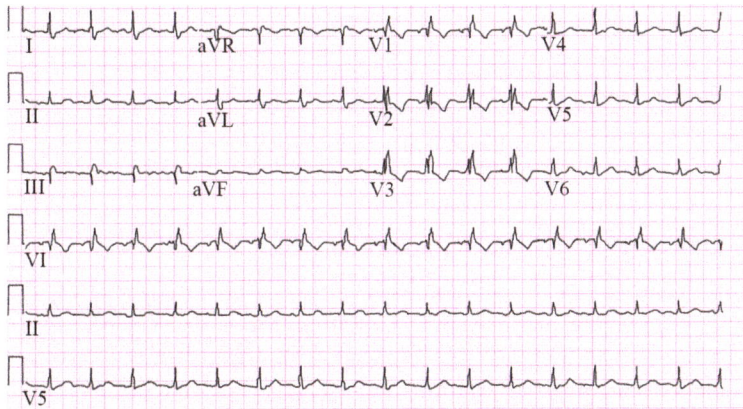

**Fig. 4:** ECG shows RBBB, right atrial enlargement, and right ventricular hypertrophy. (ECG: electrocardiogram; RBBB: right bundle branch block).

Criteria for RBBB:
- QRS complex duration of ≥120 ms
- rsR' "bunny ear" pattern in precordial leads
- Slurred S waves in leads I, V5, and V6.

*Source:* http://www.learntheheart.com/RBBB.html.

### Pulmonary Function Test
- Decreased diffusion capacity of the lung for carbon monoxide (DLCO), only mild restrictive pattern [decrease in forced expiratory volume in 1 s ($FEV_1$), rules out restrictive lung disease].

### Arterial Blood Gases (ABG) and Polysomnography (Sleep Study)
- Show decreased arterial $O_2$ concentration and saturation
- Show and increased A—a gradient
- Used to rule out hypoventilation and obstructive sleep apnea (OSA).

### Acute Vasodilatory Test
- It is performed during cardiac catheterization, and it is done to screen for responsiveness to calcium channel blocker (CCB).
- A positive acute vasodilator test response means better survival.
- It can be performed on all patients who have idiopathic pulmonary hypertension and who are candidates for long-term CCB. Medications used to perform this test include inhaled nitrous oxide, intravenous (IV) epoprostenol, and IV adenosine.
- Cardiac catheterization is contraindicated in right heart failure and if the patient is hemodynamically unstable.

## TREATMENT

The major treatment goals in pulmonary hypertension are the inhibition of vasoactive substances in lungs and prevention of right ventricular failure (Flowchart 1).

## Oral calcium Channel Blockers

Calcium channel blockers (CCBs) are a great choice for patients who have a positive acute vasoactive response. Half of all the patients will have a long-term response and a significant decrease in mortality. Side effects of CCB include hypotension and lower limb edema.

## Intravenous Prostacyclin

These medications include epoprostenol and flolan. They act by vasodilation, decreasing platelet aggregation and decreasing smooth muscle proliferation.

**Flowchart 1:** Treatment of pulmonary arterial hypertension. Initial therapy should be guided by the results of acute vasodilator challenge.

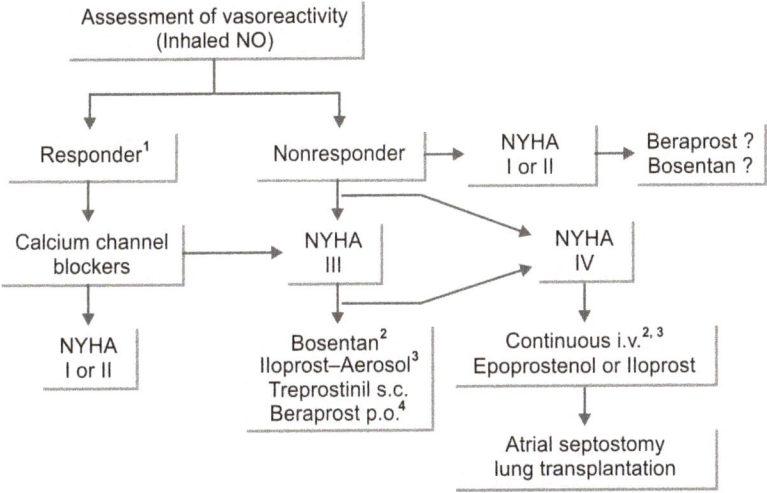

Source: http://ajrccm.atsjournals.org/content/165/9/1209/F.larage.jpg.
(1) In patients who show a fall in pulmonary arterial pressure and pulmonary vascular resistance to near-normal values, calcium channel blockers remain a reasonable therapeutic option. Nonresponders and responders who are not in NYHA Class I or II while being treated with calcium channel blockers should be offered the endothelin receptor antagonist bosentan or one of the novel prostaglandins. In case of deterioration or in patients with advanced disease, IV epoprostenol or iloprost should be started and atrial septostomy or lung transplantation should be considered. (2) The combination of epoprostenol and bosentan is currently being evaluated in clinical studies. (3) Iloprost is not available in the United States and has not received official approval for treatment of pulmonary hypertension in Europe. (4) Some of these substances have not been approved in the United States and Europe.

These benefits are thought to increase with time. They have been shown to also decrease mortality. Adverse effects include flushing, headaches, jaw or leg pain, abdominal cramps, nausea, and diarrhea.

## Prostacyclin Analogs

Iloprost (inhaled), treprostinil (IV or subcutaneous), and beraprost (per oral) have the same mechanisms as the IV prostacyclins. They are easier to adhere to and have decreased side effects. Iloprost has the most increased efficacy.

## Endothelin Receptor Antagonists

These agents include bosentan and ambrisentan. They cause a decrease in smooth muscle remodeling, increase in vasodilation, decrease in fibrosis, decrease in symptoms, and increase in 6-min walking test. However, it has no change in clinical outcomes. They have a low adverse-effect profile.

## PEARLS

- Removal of secondary causes is the mainstay treatment
- CXR and ECG are a good starting point
- Oral CCB and IV prostacyclin—only medications proven to lower mortality.

## REFERENCE

1. World Health Organization. http://www.who.int/respiratory/other/Pulmonary_hypertension/en/.

## FURTHER READING

1. Brady Pregerson, Quick Essentials Emergency Medicine 4.0 4th Edition. ER PocketBooks.com; 4th edition (January 1, 2010). https://www.amazon.com/Quick-Essentials-Emergency-Medicine-4-0/dp/0976155230.

## CASE STUDY 9: PULMONARY EMBOLISM

*"Every moment of your life is an opportunity to learn and perfect your skills to save a life."*

—Badar M Zaheer

## CASE HISTORY

The patient is a 61-year-old female refugee from Afghanistan with an unknown previous medical history. She is presented to an urgent care clinic with a chief complaint of vague abdominal pain and a long history of back pain that radiates to the back of the leg. She was seen in emergency room 1 day prior, with similar symptoms. Abdominal and pelvic X-rays are done and they show no significant pathology. Doppler ultrasounds are done in both legs and they show negative findings for deep venous thrombosis (DVT). The patient is given morphine and zofran and then sent to home.

Soon after, she says that her symptoms have not improved. The patient is given a gastrointestinal (GI) cocktail which consists of three ingredients: lidocaine 2% gel, mylanta (a solution of magnesium hydroxide and aluminum hydroxide), and dicyclomine. She then left the clinic accompanied by her family. Thirty minutes later, her family rushes back to the clinic and she is found to be gasping for air, sobbing and straddling between consciousness and unconsciousness. A pulse oximeter is quickly attached. As the patient is being taken out of the car, she loses consciousness and stops breathing. Her heart rate is still present, and her $O_2$ saturation level drops from 98% to 85%. Cardiopulmonary resuscitation (CPR) is immediately performed in the back seat of the car and an ambulance is called. Patient has become responsive and started breathing on her own within 10 min. By the time the ambulance arrived, she is able to answer questions and appears comfortable. At the emergency department (ED), patient has an elevated D-dimer.

## REVIEW OF SYMPTOMS

Vague abdominal pain, back pain, and unilateral leg pain resembling sciatica.

## Physical Examination

- *Homan's sign*: Positive—patient was not letting examiner to touch lateral leg.
- *On dorsiflexion*: Calf pain is present.
- *Lungs*: Clear to auscultation bilaterally, no obvious findings.
- *Abdominal*: Periumbilical tenderness on palpation.

## Laboratory Test

D-dimer positive.

## Imaging

Spiral computed tomography (CT) scan pending.

# DIAGNOSIS

The D-dimer and acute shortness of breath (SOB), dyspnea, alongside unilateral leg pain, strongly suggests pulmonary embolism (PE). Sometimes, PE is very difficult to diagnose unless you have high index of suspicion. Panic attacks, myocardial infarction (MI), acute pneumonias, and pneumothorax may have overlapping symptoms.

# WORKUP

## Differential Diagnosis

- *Cardiac:* Acute coronary syndrome, aortic stenosis, atrial fibrillation, cardiomyopathy, congestive heart failure, cor pulmonale, mitral stenosis, MI, myocardial ischemia, pericarditis and cardiac tamponade, sudden cardiac death, superior vena cava syndrome, and cardiogenic shock
- *Pulmonary*: Acute respiratory distress syndrome, chronic obstructive pulmonary disease, pulmonary edema, emphysema, fat embolism, extrinsic allergic alveolitis, lung arteriovenous malformation, pneumothorax, pulmonary edema, noncardiogenic, pulmonary hypertension
- *Psychological*: Anxiety disorders
- *Neurologic*: Central apnea
- *Homan's sign*: Dorsiflexion of leg while the knee is at 90° angle causes calf pain. Relatively useless, low-negative predictive value (NPV) and positive predictive value (PPV)
- *Chest X-ray (CXR)*: Initial workup in patients complaining of dyspnea and tachypnea includes a CXR to rule out pneumonia, tuberculosis,

malignancies, and pneumothorax. If CXR is abnormal but not diagnostic for any of the above, a helical CT is required. A normal CXR should be followed up with a ventilation/perfusion (V/Q) scan.
- A typical CXR will show a wedge-shaped, triangular opacity with an apex pointing toward the hilum or decreased vascularity (Westermark sign).
- Pulmonary artery will be prominent.
- *Compression ultrasound*: This is a Doppler ultrasound of the deep veins in both which looks for thrombi.
- *D-dimer test*: This is a blood test that measures the level of broken down fibrin products that are covalently bound. A positive result indicates active thrombotic events. It is currently used to rule in DVTs, PE, and disseminated intravascular coagulopathy (DIC). Normally, a D-dimer has a very high-NPV. However, if the PE is very likely and the patient has a strong story, a negative D-dimer cannot rule out a PE (Table 1).
- *CT angiography*: Spiral CT (Figs. 1A and B) can be very sensitive in showing thrombi in the lungs. PPV and NPV approach higher than 95%. However, they may show smaller thrombi with unclear clinical consequences (Figs. 2 and 3).

**Table 1:** Well's criteria.

| Variable | Point |
|---|---|
| Clinical symptoms of DVT (leg tenderness and unilateral swelling) | 3 |
| No alternative diagnosis | 3 |
| Heart rate higher than 100 bpm | 1.5 |
| Immobilization or surgery in the previous 4 weeks | 1.5 |
| Previous DVT/PE | 1.5 |
| Hemoptysis | 1.0 |
| Malignancy | 1.0 |
| *Patient risk* | |
| Low risk (<10%) | <2 |
| Moderate risk (10–40%) | 2–6 |
| High risk (40–80%) | >6 |
| *Likelihood of physical examination* | |
| PE likely | >4 |
| PE unlikely | ≤4 |

(DVT: deep venous thrombosis; PE: pulmonary embolism).
Source: Reproduced with permission from Wells PS, Anderson DR, Rodger M, et al. Derivation of a simple clinical model to categorize patients' probability of pulmonary embolism: increasing the models utility with the SimpliRED D-dimer. Thromb Haemost 2000;83(3):416–20. Available online from http://www.schattauer.de/en/magazine/ subject areas/journals a-z /thrombosis-and-haemostasis/contents/archive/manuscript/2372.html.

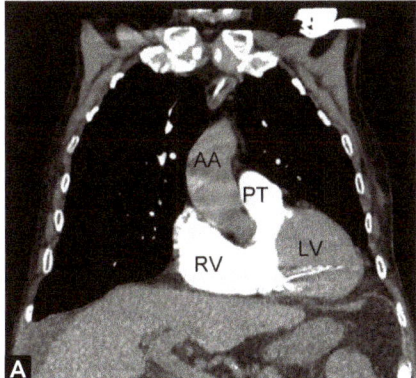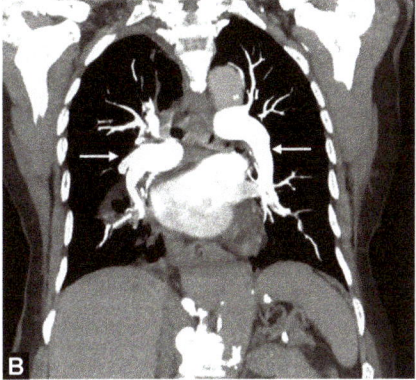

**Figs. 1A and B:** Pulmonary embolism CT. (CT: computed tomography). (A) Coronal CT image with iodinated contrast media in the right ventricle; (B) Coronal CT image
*Source:* Available online from http://www.ceessentials.net/images/pulmonaryEmbolus/image018.jpg.

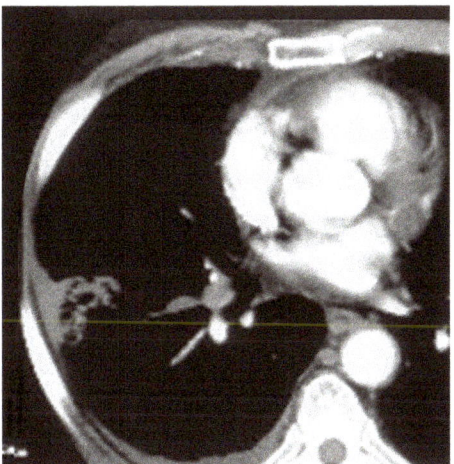

**Fig. 2:** Helical CT shows an intraluminal clot in anterior segmental artery in left upper lung.[1] (CT: computed tomography).
*Source:* Garg K. Acute pulmonary embolism (helical CT). In: Amorosa JK, et al. 2008, editors. eMedicine. MedScape; 2009. Available online from http://emedicine.medscape.com/article/361131-overview.

- *V/Q scan*: This involves a ventilation phase in which a patient inhales radioactive nucleotide gases and a perfusion phase in which the patient is injected with a radioactive albumin. A γ-camera is used during each phase to show the level of these materials in the lungs. A V/Q scan is used if CTs are unavailable or contraindicated.
- *Pulmonary angiography*: This is the gold standard, but it is invasive and expensive (Fig. 4).

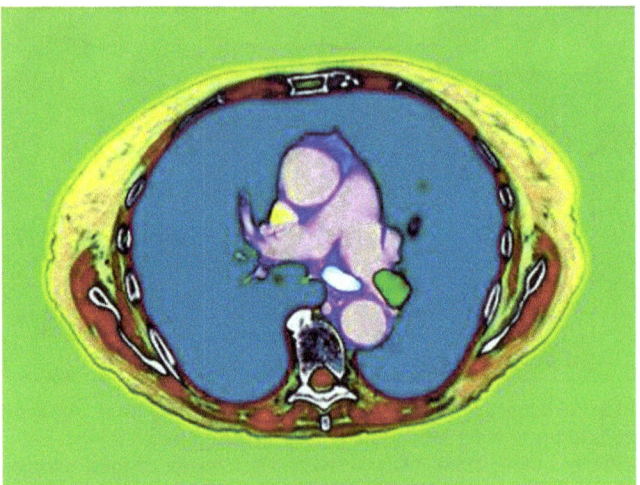

**Fig. 3:** Pulmonary embolism colored CT. (CT: computed tomography).
*Source:* Available online from http://www.images.cpcache.com/merchandise/514_400x 400_NoPeel.jpg?region=name:FrontCenter,id:71660204,w:16.

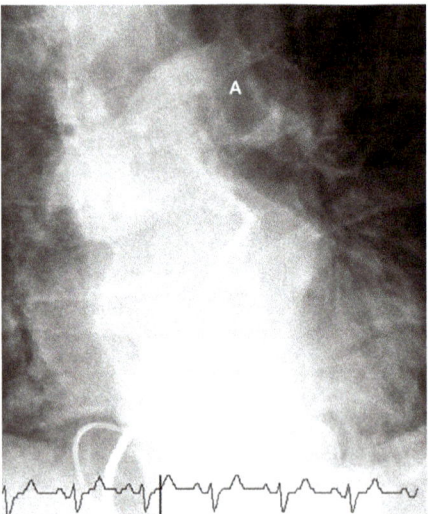

**Fig. 4:** Selective pulmonary angiogram revealing clot (labeled A) causing a central obstruction in the left main pulmonary artery. Electrocardiogram (ECG) tracing shown at bottom.
*Source:* Wikipedia.

## Therapies

- *Acute anticoagulation*
  - *Unfractionated heparin*: 80 U/kg, then changes by 18 U/kg/h to get to partial thromboplastin time of 65–80 s.

- Low molecular weight heparin (enoxaparin): It is preferred choice unless patient is obese or has renal failure.
- *Thrombolysis*
  - *Tissue plasminogen activator*: 100 mg over 2 h, reserved for massive PE
- *Catheter-directed therapy*
  - Fibrinolytic and thrombus fragmentation/aspiration
  - Used in extensive PE and in those patients in whom systemic thrombolysis is contraindicated (high risk for bleeding).
- *Thrombectomy*
  - Reserved for patients with massive or extensive PE at large centers that cannot tolerate systemic thrombolysis.
- *Long-term anticoagulation*
  - *Warfarin*: Start at the same time as heparin
  - Can be used as single agent for proximal DVT and uncomplicated PE
  - Used alongside enoxaparin for PE associated with cancer
- *Inferior vena cava filter*
  - Used for DVT at risk of embolization.

## MASSIVE PULMONARY EMBOLISM

*Definition:* Sustained hypotension, SBP <90 mm Hg (≥15 min), inotropic support, pulseless, and persistent profound bradycardia (Fig. 5).

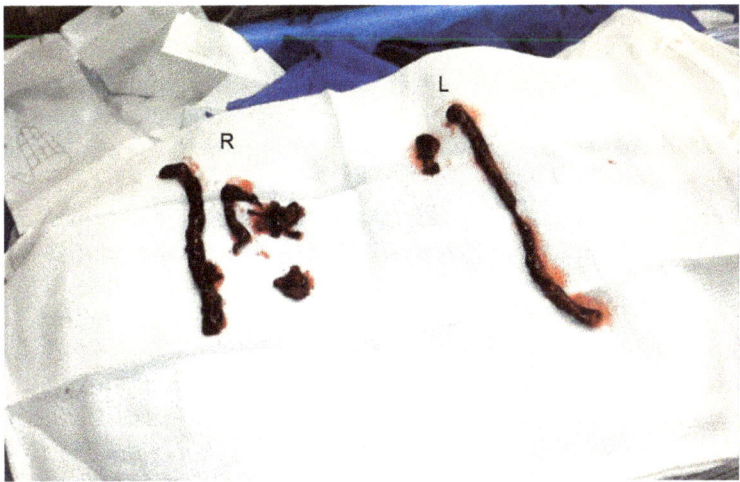

**Fig. 5:** Massive pulmonary embolism.
*Courtesy:* Michael C Bond, MD, Assistant Professor, Residency Program Director, Department of Emergency Medicine, University of Maryland School of Medicine, Maryland, USA.

## Thrombolytics

- *Thrombolytics benefits*: Rapid resolution of symptoms, stabilization of respiratory/CV function, Cochrane review: reduce mortality and recurrence
- Should not be delayed for patients with hemodynamic compromise
- Three agents FDA approved, streptokinase, urokinase, alteplase
- *Alteplase*: Bolus dose 10 mg, infusion 90 mg over 2 h. Peripheral IV
- Heparin infusion should be paused.

## REFERENCE

1. Garg K. Acute pulmonary embolism (helical CT). In: Amorosa JK, et al. 2008, editors. eMedicine. Medscape; 2009. Available online from http://emedicine.medscape.com/article/361131-overview.

## FURTHER READING

1. Bond MC, MD, Assistant Professor, Residency Program Director, Department of Emergency Medicine, University of Maryland School of Medicine.

## CASE STUDY 10: PULMONARY CONTUSION

## CASE HISTORY

An 8-year-old boy is presented to the emergency department (ED) after being hit by a car. The driver was attempting to stop when the boy rode in front of the car on his roller skates. The boy was struck with the vehicle at low speed while the vehicle was attempting to stop. The boy struck the car and then the ground. He was wearing his helmet which struck the ground with him. He did not lose consciousness at any point. Primary survey reveals intact airway, breathing, and circulation (ABC) and mental status. Secondary survey reveals multiple contusions and abrasions on his arms and legs. The boy is holding his right (R) arm close to his chest. Vitals are initially unremarkable except for tachycardia to 140 bpm. Fluids and analgesia are started. X-ray of the R-forearm reveals a R-forearm fracture. Distal pulses and sensation are intact. While waiting for further orthopedic follow-up, the boy begins to complain of difficulty in breathing. His oxygen saturation continues to slowly drop down from 100% to 97%. He is started on $O_2$ by nasal cannula but continues to worsen. Immediate chest X-ray (CXR) is ordered and reveals infiltrates on the left (L) lower lung fields. No rib fractures or pneumothorax is present. What is the diagnosis? What management steps should be considered?

## DISCUSSION

Pulmonary contusion typically occurs in younger patients without completely ossified ribs. It may occur with or without the presence of flail chest or rib fractures.[1,2] Pulmonary contusion is a common potentially fatal injury (Fig. 1). Clinically, respiratory failure may present insidiously. Contusions present with pulmonary infiltrates and hemorrhage into pulmonary tissue.

Consider intubation for patients with significant hypoxia. Preexisting conditions, such as chronic obstructive pulmonary disease (COPD) or renal failure, may warrant earlier intubation. If patients with these conditions are transferred to your institution, they will require mechanical intubation. Every patient needs to be monitored for oxygen saturation, serial electrocardiograms (ECGs), arterial blood gases (ABGs), and suctioning, if needed. Basic laboratory tests values, such as complete blood count (CBC), troponin, chest CT, or CXR should be repeated as needed.

Flail chest can often be seen with pulmonary contusions (Fig. 3). Flail chest presents with multiple rib fractures and paradoxical breathing, which is when the chest bulges out on expiration and caves in on inspiration. Flail chest presentation is very sensitive to fluid overload. So, in treatment, we must restrict fluid intake.

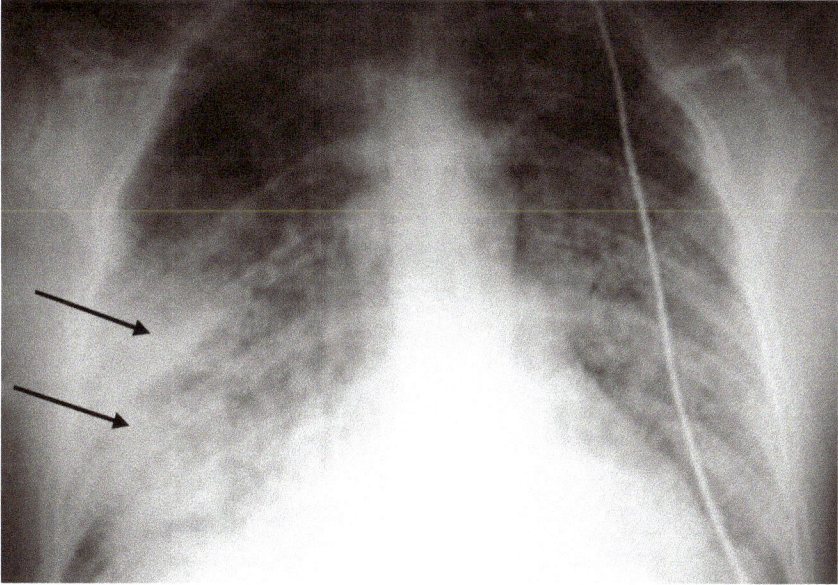

**Fig. 1:** White-out appearance with rib fractures (arrows).
*Source:* http://en.wikipedia.org.

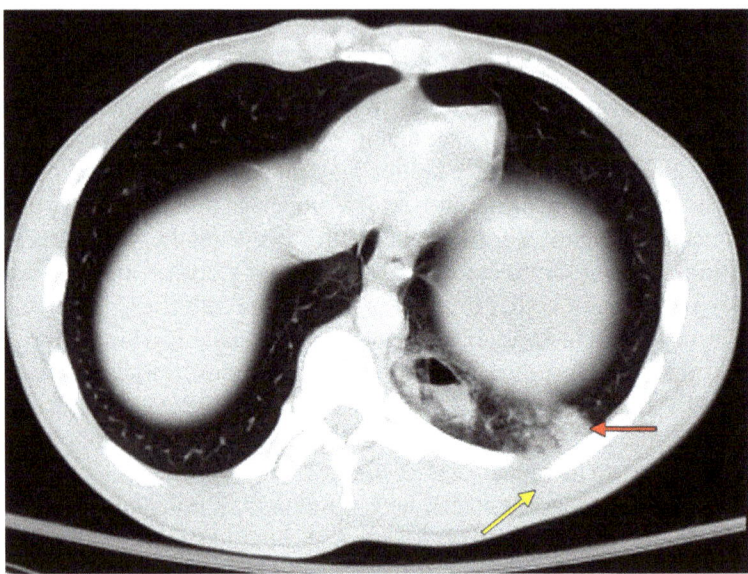

**Fig. 2:** CT chest with rib fractures (yellow arrow) and pulmonary contusion (red arrow).
*Source:* NIH & Medscape, Bethesda, USA.

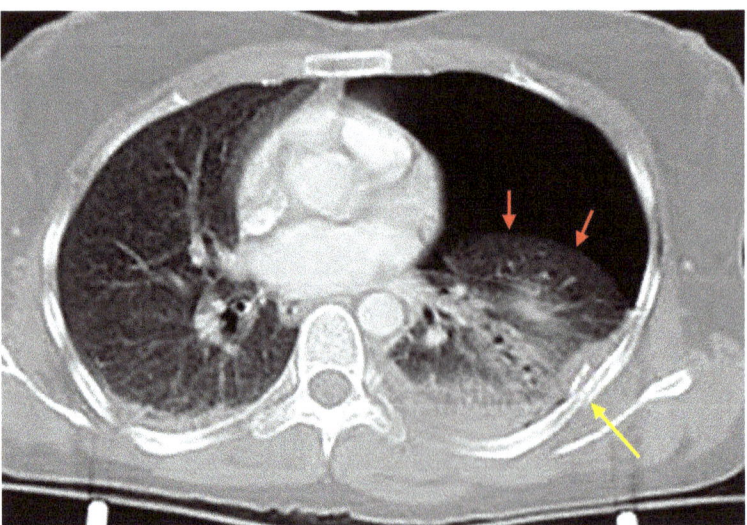

**Fig. 3:** CT chest of flail chest
*Source:* Medscape, New York, USA

Chest contusion may present with a white-out appearance on CXR (Fig. 1). We will need to continue monitoring because 50% of patients after trauma show the signs and symptoms of pulmonary contusion (Fig. 2).

## TREATMENT

- Judicious use of fluids. Use colloids for resuscitation if needed, avoid crystalloids
- Diuretics
- Intubation with positive end-expiratory pressure (PEEP) and cardiopulmonary monitoring in intensive care unit
- Early intervention of a pulmonologist will have a better outcome.

## REFERENCES

1. Mancini MC. Blunt chest trauma 2016; Available online from http://emedicine.medscape.com/article/428723-overview#a7.
2. ATLS Subcommittee, Atls Student Course Manual: Advanced Trauma Life Support 9th ed. Edition, American College of Surgeons; 9th ed. edition (September 1, 2012), https://www.amazon.com/Atls-Student-Course-Manual-Advanced/dp/1880696029?crid=11S7PIVW7Y3E9&keywords=advanced+trauma+life+support+9th+edition&qid=1538512530&sprefix=advanced+trauma+life+support+9th+edition%2Caps%2C213&sr=8-1&ref=sr_1_1

## CASE STUDY 11: TENSION PNEUMOTHORAX

*"Preparation is everything."*

—Badar M Zaheer

## CASE HISTORY

A 17-year-old boy was crushed between the garage door and the bumper of a car while his younger brother started the car and was trying to backup. This was his first driving experience without supervision. He was presented to the emergency department in a semi-rigid cervical collar and immobilized on a long back board on 10 L/min of oxygen via mask.

Physical examination shows a child who is alert but in severe distress. His vital signs are temperature 98.8°F, pulse rate 144 bpm, respiratory rate 40 breaths/min, and blood pressure 150/70 mm Hg. His airway is patent but respirations are rapid and shallow and he is cyanotic. There is decreased movement of the left hemithorax and there are absent breath sounds on left. There is mild subcutaneous emphysema over the left chest wall and neck but no tracheal deviation. Cardiac examination reveals tachycardia with a regular rhythm and jugular venous distension.

Chest X-ray is consistent with a left-sided pneumothorax.

## PNEUMOTHORAX

A pneumothorax is a collection of air around the lungs which subsequently puts pressure on the lungs so that they cannot expand during inspiration.

Pneumothorax presents initially as respiratory distress, often with tachypnea and shallow breathing. On physical examination, there will be decreased movement of the hemithorax and absent breath sounds on the affected side. In more severe cases, there may also be subcutaneous emphysema of the chest wall and neck on the injured side as well as tracheal deviation toward the unaffected side.

## TREATMENT

The first step in management in a person with a pneumothorax is evaluation of the airway, breathing, and circulation (ABC). Determination of airway patency and evaluation of the quality of the breathing should be done. Administration of oxygen via nasal cannula or mask is the first step. If the patient continues to experience respiratory distress despite supplemental oxygen, intubation should be considered. It is critical to recognize a pneumothorax quickly in order to initiate treatment and relieve the pressure. Once the patient is stabilized, immediate decompression is needed; the first step is to insert a large caliber needle into the second intercostal space on the midclavicular line of the affected pneumothorax (Fig. 1). An immediate release of air will occur. A chest tube is inserted with a 20–26 French chest tube in the fourth or fifth intercostal space in the anterior axillary line (Fig. 2). A chest X-ray should be repeated at this time to confirm chest tube placement and improvement of the pneumothorax. The patient should also be placed on continuous pulse oximetry to monitor oxygen levels. Circulatory status

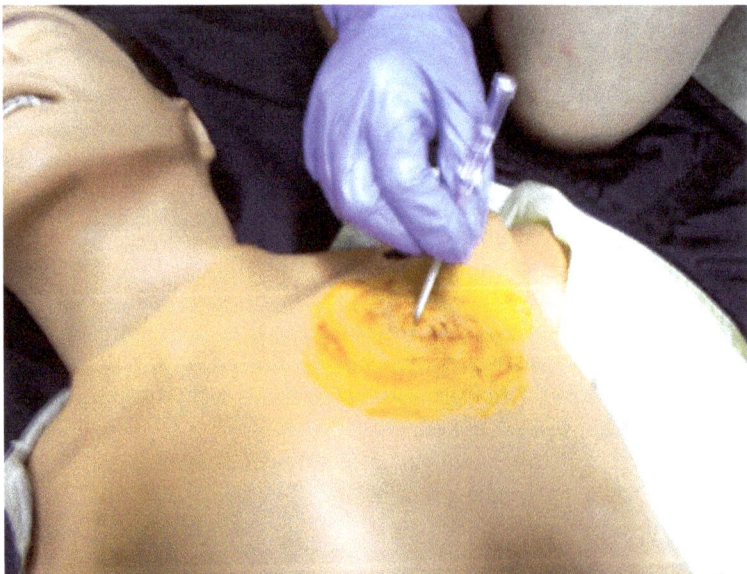

**Fig. 1A:** Angiocath is inserted at a 90° angle and advanced till air escaping is heard.
*Source:* http://www.civiliandefenseforce.com/needledecompression.html.

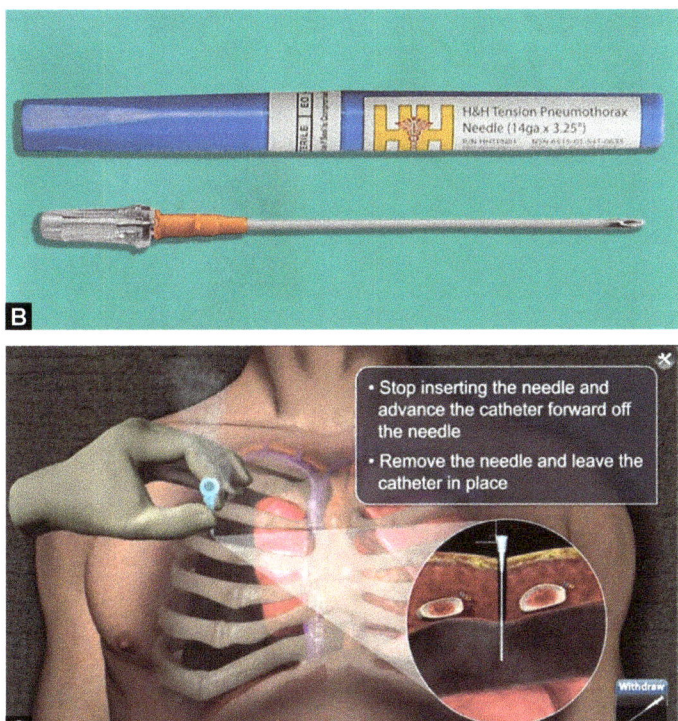

**Figs. 1B and C:** (B) High-tension pneumothorax needle; (C) Catheter insertion.
*Courtesy:* Foam EM RSS.

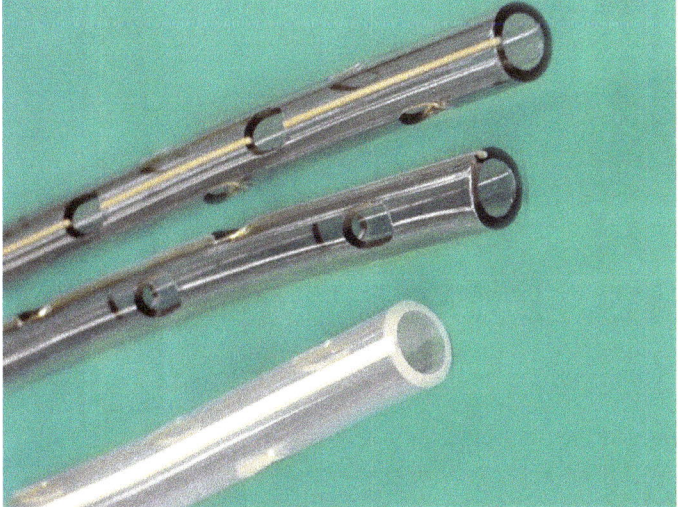

**Fig. 2:** Chest tube.
*Source:* http://en.wikipedia.org/wiki/chest_tube.

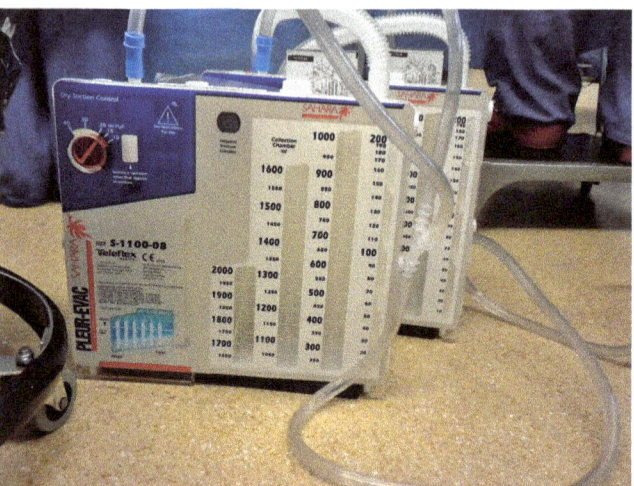

**Fig. 3:** Drainage canisters Pleur-evac.
*Source:* http://en.wikipedia.org/wiki/Chest_tube.

should be maintained with two large bore IVs and normal saline infused to maintain intravascular volume.

**Remember:**
- Chest tube should be directed above for air (pneumothorax) or below for blood (hemopneumothorax) and connected to drainage canisters shown in Figure 3.
- "A" for air and "B" for blood
- Always remember not to insert the needle or chest tube below the rib to avoid bleeding from intercostal vasculature.

## FURTHER READING

1. http://www.ncbi.nlm.nih.gov/pubmed/16825880.
2. http://en.wikipedia.org/wiki/Hemopneumothorax.
3. http://www.foamem.com/author/valerio-pisano-brasca/.

## CASE STUDY 12: HEMOPNEUMOTHORAX

### CASE HISTORY

A 15-year-old boy was crushed between a wall and the back of a van that was reversing. He is lying on the parking in severe respiratory distress. He is breathing at 40 breaths/min, labored and shallow. He is alert and moves all of his extremities. The patient's blood pressure is 160/70 mm Hg and he is transported on a rigid board with a C-collar on with supplemental oxygen.

## PREHOSPITAL TREATMENT

On arrival to the emergency room, the patient is in severe respiratory distress. He has absence of breath sounds on the left side of chest and tracheal shift to the right side.

## Respiration

Crepitus is heard over left chest wall and is extending up to the neck.

## Abdominal Findings

Abdomen is distended and tender on palpation. Bowel sounds are absent.

## Imaging

Chest X-ray findings include left tension pneumothorax, right lung contusion, and acute gastric dilatation (Fig. 1).

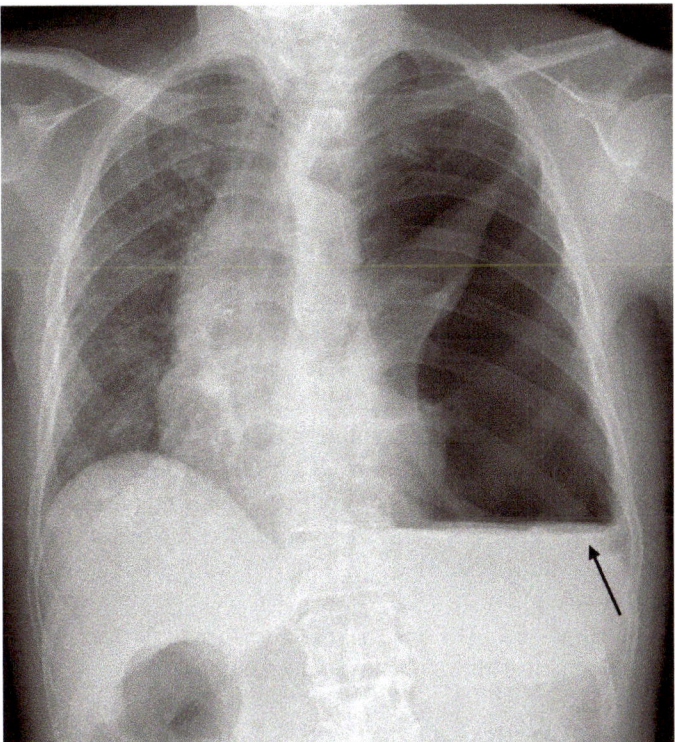

**Fig. 1:** Chest X-ray for hemopneumothorax blood/fluid level (arrow).
*Source:* Postgrad Med J© 2012 The Fellowship of Postgraduate Medicine.

## TREATMENT

- *Primary survey*: Carrying out the airway, breathing, circulation, disability, and exposure (ABCDE) is important. Remove all clothing
- A = assess the airway (respiratory distress at 40 bpm)
  - Airway suction and lifting of chin is done
  - If pulse oximeter has saturation of 80%, switch to nonbreathing mask (cyanosis present)
  - If patient becomes increasingly lethargic, anxious and shows increased respiration rate, then assess the breathing adequacy.
- Intubation is not required at this point, but chest tube placement is our priority.

## PHYSICAL FINDINGS

It includes the following:
- Tension pneumothorax on left chest wall
- Hyperresonance and absence of breathe sounds on left chest
- Subcutaneous emphysema on left side
- Tracheal deviation on the right chest wall (opposite of the pneumothorax).

### Difficulty in Using Bagwell Mask

*Treatment*: A large caliber needle is inserted over the second intercostal space at midclavicular line (always put needle on top of rib). You hear a gush of air and the patient immediately feels better.

### Improvement of Symptoms

- Child becomes more alert; color improves; breath sounds are less diminished on the right chest wall; and trachea begins to return to midline.
- This procedure is followed by a chest-tube insertion to replace the needle.
- A chest tube (size 24 French) is inserted and chest X-ray (CXR) is ordered.
- Saturation improves and arterial blood gas (ABG) comes back to normal.
- *Circulation*: Warm crystalloid solution is started in both arms.
- Cardiac monitor shows heart rate (HR) of 120 bpm.
- Because of possibility of abdominal trauma, a rectal examination was performed. A urinary catheter was placed after the rectal examination.
- Maintenance fluid is infused at a rate of 1 mL/kg/h. Patient is 40 kg, so 40 mL/h is used.
- Glasgow coma scale (GCS) = 12 (Child is opening his eyes, pupils are equal and reactive, and is obeying commands).

## FURTHER READING

1. http://www.ncbi.nlm.nih.gov/pubmed/16825880.
2. http://en.wikipedia.org/wiki/Hemopneumothorax.

## CASE STUDY 13: SPONTANEOUS PNEUMOTHORAX

*"Listen if you can, bear listening ... keep silence where visions are expressed."*
—**Rumi**

## CASE HISTORY

A 29-year-old male is presented to the emergency department (ED) with difficulty in breathing and a dull chest pain. The patient reports that the symptoms started all of a sudden 7 h prior to coming in. At the time, the chest pain on the right chest was more like a "stabbing" and now it has a vague and dull sensation. The pain is worse with inspiration. The patient has no past medical history except for smoking one packet per day of cigarettes for the last 10 years. On physical examination, his vital signs are blood pressure 150/80 mm Hg, heart rate 110 bpm, respiratory rate 40 breaths/min, and $O_2$ saturation of 90%. Patient is a tall thin appearing male in significant respiratory distress. He is started on nonrebreather oxygen mask at 12 L and intubation cart is prepared. Electrocardiography (ECG) and chest X-ray (CXR) are ordered.

## DISCUSSION

This patient is in severe respiratory distress and action must be taken quickly in order to reverse the effects. The differentials include pleurisy, pulmonary embolism, myocardial infarction, pericarditis, asthma, pneumonia, and pneumothorax. The first goal of treatments should be to stabilize the airway, breathing, and circulation. In severe cases, early definitive management should include needle aspiration or chest-tube placement.

Spontaneous pneumothorax is usually confirmed by upright CXR (Figs. 1 and 2).[1] On CXR, a white-visceral pleural line with the absence of vessel markings peripheral to this line must be searched. If the lateral width is >10%, a diagnosis of pneumothorax is made. The most sensitive position for detecting a pneumothorax is the left lateral decubitus with the least sensitive being supine. Even higher sensitivity may be obtained by obtaining both inspiratory and expiratory films. Computed tomography (CT) may be used to further classify or detect hard to see pneumothoraces. Furthermore, CT may detect underlying causes for secondary pneumothoraces. Bedside ultrasounds are equally effective in diagnosis.

This management differs from a suspected tension pneumothorax which is always a medical emergency and in fact should be detected by CXR or it may be too late to intervene. Tension pneumothorax must be suspected when the patient is hemodynamically unstable or when contralateral tracheal or mediastinal deviation is present (Table 1).

One goal of treatment after stabilization is prevention since the overall recurrence rate is estimated at 5%. A current mainstay of treatment is video-assisted thoracoscopy (VATS) with an aim to excise the associated bullae or perform guided pleurodesis. Talc has frequently been indicated as a sclerosing agent. However, patients with small pneumothoraces, <20%, may be observed with repetition of CXR. Regardless, definitive management is usually done after the first recurrence except in cases with high-risk occupations such as divers or pilots.

**Table 1:** The pathophysiology, presentation, and progression diagnosis and treatment of spontaneous and tension pneumothorax.

|  | Spontaneous pneumothorax | Tension pneumothorax |
|---|---|---|
| Pathophysiology | • Primary = rupture of small blebs near apex of lungs<br>• Secondary = due to COPD (most common), pneumonia, bronchogenic carcinoma, mesothelioma, sarcoidosis, tuberculosis, and cystic fibrosis | • Usually, traumatic event causes the formation of a check valve mechanism that lets air into the pleural space but it does not let it out |
| Presentation and progression | • Pleuritic chest pain that starts as sharp and turns dull (90%)<br>• 5% of patients have no symptoms and can delay treatment up to a week | • Rapid progression of dyspnea and tachypnea<br>• Emergency |
| Diagnosis | • CXR (Fig. 1) | • Tracheal deviation away from pneumothorax<br>• CXR (Fig. 2) |
|  | **Fig. 1:** Tracheal deviation towards pneumothorax | **Fig. 2:** Tracheal deviation away from pneumothorax |
|  | CT can be used if CXR is not conclusive | |
| Treatment | • 100% $O_2$: Increases the absorption of pneumothorax and should be administrated to all patients with pneumothorax<br>• Observation alone in asymptomatic patient with a small (<3 cm between lung and chest wall on CXR) | • 100% $O_2$<br>• Needle aspiration needed in patient with rapidly deteriorating condition and >3 cm between lung and chest wall<br>• Needle aspiration can be done using a large-bore angiocatheter needle. The needle is introduced in the |

*(Contd...)*

*(Contd...)*

| Spontaneous pneumothorax | Tension pneumothorax |
|---|---|
| pneumothorax. However, a repeat CXR is necessary to demonstrate the stability of the condition, which requires close monitoring. | second intercostal space of midclavicular line. The catheter is left in place and attached to a three-way stopcock and a large syringe. Air is aspirated until resistance is met or the patient experiences significant coughing<br>• Repeat CXR is done immediately after aspiration and again in 4–24 h to document re-expansion of the lung<br>• If the pneumothorax fails to resolve with aspiration, a chest tube should be placed. |

COPD: chronic obstructive pulmonary disease; CXR: chest X-ray.

## REFERENCE

1. Ferri FF. Ferri's Clinical Advisor 2013. 1st edn. Elsevier, Mosby; 2012. [Online]. Available online from www.mdconsult.com/books/page.do.

## CASE STUDY 14: DEEP VEIN THROMBOSIS

## CASE HISTORY

Patient is a 43-year-old female who is presented with right leg pain associated with redness and swelling of the calf area. Patient has a history of a similar episode 2 years ago for which she took Coumadin until 4 months ago. She took oral contraceptives for a few years in her 30s. She has no other medical problems except the history of *deep venous thrombosis* (DVT) in the past. She is not currently taking any medication. She has no recent immobilization. No symptoms of fever or shortness of breath were noticed. On physical examination, she has a temperature of 98.6°F, pulse rate 80 bpm, respiratory rate 18 breaths/min, and blood pressure 120/70 mm Hg. There is tenderness in the right lower extremity and the calf is slightly warm to palpation as compared to the left leg. Homan's sign, pain in the calf muscles with forced dorsiflexion of the foot, is absent. Laboratory workup shows complete blood count (CBC) within normal limits and D-dimer is elevated. Doppler ultrasound shows a high clinical probability of DVT.[1]

## CAUSES

Medical students remember the mnemonic THROMBOSIS:
- Trauma
- Hormones (OCPs)
- Road traffic accidents
- Operations
- Malignancy
- Blood disorders (polycythemia)
- Obesity
- Serious illness
- Immobilization
- Splenectomy.

## DISCUSSION

In cases of leg pain and swelling, several diagnoses should be considered, such as congestive heart failure (CHF) exacerbation, cellulitis, venous stasis without thrombosis, musculoskeletal injuries, vasculitis as well as DVT. Given the patient's history of DVT in the past, unilateral leg pain and swelling, elevated D-dimer, and absence of signs of heart failure or injuries, she likely has a recurrent DVT.

The classical signs and symptoms of a DVT include calf or leg pain, redness, swelling, and warmth (Fig. 1). Unfortunately, these are present in only

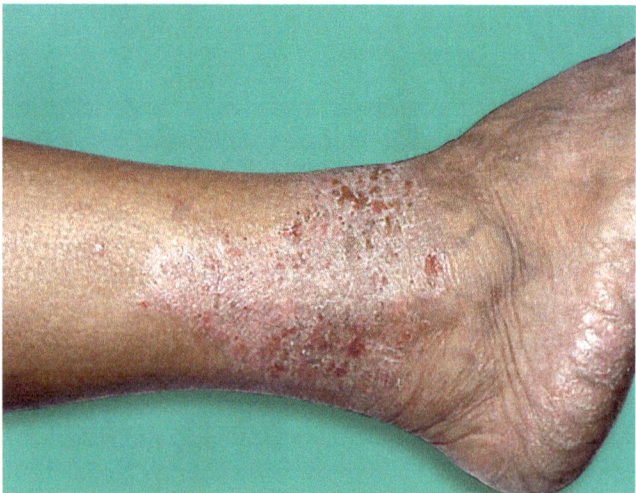

**Fig. 1:** Venous eczema.
*Source:* Available online from http://www.healthhype.com/deep-venous-thrombosis leg-vein-clot-dvt-pictures-symptoms.html [accessed June, 2012].
*Courtesy:* da Silva SF, Dermatology Atlas.

Chest

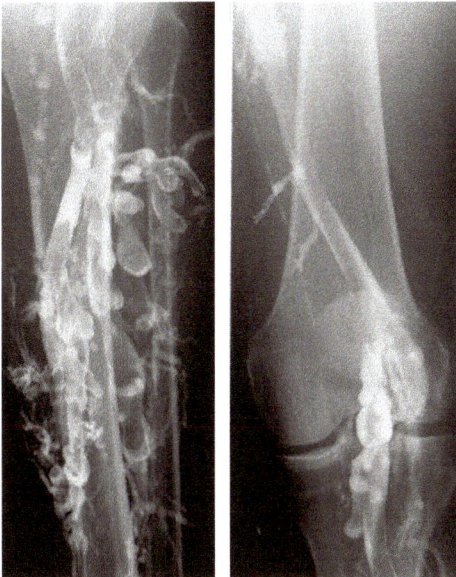

**Fig. 2:** Venograms of deep venous thrombosis.
*Source:* Wikipedia.

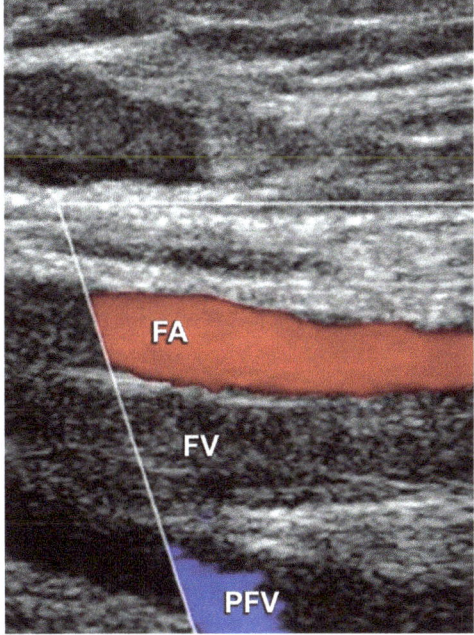

**Fig. 3:** Doppler ultrasound of deep venous thrombosis, femoral artery (FA), femoral vein (FV) and profunda femoris vein (PFV).
*Courtesy:* Dr Samir Haffar, Morgan Hill, California, USA.

> **Box 1:** Well's score or criteria (Possible score—2–9).
>
> - Active cancer (treatment within last 6 months or palliative): +1 point
> - Calf swelling ≥3 cm compared to other calf (measured 10 cm below tibial tuberosity): +1 point
> - Collateral superficial veins (nonvaricose): +1 point
> - Pitting edema (confined to symptomatic leg): +1 point
> - Previous documented deep vein thrombosis: +1 point
> - Swelling of entire leg: +1 point
> - Localized pain along distribution of deep venous system: +1 point
> - Paralysis, paresis, or recent cast immobilization of lower extremities: +1 point
> - Recently bedridden ≥3 days, or major surgery requiring regional or general anesthetic in past 4 weeks: +1 point
> - Alternative diagnosis at least as likely: −2 points.

about 50% of patients who present with a DVT. Homan's sign is an unreliable diagnostic test for DVT. For these reasons, criteria have been developed to determine the probability of whether or not a patient has a DVT, of which the most universally used is the Well's criteria.[2] Box 1 shows the list of Well's criteria and the scoring system.

A score of 3 or more indicates a high probability of DVT, a score of 1–2 indicates at moderate probability, and a score of ≤0 indicates a low probability. The need for further workup is determined by the score on these criteria. D-dimer assay is one option for testing; however, this test has a very low sensitivity of about 80% and therefore is not useful in ruling out DVT. Duplex ultrasonography has a sensitivity of 97% and specificity of 94% and is considered a reliable method of diagnosis (Figs. 2 and 3). For patients with a high probability of DVT but a negative Doppler, the test should be repeated in 1 week. After two consecutive negative Doppler ultrasounds 1 week apart, the risk of symptomatic DVT or pulmonary embolism (PE) within the next 3 months is <1%.

Treatment includes anticoagulation to prevent extension of the clot and decrease risk for PE and allow the natural fibrinolytic system to function. The treatment should begin with a low-molecular weight heparin (LMWH), such as dalteparin, enoxaparin, or tinzaparin, with a dose given every 24 h. Unfractionated heparin can be used when LMWH is contraindicated and lepirudin can be used for patients with a history of heparin-induced thrombocytopenia. Warfarin should be started concurrently at a dose of 5 mg/day with a goal international normalized ratio (INR) of 2.0–3.0. Bridging with heparin should be continued until the aimed INR is reached. In cases in which anticoagulation is contraindicated, inferior vena cava (IVC) filter can be placed to prevent the development of a PE. Most patients can be discharged safely with close follow-up if a dose of LMWH is given except for patients with complicated cases or patients with lack of follow-up.

# REFERENCES

1. Kabrhel C. McGraw-Hill Professional; 6th edition (2003), Peripheral vascular disorders. In: Emergency medicine manual. 6th ed. p. 166-8.
2. Well's criteria used. No copyright needed.

## CASE STUDY 15: ASTHMA

### CASE HISTORY

A 32-year-old man who has a history of asthma is presented to emergency department (ED) in severe respiratory distress. He was wheezing and using accessory muscles of respiration. His vital signs are blood pressure 120/90 mm Hg, heart rate 120 bpm, respiratory rate 40 breaths/min, temperature 97°F, and $O_2$ saturation 88% on room air (RA). This patient was brought to emergency room (ER) by ambulance. His $O_2$ saturations remain 88% on RA. Even with $\beta_2$ agonist, the patient still remains in respiratory distress, and with ipratropium treatment, the saturation improves slightly, patient stating 90% $O_2$ saturation. Initial peak flow was <200 L/min. Dexamethasone 4 mg IV is given at this time.

### DISCUSSION

This patient is obviously in respiratory distress and needs immediate coordination from physicians, respiratory therapist, and nursing staff. The objective of the treatment is to prevent the patient from going to respiratory failure. Asthma is a complex disorder that results from airway inflammation, airflow obstruction, and bronchial hyperresponsiveness. Many factors may contribute to the hyperreactivity, including environmental allergens, exercise, occupational exposure, emotional factors, gastroesophageal reflux disease (GERD), chronic sinusitis, and many more. The differential is broad and includes vocal cord dysfunction, tracheal and bronchial lesions, foreign bodies, pulmonary migraine, congestive heart failure, diffuse panbronchiolitis, aortic arch anomalies, sinus disease, cystic fibrosis, and pulmonary embolism.

When assessing asthma, it is important to determine precipitating factors: rapidity of onset, associated illness, number of exacerbations in the last year, need for ED visits, hospitalizations, intensive care unit admissions, intubations, and missed days from work or school/activity limitation. Asthma presents with wheezing as a very common symptom.[1] Wheezing may vary from mild, only at the end of expiration to severe, lasting throughout expiration. In extremely severe cases, wheezing may be absent from severe outflow obstruction. Other symptoms include cough or chest tightness. With worsening episodes, patients will be unable to lie flat and may even be hunched forward, only able to talk short words or phrases, and may be agitated. Use of accessory muscles may be seen. Respiratory rate is high and often >30 breaths/min. Heart rate is generally >120 bpm.

Initial evaluation should include electrocardiography (ECG), pulse oximetry, and chest X-ray. In cases of asthma, chest X-ray may indicate hyperinflation but will also be used to investigate other sources for respiratory distress. Peak expiratory flow may be used easily in the ED to compare to patient's baseline and response to treatment. Optimization of care should be done on outpatient basis.

In the ED, the most common treatment will be the use of $\beta_2$ agonists which may be administered via inhaled or nebulized forms. The main side effect is tachycardia, which is well tolerated in children but must be carefully monitored in adults with comorbid illnesses.

Ipratropium may also be used as a bronchodilator. Steroids should be used in moderate-to-severe cases. There is no explicit benefit of using oral versus intravenous steroids other than the possible ease of administration. The mainstay of treatment is to use enough bronchodilators to allow the steroids to take effect to diminish the bronchial inflammation. Heliox is also shown to provide relief to patients in the ED. Intubation should be considered in patients who fail to respond to treatment. Additionally, recent studies have shown that IV magnesium has therapeutic benefits in acute refractory asthma. The recommended does is 45 mg/kg IV.

Considerations for admission should be made on a case-by-case basis given history of frequent exacerbations, comorbid illness, and response to treatment. In severe cases, intensive care unit admission should be considered for patients who may be somnolent, have significant hypoxemia, hypercapnia, or who require intubation. Patients who are on RA, maintaining their saturation, and are no longer symptomatic while walking, may be discharged home.

| Classification | Days with symptoms | Nights with symptoms | For children >5 years who can use a spirometer or peak flow meter | |
|---|---|---|---|---|
| | | | FEV or PEF (% predicted normal) | PEF Variability |
| Severe persistent | Continual | Frequent | ≤60% | >30% |
| Moderate persistent | Daily | ≥5/month | >60% to <80% | >30% |
| Mild persistent | >2/week | 3–4/month | ≥80% | 20–30% |
| Mild intermittent | ≤2/week | ≤2 month | ≥80% | <20% |

NIH/National Asthma Education and Prevention Program Classification of Asthma Severity.

## REFERENCE

1. Morris MJ. Asthma. 2017. [Online]. Available from emedicine.medscape.com article/296301. [Accessed June, 2012].

## CASE STUDY 16: ACUTE RESPIRATORY DISTRESS SYNDROME

### CASE HISTORY

A 78-year-old Caucasian male was noted to be very lethargic for the past 4 days by his family members. His family called the emergency number and brought him to nearest hospital by emergency medical services (EMS). Patient was on nonrebreather (NRB) mask during transport to the nearest hospital. His vital signs are heart rate 123 bpm, temperature 101.2°F, respiratory rate 40 breaths/min and shallow, blood pressure 70/50 mm Hg, and $O_2$ saturation 78% on NRB mask. His past medical history (PMH) includes asthma, hypertension, and diabetes mellitus. Upon arrival, patient is intubated by emergency department (ED) physician and placed on 100% fraction of inspired oxygen ($FiO_2$); he is given 2 L fluid boluses. Laboratory data include WBC count of 22,000/µL, bands 5%, lactic acid 9 mmol/L, and sputum cultures were sent. Portable chest X-ray (CXR) shows left lower lobe (LLL) infiltrates and computed tomography (CT) scan of head negative for acute intracranial process or bleed. CT scan of chest shows negative results for pulmonary embolism. Patient is admitted to intensive care unit for acute respiratory distress syndrome (ARDS) from pneumonia. He is placed on sepsis protocol as per intensive care unit routine and he continued to receive 1 L fluid bolus and 0.09 normal saline (NS) placed at 150 cm³/h after. He has given injection Rocephin 2 g intravenous piggyback [IV short-term infusion (IVPB)] q 24 h. Tylenol supplement is used for fever. Ventilator settings in intensive care unit are given as follows: assist control (A/C) mode = 12 h, tidal volume (TV) = 450 cm³, pressure support = 10 cm $H_2O$, positive end-expiratory pressure = +5 cm$H_2O$, fraction of inspired oxygen ($FiO_2$) = 100%, and taped 23 at the lip. Patient is given propofol drop (gtt) for Richmond Agitation–Sedation Scale (RASS) of −2 or 15 µg/kg/min.

### DISCUSSION

ARDS (Table 1) includes an abrupt onset of diffuse lung injury accompanied by severe hypoxemia and bilateral pulmonary infiltrates.[1] Having a $PaO_2/FiO_2$

**Table 1:** The Berlin definition of acute respiratory distress syndrome.

| | Acute respiratory distress syndrome |
|---|---|
| Timing | Within 1 week of a known clinical insult or new or worsening respiratory symptoms |
| Chest imaging* | Bilateral opacities—not fully explained by effusions, lobar/lung collapse, or nodules |
| Origin of edema | Respiratory failure not fully explained by cardiac failure or fluid overload. Need objective assessment (e.g., echocardiography) to exclude hydrostatic edema if no risk factor present |
| Oxygenation† | |
| Mild | 200 mm Hg < $PaO_2/FiO_2$ ≤300 mm Hg with PEEP or CPAP ≥ 5 cm $H_2O$‡ |
| Moderate | 100 mm Hg < $PaO_2/FiO_2$ ≤200 mm Hg with PEEP ≥ 5 cm $H_2O$ |
| Severe | $PaO_2/FiO_2$ ≤100 mm Hg with PEEP ≥5 cm $H_2O$ |

CPAP: continuous positive airway pressure; $FiO_2$: fraction of inspired oxygen; $PaO_2$: partial pressure of arterial oxygen; PEEP: positive end-expiratory pressure.
*Chest radiograph or computed tomography scan.
†If altitude is higher than 1,000 m, the correction factor should be calculated as follows: [$PaO_2/FiO_2$ × (barometric pressure/760)].
‡This may be delivered noninvasively in the mild acute respiratory distress syndrome group.

of <200 is suggestive of ARDS. Having a $PaO_2/FiO_2$ of <300 is suggestive of patients with significant hypoxemia or acute lung injury (ALI).

Every year, there are 45–75 cases/100,000 people. Risk factors include severe infection, aspiration, shock, lung contusion, nonthoracic trauma, toxic inhalation, near drowning, and multiple blood transfusions.

Pathophysiology includes an inflammatory response consisting of an acute exudative phase, followed by a fibrosing alveolitis phase lasting 1–2 weeks during recovery, and finally resolution requires anywhere between 6 and 12 months.

Historical factors include absence of heart disease and history of any precipitating event. Physical examination demonstrates tachypnea, tachycardia, respiratory distress, lethargy, obtundation, flat neck veins, hyperdynamic pulses, physiologic gallop, absence of edema, moist and cyanotic skin, and manifestations of underlying disease. Arterial blood gas (ABG) will show severe hypoxemia. As described above, $PaO_2/FiO_2$ will be <200. Electrocardiography (ECG) may show sinus tachycardia or nonspecific ST changes. Pulmonary artery wedge pressure will be <15 mm Hg, and cardiac index will be >3.5 L/min/m². Initial imaging should include CXR and CT chest followed by serial CXRs. CXR will show fluffy bilateral infiltrates and CT chest will show diffused interstitial opacities and bullae. Differential diagnosis includes left ventricular failure, interstitial and airway disease, veno-occlusive disease, and mitral stenosis.

Patients with ARDS should be admitted to the intensive care unit. Overall, treatment goal is supportive with management directed at the underlying cause. Patients should be given supplemental oxygen and placed on ventilatory support. Ventilation settings should include lower TVs and optimization of positive end-expiratory pressure (PEEP). Other treatment goals are directed toward sepsis protocol including use of ionotropic agents such as dobutamine to maintain blood pressure support. Corticosteroid use is controversial, but sustained therapy in severe ARDS may be beneficial. Inhaled nitric oxide is no longer indicated. Some evidence suggests that pulmonary surfactant may be used in neonatal cases. Bronchodilators may be helpful while recovering. Data for antioxidants are controversial. Other supportive measures include deep vein thrombosis prophylaxis, ulcer prophylaxis, and parenteral nutrition. Invasive monitoring of vital signs, cardiac function, and pulmonary wedge pressure is also controversial. Large clinical trials have called the utility of these measures into question.

Overall, prognosis is poor with a mortality rate of 47%. Those that do survive often have multiple complications such as pulmonary lung disease, oxygen toxicity, barotrauma, superinfection, and multiorgan dysfunction (Figs. 1 and 2).

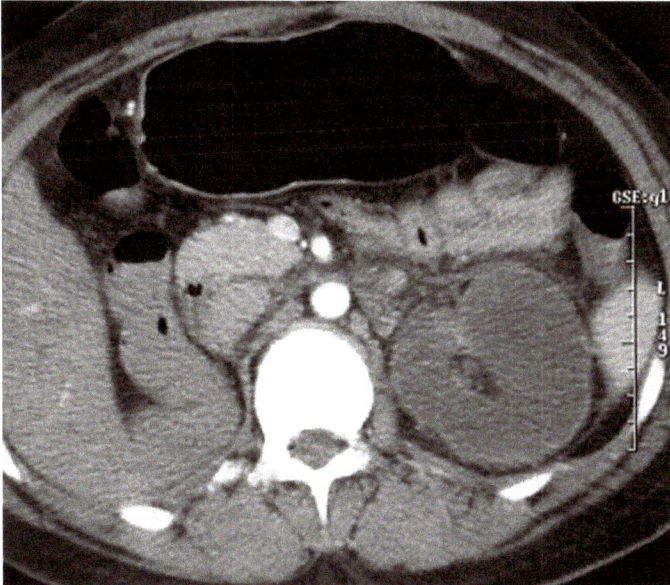

**Fig. 1:** CT abdomen in ARDS. (CT: computed tomography; ARDS: acute respiratory distress syndrome).

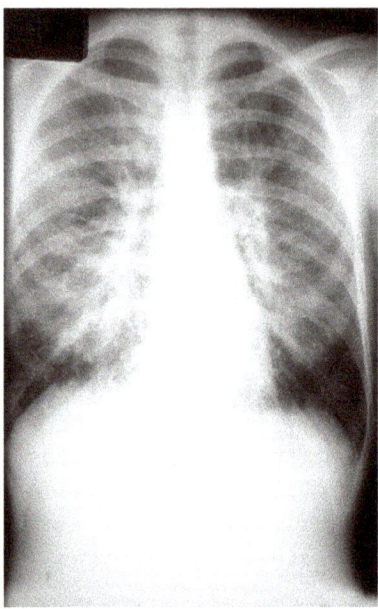

**Fig. 2:** Marked interstitial edema with hilar indistinctness, Kerley B lines, in HPS. (HPS: hantavirus pulmonary syndrome.)
*Source:* Available online from http://www.cdc.gov/hantavirus/technical/hps/clinical-manifestation.html. [Accessed June, 2012].
*Courtesy:* Ketai DL, Albuquerque, New Mexico, USA.

## REFERENCE

1. Mary C. Respiratory distress syndrome, acute (ARDS). In: Domino FJ, editor. The 5-Minute Clinical Consult. 20th edn. Philadelphia, PA: Lippincott Williams & Wilkins; 2012. p. 1130-1.

## CARDIOVASCULAR

### CASE STUDY 17: ACUTE CORONARY SYNDROME—ST-SEGMENT ELEVATION MYOCARDIAL INFARCTION

## CASE HISTORY

A 75-year-old man is seen in the emergency room (ER) for chest pain and lightheadedness for the past 4 h. His past history includes hypertension (HTN), hyperlipidemia, and diverticulosis. Current medications included atenolol 50 mg, aspirin 325 mg, and lovastatin 20 mg. His vital signs are pulse rate of 70 bpm regular, blood pressure 90/70 mm Hg, and chest and cardiac examinations are normal. Electrocardiogram (ECG) showed normal sinus rhythm with diffuse ST-T wave abnormalities. Initial troponin level is within normal limits, but after 6 h, his troponin level has reached 9 ng/mL.

# Chest

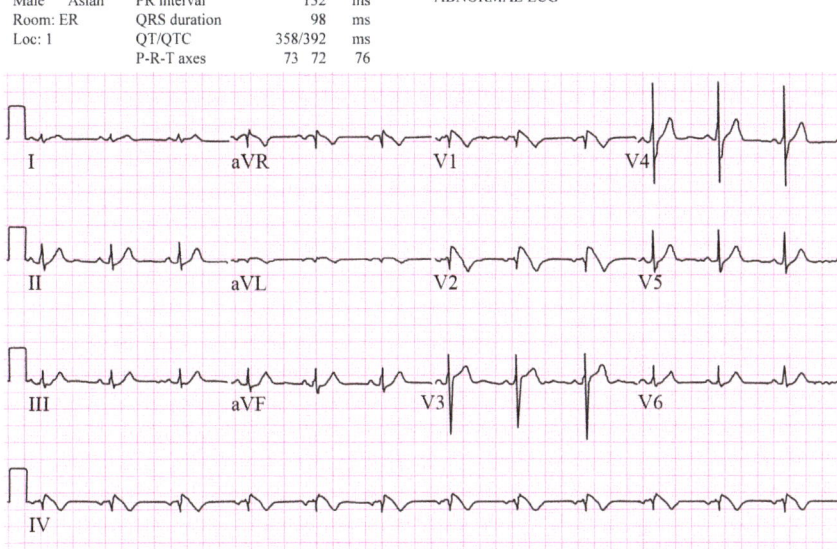

**Fig. 1:** ECG showing diffuse ST changes. (ECG: electrocardiography).
*Courtesy:* Badar M Zaheer, MD, Chicago, USA.

His hematocrit is 26%. Rectal examination is hemoccult positive. Repeat ECG was ordered to determine further management (Fig. 1).

## INTRODUCTION

Given that the patient has chest pain with a positive troponin, he likely has an acute coronary syndrome (ACS). ACS includes both myocardial infarction (MI) and unstable angina. MI results from an imbalance between myocardial oxygen supply and demand. Oxygen supply can be disrupted by atherosclerotic lesions, vasospasm, platelet aggregation, and thrombus formation. There are seven major risk factors for coronary artery Disease including age, male sex, family history, cigarette smoking, HTN, hypercholesterolemia, and diabetes.

## APPROACH TO CHEST PAIN (FLOWCHART 1)

Chest pain may have many causes. It is important to have an approach to chest pain to first ensure that the deadly causes of chest pain are ruled out before pursuing more benign causes. The five deadly causes of chest pain are MI, pulmonary embolism, esophageal rupture, pneumothorax, and aortic dissection. Nonlife-threatening causes of chest pain may include panic attack, costochondritis, pneumonia, and referred abdominal pain, such as gastroesophageal reflux disease (GERD) or cholecystitis.

Typical presentation for cardiac causes of chest pain includes pain that is retrosternal and is either squeezing, tightening, crushing, or pressure-like

**Flowchart 1:** Causes of chest pain.

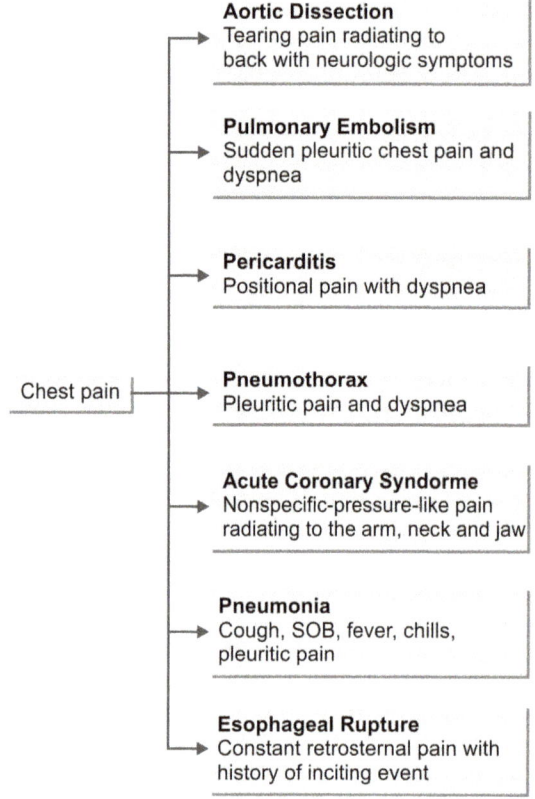

*Courtesy:* Badar M Zaheer MD.

in nature. Typically, sites of radiation include the left shoulder, jaw, arm, or hand. Presentations in the elderly, diabetics, or women may not include chest pain at all but will present with extreme fatigue. In the elderly, the chief complaint may be dyspnea, diaphoresis, nausea, light-headedness, or profound weakness. This is why there should be a low threshold for ordering an ECG. Symptoms lasting <2 min or over several days are less likely to be ischemic in origin.

Physical examination may vary from normal to extremely abnormal hemodynamics. Stable angina presents in episodes anywhere from 5 to 10-min long. Pain is worse with exertion and relieved with rest and nitroglycerin. Unstable angina has symptoms at rest. Prinzmetal angina occurs at rest and it is often associated with tobacco or cocaine use.

Aortic dissection presents with sudden onset and tearing pain that radiates to the back. Patients are typically hemodynamically unstable with either HTN or hypotension. If suspected, chest X-ray, computed tomography (CT), transesophageal echo, or angiography may be used to diagnose a dissection. Patients with pericarditis will complain of chest pain that radiates to the jaw, back, or neck and is alleviated by leaning forward. ST segment changes will be diffused. Patients with pulmonary embolism will complain of sudden onset, pleuritic chest pain associated with dyspnea, tachypnea, tachycardia, or hypoxemia. Chest wall tenderness supports a diagnosis of costochondritis but does not rule out acute MI. Gastrointestinal causes of pain may be associated with meals and relieved by antacids. GERD should be a diagnosis of exclusion. Cholecystitis should be considered in cases of atypical chest pain, especially in women.

All patients should be placed on oxygen, cardiac monitors, and start IV lines. Patients should be questioned about cardiac risk factors and careful history should be elicited. Serial ECGs should be obtained when considering cardiac causes of chest pain. Moderate-to-high-risk patients should be admitted for further observation, serial ECGs, serial enzymes, and possible stress testing.

## MANAGEMENT OF ACUTE CORONARY SYNDROME

Treatment depends on symptoms, history, physical, and ECG findings. The overall goal is to restore perfusion and limit infarction. This may be done in several ways: mechanical fibrinolytics, angioplasty, or coronary artery bypass graft (CABG). Initially, all patients should be placed on a cardiac monitor, given an IV line, and placed on oxygen. An ECG should be obtained within 5 min. Acetylsalicylic acid (ASA) or aspirin 160–325 mg should be given as soon as possible. Chewable form should be administered for more rapid onset. ASA has been shown to reduce death by up to 23%. Next, nitroglycerin also reduces mortality by up to 35%. Nitroglycerin may be given sublingually and repeated up to three times at 2–5-min intervals. If no improvement is noticed, a nitro drip should be started. The exception is the case of preload-dependent right ventricular infarction. Headache is a common side effect of nitroglycerin. Morphine may be used effectively to control pain.

Beta blockers have also been shown to reduce mortality and therefore cardioselective agents, preferably, should be used for ST-segment elevation MI (STEMIs), recurrent ischemia, tachydysrhythmia, and non-STEMI (NSTEMIs). Relative contraindications are heart rate (HR) slower than 60 bpm, systolic BP < 100 mm Hg, moderate-to-severe congestive heart failure (CHF), signs of peripheral hypoperfusion, pulse rate (PR) interval longer than 0.24 s, second- or third-degree atrioventricular block (AVB), severe chronic obstructive pulmonary disease (COPD), history of asthma, severe diabetes mellitus, and severe peripheral vascular disease.

Unfractionated heparin may be used with ASA to control the thrombus. In patients with unstable angina, this combination may reduce mortality. Low-molecular-weight heparins such as enoxaparin are preferred for unstable angina or NSTEMI patients, unless percutaneous intervention or CABG is scheduled in the next 24 h. Enoxaparin is not reversible, but unfractionated heparin has a shorter half-life and may be emergently reversed with protamine sulfate.

With ECG findings of ≥1 mm ST-segment elevation in two or more contiguous leads, the patient requires intervention for STEMI. The preferred method is percutaneous coronary intervention (PCI), but distance to centers and time delays limit this practice to be administered to every patient. Fibrinolytics may be considered as an alternative to either angioplasty or stent placement. Fibrinolytics should be administered within 6–12 h. If there is access to a cardiology consult, one should be obtained before administering. Patients should be selected carefully because fibrinolytics carry significant risk. Elderly patients over 75 years of age have been shown to have significant complications. Alteplase or tissue plasminogen activators (tPAs) have been shown to have good rate of reperfusion and minimal risk within 90 min given a front-loaded dose. Hemorrhage, especially intracranial bleeding, is the most feared complication. Clopidogrel in combination with ASA is considered for unstable angina (UA)/NSTEMI patients since it reduces the composite risk of cardiovascular (CV) death, MI, or stroke. Glycoprotein IIb/IIIa may be used as an adjunct to angioplasty, medical stabilization of ACS, and in combination with low-dose fibrinolytics.

Right ventricular infarcts have special considerations. These types of infarcts are preload dependent to maintain cardiac output; therefore, diuretics and nitroglycerin should be avoided. Cardiac output may need to be maintained with volume infusion. Dobutamine should be used if an inotropic agent is needed. Nitroprusside or intra-aortic balloon counterpulsation is available in refractory cases.

STEMI Alert criteria: ST elevation MI with symptom onset >30 min and <12 h
- Call your transfer services
- Activate code "STEMI Alert" and give patient's weight
- Air ambulance/helicopter dispatched
- Call the cardiologist on call and discuss the plan and activate cardiac catheterization laboratory.

Primary PCI protocol
- ECG (within 10 min of arrival)
- Communicate with cardiology
- Oxygen
- Laboratories: CBC, INR, aPTT, BMP, BNP, magnesium, cardiac specific troponin, CK-MB
- Non-enteric-coated ASA; 81 mg (four chewable) po
- Ticagrelor (Brilinta) 180 mg po loading dose (two tabs), if already on Brilinta continue regular dosing OR if ticagrelor is not available, give clopidogrel (Plavic) 600 mg po (75 mg × 8 tabs)
- Beta blocker—consider for hypertension; Lopressor 5 mg IV every 5 min × 3 (hold for heart rate <50 AV block, SBP < 100)
- Nitroglycerin 0.4 mg SL (repeat as needed)—use with caution in inferior MI with hypotension
- Nitroglycerin paste—2 in—use with caution inferior MI with hypotension

- Heparin bolus 4,000 units (no GTT)
- Assess patient for dye allergy, if yes, pretreat with Solu-Medrol 100 IVP and Benadryl 50 mg po
- Morphine sulfate: 2–4-mg IV q 5–15 min as needed for pain
- Fax laboratories and other pertinent for MD to review prior to patient arrival
- Call report to cardiac intensive care unit.

## ASSESSMENT

### Tests

*Electrocardiogram*
- Persistent ST-segment elevation 2 mm in two contiguous limb leads
- ST-segment elevation 3 mm in two contiguous chest leads
- *New left bundle branch block pattern*: QRS 130 ms V1: rS complex. V6: RsR'
- *Cardiac biomarkers*: Elevation of biomarkers such as troponin, creatine kinase muscle and brain (CK-MB) 24 h postonset of symptoms.

## MANAGEMENT

Following measures should be taken as soon as possible (ASAP):
- Cardiac monitoring
- $O_2$ therapy
- IV line should be established ASAP
- Chew aspirin
- Nitroglycerin
- Pain control by morphine
- Reperfusion strategy ASAP, fibrinolytic therapy, or PCI
- *ER reperfusion*: Restores coronary patency
- *Percutaneous coronary intervention*: Best if promptly provided
  - Short- and long-term benefit if done within 12 h of symptom onset versus thrombolysis
  - Less than 90 min from first medical encounter to PCI
  - Transfer to facility capable of performing PCI if can be done within 90 min.
- If PCI is not available, thrombolysis/fibrinolysis
  - Streptokinase or tPA
    - Restore perfusion to ischemic area
    - Lyse clot, reduce infarct size, and improve survival
    - Most beneficial for anterior infarction
    - Early implementation is better
    - Greatest benefit recorded is for ST elevation or bundle branch block (BBB) with symptom onset within 12 h
  - IV streptokinase and alteplase
  - *Rapid bolus injection*: reteplase, tenecteplase
  - *tPA*: most common agent.

## Contraindications of Streptokinase

- Prior use <12 months due to antibody persistence
- Consider thrombolytic as alternative to PCI in patient with STEMI with >1 mm ST elevation in two contiguous leads
- New LBBB.

### Absolute Contraindications

- Active bleeding, bleeding diathesis
- Significant closed head or facial trauma <3 months
- Suspected aortic dissection
- Prior intracranial hemorrhage
- Ischemic stroke within 3 months.

### Relative Contraindications

- Active peptic ulcer
- Severely, poorly control HTN
- Ischemic stroke within 3 months
- Late presentation
- *Reperfusion with PCI or fibrinolysis*: Not recurrent if >12 h after symptoms onset, asymptomatic versus stable angina.
    - CABG more appropriate
    - Cardiogenic shock with mechanical repairing.

## Adjuvant Therapy

- *Antiplatelet therapy*: Aspirin 300 mg. Low dose followed on long-term basis
    - Clopidogrel
        - 300–600 mg loading dose if PCI with stent is planned
        - 300 mg with aspirin if used for fibrinolysis
        - withhold if CABG is required acutely
        - 75 mg daily
        - 1 month after thrombolysis
        - 9–12 months after stent
- *Antithrombin therapy*
    - *With PCI*: Unfractionated heparin (UFH) and glycoprotein (GP) IIb/IIIa inhibitors
    - *With fibrinolysis*: UFH
    - Recommended dose of UFH is an initial bolus of 60 units/kg body weight (maximum 4,000 units) followed by an initial infusion of 12 units/kg/h, maximum units 1,000/h
    - Adjusted to attain activated partial thromboplastin time (aPTT) at 1.5–2 times the control value

- Enoxaparin in conjunction with fibrin-specific fibrinolytic agent can be used
- If <75 years, no renal dysfunction
- *GP IIb/IIIa inhibitors*: abciximab and primary PCI with full-dose fibrinolytic therapy.

## Cardiac Surgery

- Coronary artery bypass surgery (CABG) is performed if PCI fails with pain or hemodynamic instability and coronary anatomy is suitable
- Persistent/recurrent ischemia refractory to medical therapy.

## Differential Diagnosis

- Costochondritis
- Hiatal hernia
- GERD
- Peptic ulcer disease
- Gallbladder disease
- STEMI
- Aortic stenosis
- Myocarditis
- Pericarditis
- Pleuritis
- Dissecting aortic aneurysm
- Mitral valve prolapse
- CHF
- Pulmonary embolism
- Pulmonary HTN
- Pneumothorax.
- *Diagnosis*: STEMI.

## PLAN

- Discharge medications after ACS
- *Aspirin*: 75–325 mg po daily
- *Clopidogrel*: 75 mg po daily for 9–12 months after ACS if aspirin is contraindicated
- *Beta blockers*: Metoprolol or carvedilol po daily lifelong 50 mg po daily
- *Angiotensin converting enzyme inhibitors*: Used in ACS patient in CHF left ventricular (LV) dysfunction with ejection fraction (EF) <40%. Discharge if heart failure resolves
- *Statin*: Initiate in hospital
- *Nitrates*: Short-acting nitrates are used

- *Warfarin*: Used only if high-risk thromboembolism is present because of atrial fibrillation, mural thrombus, and CHF
- *Address risk factors*: Hyperglycemia, HTN control, tobacco cessation, physical inactivity, and alcohol
- Exercise ECG testing
- *Submaximal testing*: 4–7 days postinfarction, *maximum*: 3–6 weeks postinfarction
- Identify patient with recurrent ischemia, who needs angiogram to assess CABG
- *Myocardial perfusion imaging*
  - It assesses the residual ischemia extent
  - It should be done before cardiac catheterization and angiography.

## DISCUSSION

Acute Coronary Syndrome
*These are of three types*: (1) unstable angina, (2) NSTEMI, and (3) STEMI.

## Causes

Coronary versus atherosclerotic obstruction, superimposed thrombotic occlusion.

## Site

*Infarction in areas of nonlimited blood flow at rest*: Noncritical coronary stenosis.

## Pathophysiology

- Periods of relative quiescence
- Interposed with episodes of rapid and abrupt plaque development and changes
- Plaque disruption and mural thrombosis
- *Rate-limiting mechanisms*: Acute thrombosis—resultant obstruction of coronary lumen.

## Angiography

- Noncritical lesions account for majority of ACS
- "Red" thrombi, fibrin rich for STEMI.

## Duration

- Symptoms remain for >20 min and do not respond completely to nitroglycerin
- Symptoms may resolve completely after a few hours or persist for >24 h.

## Comorbidities
- Elderly, diabetes mellitus
- One-fifth MIs are "silent" and may not seek medical treatments.

## Presentation
- Anxiety and pain
- Diaphoresis
- *Pulse rate*: Normal; *bradycardic*: inferior infarction; *tachycardic*: large infarction
- *BP*: Elevated
- Cardiac activity: Usually normal
- *Large infarction*: Ventricular failure, valve dysfunction
- *S4*: Stiffened ventricle
- *Mitral regurgitation*: Papillary muscle malfunction
- S2 paradoxically split at LV control time increases due to LBBB, weakened LV
- Progression
  - *Later*: Mild fever
  - Pericardial friction rub
  - Ventricular septal defect murmur due to septal rupture
  - Severe mitral regurgitation due to papillary muscle rupture.

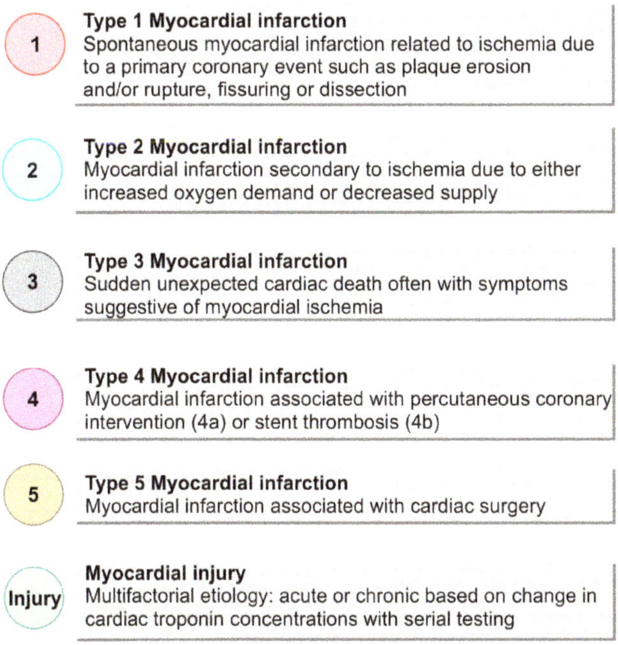

**1 — Type 1 Myocardial infarction**
Spontaneous myocardial infarction related to ischemia due to a primary coronary event such as plaque erosion and/or rupture, fissuring or dissection

**2 — Type 2 Myocardial infarction**
Myocardial infarction secondary to ischemia due to either increased oxygen demand or decreased supply

**3 — Type 3 Myocardial infarction**
Sudden unexpected cardiac death often with symptoms suggestive of myocardial ischemia

**4 — Type 4 Myocardial infarction**
Myocardial infarction associated with percutaneous coronary intervention (4a) or stent thrombosis (4b)

**5 — Type 5 Myocardial infarction**
Myocardial infarction associated with cardiac surgery

**Injury — Myocardial injury**
Multifactorial etiology: acute or chronic based on change in cardiac troponin concentrations with serial testing

**Fig. 2:** New Classification of MI. (MI: myocardial infarction).
*Source:* Thygesen K, Alpert JS, Jaffe AS, *et al*. Third universal definition of myocardial infarction. Eur Heart J 2012;**33**:2551–67.

## PRACTICE PEARL AND PITFALL

Women are at a greater risk for misdiagnosis because they tend to have atypical symptoms and false-negative stress tests. Consider any extreme fatigue in a young woman an MI unless proved otherwise. Painless MIs are associated with higher mortality than painful MIs.

## FURTHER READING

1. Cardiovascular medicine. Medical Knowledge Self-assessment Program (MKSAP 13), 2009, Item 31. p. 152.
2. Thomas R. Approach to chest pain and ischemic equivalents. In: Emergency Medicine Manual. 6th edn. McGraw-Hill Professional; 6th edn. 2003. p. 123-8.
3. Jim Edward W. Acute coronary syndromes: management of myocardial infarction and unstable angina. In: Emergency Medicine Manual. McGraw-Hill Professional; 6th edn. 2003. p. 129-36.
4. Coven DL. Acute coronary syndrome medication. [Online]. Available from emedicine.medscape.com/article/1910735-medication#2. [Accessed June, 2012].

## CASE STUDY 18: ACUTE CORONARY SYNDROME—NON-ST-SEGMENT ELEVATION MYOCARDIAL INFARCTION

## CASE HISTORY

Patient is a 60-year-old Caucasian female who presents with chest pain for 1 h. Patient states that "it feels like a heavy weight on my chest. It would not go away." Pain is constant, substernal/epigastric radiating to her neck, left shoulder, and left arm. She has a past history of hypertension (HTN), diabetes, coronary artery disease (CAD), and stroke for which she takes acetylsalicylic acid (ASA), humalog, metformin, enalapril, and atenolol. She has smoked two packs of cigarettes per day for the past 40 years and drinks a glass of wine daily. She used cocaine regularly in the past but has been in remission for 30 years. Her vital signs are temperature of 36°C, blood pressure 95/65 mm Hg, pulse rate 110 bpm, and respiratory rate 20 breaths/min. On physical examination, skin is pale and cool. Cardiac examination reveals tachycardia with an S3. Bibasilar pulmonary rales are present on lung examination. Remainder of examination is unremarkable. Electrocardiogram (ECG) reveals dynamic ST-segment depression of 0.6 mm with a new T-wave inversion of 3 mm as well as sinus tachycardia. Cardiac markers are negative. Patient has a presumed non-ST-segment elevation myocardial infarction (MI) (NSTEMI) and medical management is initiated (Fig. 1). Patient is admitted for further evaluation.

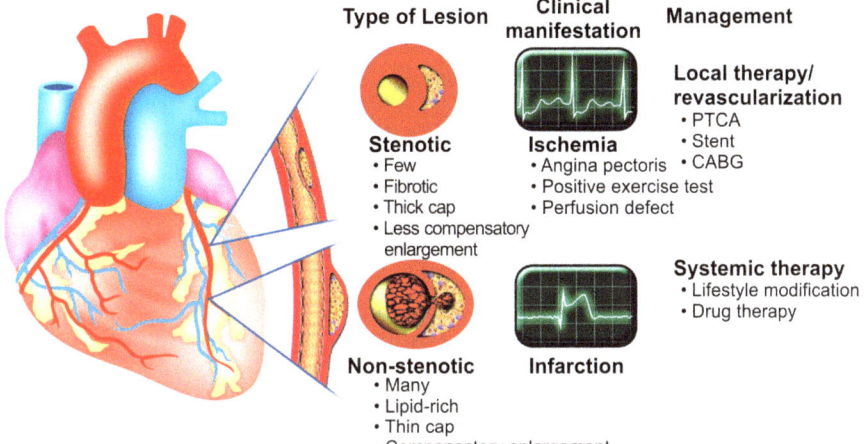

**Fig. 1:** Clinical management of NSTEMI. (NSTEMI: non-ST-segment elevation myocardial infarction; PTCA: percutaneous transluminal coronary angioplasty; CABG: coronary artery bypass grafting).

## DISCUSSION

Differential diagnosis includes costochondritis, hiatal hernia, gastroesophageal reflux disease (GERD), peptic ulcer disease, gallbladder disease, aortic stenosis, mitral valve prolapse, myocarditis, pericarditis, dissecting aortic aneurysm, pleuritis, congestive heart failure (CHF), pulmonary embolism, pulmonary HTN, and pneumothorax.

Initially, unstable angina (UA) and NSTEMI have similar presentations. UA or ischemic equivalent has one of the three features:
1. Occurs at rest or with minimal exertion, lasting >10 min.
2. Severe and of new onset, prior within 4–6 weeks.
3. Occurs with crescendo pattern, more severe, prolonged, and frequent than before. NSTEMI has the clinical features of UA but develops evidence of myocardial necrosis with elevated cardiac biomarkers, creatine kinase muscle and brain (CK-MB), and troponin over time.

A list of acute coronary syndromes as they increase in severity includes UA occurring without serologic evidence of myocardial necrosis; new-onset angina, severe and lasting longer than 2 months; increasing (crescendo) angina which is gaining in severity, length, or frequency. Angina pectoris usually occurs at rest, prolonged pain for >20 min and within 1 week of presentation. Postinfarction angina occurring 2 weeks after an acute MI (AMI).[1] Acute MI is next which includes the following: non-ST-elevation (non-Q-wave) MI and a transient thrombotic occlusion with early spontaneous reperfusion, also the ST-elevation (Q-wave) MI, a total thrombotic occlusion which is associated with a larger infarct size and higher in-hospital mortality rate. As in all cases, earlier the reperfusion therapy begins, the better is the probability of preventing sudden death and also decreases infarct size. "Time is Muscle." Sudden ischemic cardiac death, secondary to malignant ventricular tachyarrhythmias, is the most severe type of acute coronary syndrome.

All patients with suspected acute coronary syndrome should be administered aspirin 325 mg. NSTEMI management differs from STEMI. Patients with a suspected NSTEMI should initially be medically managed. They are still candidates for percutaneous coronary intervention (PCI), but likely during hospital admission rather than immediately. Patients should be given anticoagulants. Generally, patients are administered Plavix and Lovenox unless surgical intervention is planned within 24 h. Nitrates and/or morphine may be used for pain control. Patients should also be given an angiotensin-converting enzyme (ACE) inhibitor and beta-blocker in the first 24 h.

The cause of acute coronary syndrome regardless is a reduction in oxygen ($O_2$) supply and increase in myocardial $O_2$ demand. The cause may be superimposed on an atherosclerotic coronary plaque with varying degrees of obstruction. There are several pathophysiologic possibilities. First, there may be plaque rupture/erosion with superimposed nonocclusive thrombus causing an NSTEMI downstream embolization of platelet aggregation/atherosclerotic debris. Second, there may be dynamic obstruction causing coronary spasm and Prinzmetal's variant angina. Third, there may be a progressive mechanical obstruction causing rapidly advancing coronary atherosclerosis/restenosis after PCI. Finally, there may be secondary UA relative to increased myocardial $O_2$ demand or decreased supply.

The common findings on coronary angiography are 5% left main stenosis, 15% three-vessel (CAD), 30% two-vessel disease, 40% single-vessel disease, and 10 without critical coronary stenosis. Prinzmetal's variant *culprit lesion* may show an eccentric stenosis with scalloped/overhanging edges and narrow neck white thrombi platelets with rich multiple plaque vulnerable to disruption.

High-risk features for patients with suspected UA/NSTEMI are repetitive or prolonged chest pain lasting >10 min, elevated cardiac biomarkers, persistent (ECG) changes, hemodynamic instability with systolic blood pressure <90 mm Hg, sustained ventricular tachycardia, syncope, left ventricular ejection fraction (LVEF) below normal 40%, prior percutaneous transluminal coronary angioplasty (PTCA) or coronary artery bypass graft (CABG), diabetes, and chronic kidney disease.

## REFERENCE

1. Zafari AM. Myocardial infarction treatment & management. [Online]. Available online from emedicine.medscape.com/article/155919-treatment; 2012 [accessed June, 2012].

# CASE STUDY 19: UNSTABLE ANGINA

## CASE HISTORY

Patient is a 63-year-old male with past medical history (PMH) of hypertension and hyperlipidemia who presents with worsening chest pain. He has had chest pain in the past while working in the yard, but in the past, it always went away after a few minutes when he sat down to rest. This morning he was mowing the lawn and started experiencing a pressure-like pain in his chest that radiated to his left arm. He sat down to rest, but the pain did not go away so his wife called for an ambulance. He was given two nitroglycerin tablets en route which have not alleviated the pain. He also received four baby aspirins while en route. Pain has now lasted approximately 40 min. His vital signs on arrival are temperature of 38.6°C, blood pressure 160/90 mm Hg, pulse rate 105 bpm, respiratory rate 20 breaths/min, and $O_2$ saturation of 96% on 2 L nasal cannula. Intravenous (IV) lines are started and patient is placed on the cardiac monitor. Electrocardiogram (ECG) and chest X-ray (CXR) are ordered which are shown in Figures 1 and 2. Patient is given morphine which temporarily relieves the pain, but it returns again after approximately 20 min. Serial ECGs and cardiac enzymes are ordered. Pain is thought to be cardiac in origin with possible unstable angina.[1] How should this patient be managed?

## DISCUSSION

Please see approach to chest pain discussion in Case Study 17: Acute Coronary Syndrome—ST-segment Elevation Myocardial Infarction.

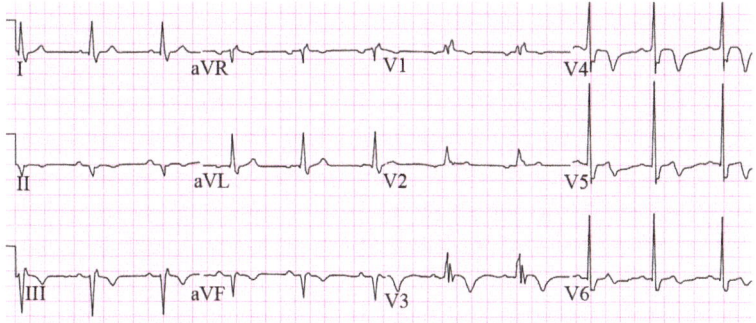

**Fig. 1:** Electrocardiogram.
*Source:* EMT Emergency Medicine Tutorials. [Online] Available from http://www.emergency-medicine-tutorials.org/Home/medical-3/cardiovascular/ecgs-1/wellen-s- syndrome-sign-warning. [Accessed June, 2012].

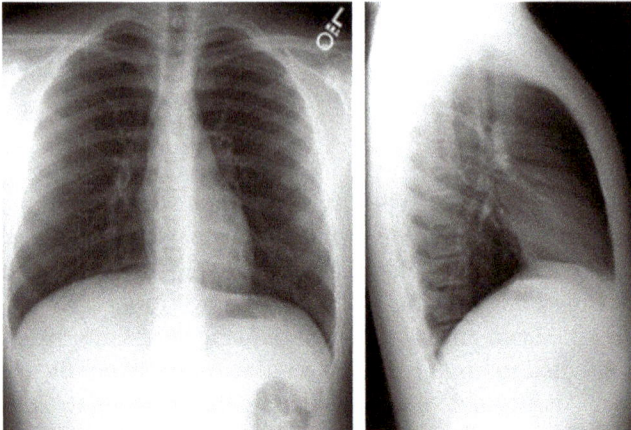

**Fig. 2:** Chest X-ray of a 63-year-old male patient.

Unstable angina is a type of acute coronary syndrome in which the patient does not experience a release of cardiac enzymes. Causes may include unstable or disrupted atherosclerotic plaques. Other factors may include supply–demand mismatch, plaque disruption or rupture, thrombosis, vasoconstriction, or cyclical flow.

Overall, the number of patients with coronary unstable angina is rising. The trends are slightly different depending on age and sex. Women tend to be older and have higher rate of hypertension, diabetes, congestive heart failure (CHF), and family history of coronary artery disease (CAD) when compared to men, whereas men tend to have higher rate of previous myocardial infarction (MI), more positive cardiac enzymes, and higher rate of catheterization. Overall, patients tend to range in age from 23 to 100 years with a median age of 62 years.

Several factors have been shown to suggest a poor outcome including ongoing CHF, poor left ventricular ejection fraction (LVEF), hemodynamic instability, recurrent angina, new or worsening mitral regurgitation, and sustained ventricular tachycardia.

A rapid but thorough history should be obtained with a focus on the symptoms and coronary risk factors. ECG should be rapidly obtained. Physical examination should include assessment of vital signs and consideration of other illnesses including aortic dissection, leaking or ruptured thoracic aneurysm, pericarditis with tamponade, pulmonary embolism, and pneumothorax.

Unstable angina is generally more intense than stable angina. Pain is ischemic in nature with either a sensation of heaviness, tightness, aching,

**Table 1:** Braunwald classification of unstable angina.

| Characteristic | Class/Category | Details |
|---|---|---|
| Severity | I | Symptoms with exertion |
| | II | Subacute symptoms at rest (2–30 days prior) |
| | III | Acute symptoms at rest (within prior 48 h) |
| Clinical precipitating factor | A | Secondary |
| | B | Primary |
| | C | Postinfarction |
| Therapy during symptoms | 1 | No treatment |
| | 2 | Usual angina therapy |
| | 3 | Maximal therapy |

*Note:* Patients in Class I have new or accelerated exertional angina, whereas those in Class II have subacute (>48 h since last pain) or Class III acute (<48 h since last pain) rest angina. The clinical circumstances associated with unstable angina are categorized as (A) secondary (anemia, fever, and hypoxia), (B) primary, or (C) postinfarction (<2 weeks after infarction). Intensity of antianginal therapy is subclassified as (1) no treatment, (2) usual oral therapy, and (3) intense therapy, such as IV nitroglycerin.
*Source:* Tan WA. Unstable angina. [Online]. Available from emedicine.medscape.com/article/159383-overview#showall; 2011 [accessed June, 2012].

fullness, or burning in the chest, epigastrium, and/or arm or forearm. Associated symptoms might be dyspnea, generalized fatigue, diaphoresis, nausea and vomiting, flu-like symptoms, lightheadedness, or abdominal pain (Table 1).

The thrombolysis in MI (TIMI) risk score may be used as a clinical prediction of severity. The risk increases greatly after a score of 3. Patients with scores of 3–7 should be considered for anticoagulation. Each of the following represents one point:
- Aged 65 years or older
- Use of aspirin in the last 7 days
- Known coronary stenosis of 50% or greater
- Elevated serum cardiac markers
- At least three risk factors for CAD (diabetes, smoking, family history of CAD, hypertension, hypercholesterolemia)
- Severe anginal symptoms (two or more anginal events in the last 24 h)
- ST deviation on ECG.

Workup in the first 24 h should include serial cardiac biomarkers, hemoglobin, chemistry, and lipid panel. Stress testing should not be performed in the acute phases of unstable angina (Fig. 3).

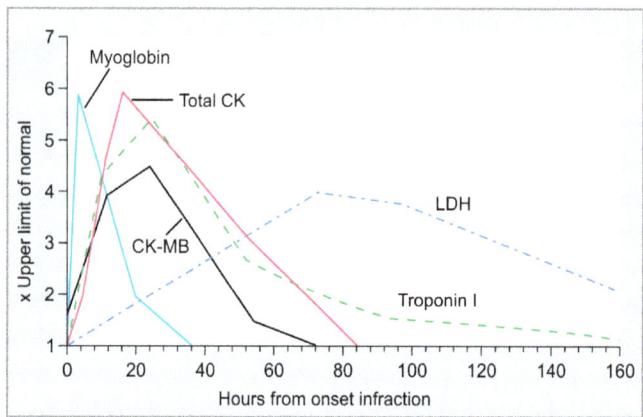

**Fig. 3:** Time course of elevations of serum markers after acute myocardial infarction.
*Source:* Tan WA. Unstable angina. [Online]. Available from emedicine.medscape.com/article/159383-overview#showall; 2011 [accessed June, 2012].

**Flowchart 1:** Algorithm for initial invasive strategy.

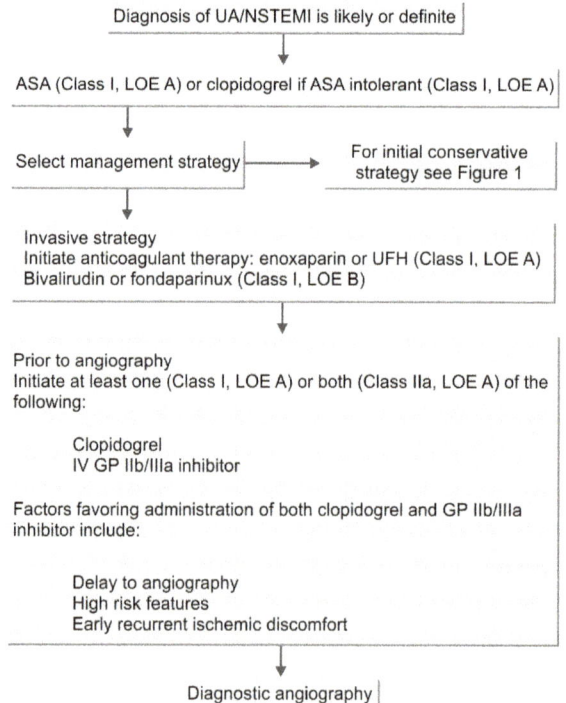

*Source:* Adapted from 2007 ACC/AHA UA/NSTEMI guidelines.

Algorithms shown in Flowcharts 1 and 2 are helpful in determining management.

**Flowchart 2:** Algorithm for initial conservative strategy.

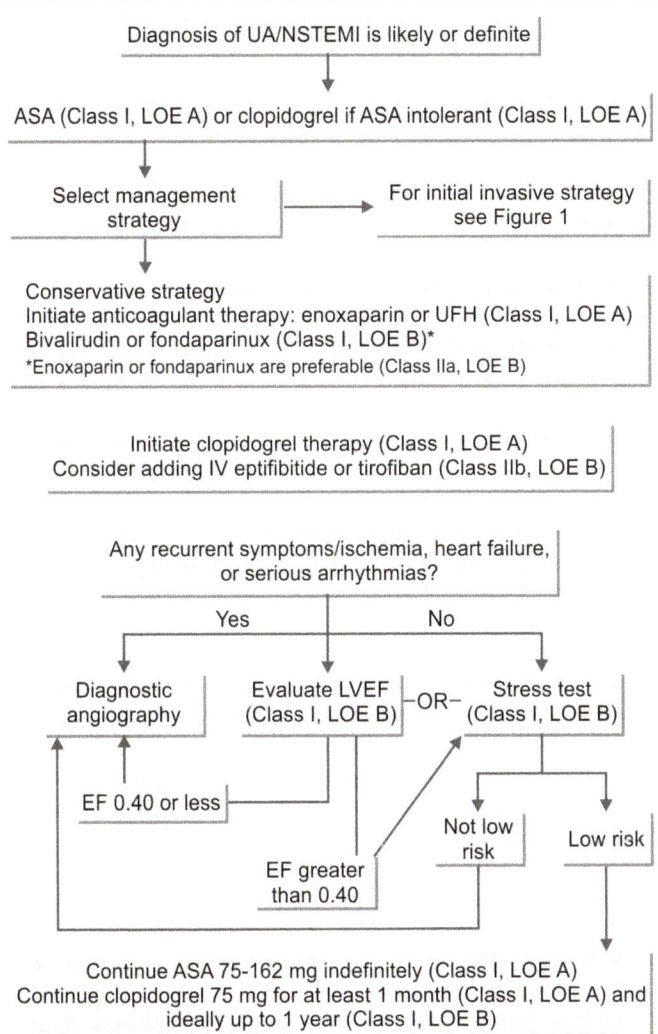

Source: Adapted from 2007 ACC/AHA UA/NSTEMI guidelines.

# REFERENCE

1. Tan WA. Unstable angina. [Online]. Available from emedicine.medscape.com/article/159383-overview; 2011 [accessed June, 2012].

## CASE STUDY 20: ABDOMINAL AORTIC ANEURYSM

### CASE HISTORY

Patient is a 70-year-old male with a 50-year smoking history who presents to the emergency department (ED) after passing out while sitting on the couch watching TV. Right before passing out, he complained to his daughter that he had a sudden onset, intense abdominal pain that radiated to his back. Patient's daughter denies recent trauma. However, he recently experienced some stomach discomfort and has had multiple episodes of nausea and vomiting in the last couple of days. The daughter denies that the patient had chest pain, shortness of breath (SOB), fever, diarrhea, or constipation. He has a 20-year history of hypertension, coronary artery disease (CAD), and dyslipidemia as well as a 10-year history of non-insulin-dependent diabetes mellitus (NIDDM). His vital signs on admission are insignificant except for a blood pressure (BP) of 140/90 mm Hg. On physical examination, patient is now awake and alert but still appears drowsy. Heart examination reveals systolic murmur 2/6 near mitral area with S1, S2, and S4. Respiratory examination reveals wheezing. Abdominal examination reveals pulsatile abdominal mass.

Electrocardiogram (ECG) shows left ventricular hypertrophy. Abdominal ultrasound is done immediately and shows enlarged aorta without free peritoneal fluid (*see* Fig. 7B).

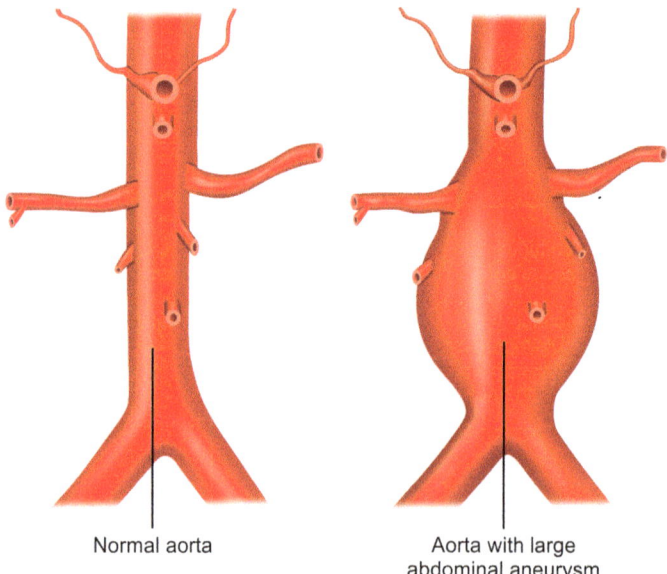

Normal aorta      Aorta with large abdominal aneurysm

**Fig. 1:** Abdominal aortic aneurysm.
*Source:* Available online from http://www.drfansler.com/images/abdominal/aortic/aneurysm-320.jpg.

## DISCUSSION

The immediate concern with this elderly patient with a history of smoking is a ruptured abdominal aortic aneurysm (AAA) versus a myocardial infarction.[1] These must be ruled out immediately. The history of syncope is concerning, but it is reassuring that the patient is not significantly hypotensive, although, given his history of hypertension, this BP may be relatively hypotensive compared to his baseline. A broader differential includes myocardial infarction, appendicitis, cholelithisasis, diverticular disease, gastritis and peptic ulcer disease, large bowel obstruction, pancreatitis, small-bowel obstruction, gastrointestinal (GI) bleeding, ischemic bowel, perforated ulcer, *urinary tract infection* (UTI), nephrolithiasis, pyelonephritis, and musculoskeletal pain. Please see Figure 1 to understand the anatomy of AAA.

A good initial step to check for an enlarged abdominal aorta is by bedside ultrasound (Fig. 2). Limitations of the study are few but include inability to detect leakage, rupture, branch artery involvement, and suprarenal involvement. In addition, the ability to image the aorta is reduced in the presence of bowel gas or obesity. Visualization may be further limited if patients are non-fasting. Other early studies should include ECG, chest X-ray (CXR), complete blood count (CBC), *basic metabolic panel* (BMP), and type and screen.

Other causes of abdominal pain may be investigated using abdominal radiography (Fig. 3).

A secondary study to evaluate and detect AAA is an abdominal computed tomography (CT) scan with a sensitivity of almost 100% (Fig. 4). CT may

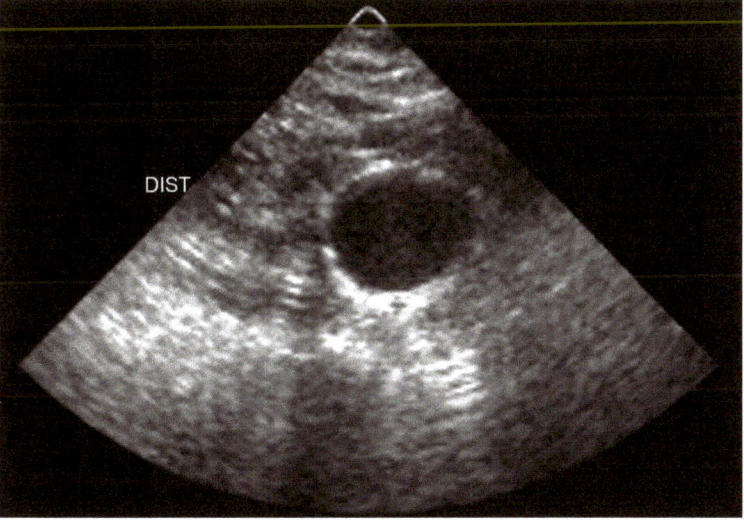

**Fig. 2:** A bedside ultrasound of an enlarged abdominal aorta.
*Courtesy:* Dr Beatrice Hoffman at John Hopkins University www.sonoguide.com, Baltimore, USA.

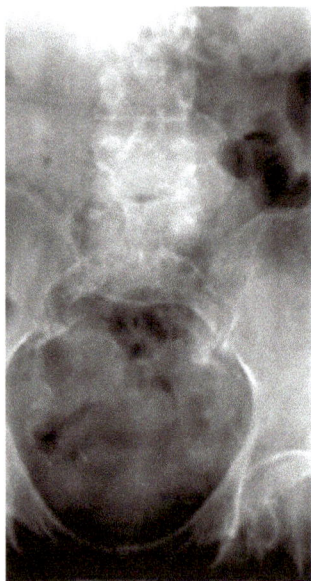

**Fig. 3:** Radiograph shows calcification of the abdominal aorta. The left wall is clearly depicted and appears aneurysmal; however, the right wall overlies the spine.

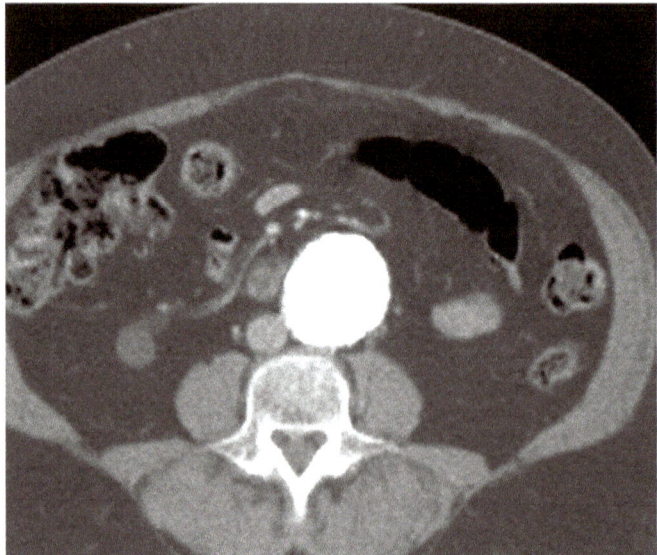

**Fig. 4:** Computed tomography (CT) scan demonstrate an abdominal aortic aneurysm (AAA). The aneurysm was noted during workup for back pain, and CT was ordered after the AAA was identified on radiographs. No evidence of rupture is seen.

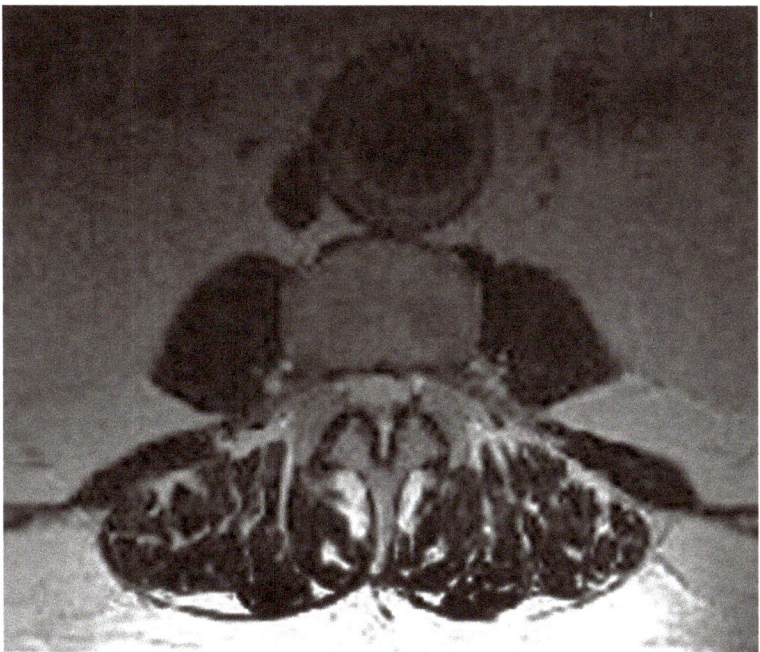

**Fig. 5:** Magnetic resonance imaging of a 77-year-old man with leg pain believed to be secondary to degenerative disk disease. During evaluation, an abdominal aortic aneurysm was discovered.

visualize the entire aorta as well as branches and the retroperitoneum. The limitations are time, cost, and exposure to radiation.

Magnetic resonance imaging (MRI) is similar in benefits to CT scan. However, MRI is even more limited in access and is more expensive (Fig. 5).

Finally, angiography is the gold standard, but widespread use is limited by its invasiveness, cost, lack of operator availability, time involved, and risk of complications such as bleeding, perforation, or embolism (Fig. 6). Therefore, ultrasound and CT are the most highly recommended studies for evaluating abdominal aneurysms.

Treatment initially depends on the hemodynamic stability of the patient. Unstable patients require immediate surgical intervention. Mortality rate for ruptured aneurysms is extremely high even with intervention that is initiated in a timely fashion. BP control is important as not to exacerbate the bleed. A short-acting beta blocker, such as esmolol, is ideal. Stable but symptomatic patients should be admitted especially when comorbid conditions are present such as chronic obstructive pulmonary disease (COPD), CAD, and congestive heart failure (CHF).

Stable patients can be monitored on a yearly basis. If the aneurysm grows to >5.5 cm or is growing at a rate of 1 cm/year, then surgical intervention

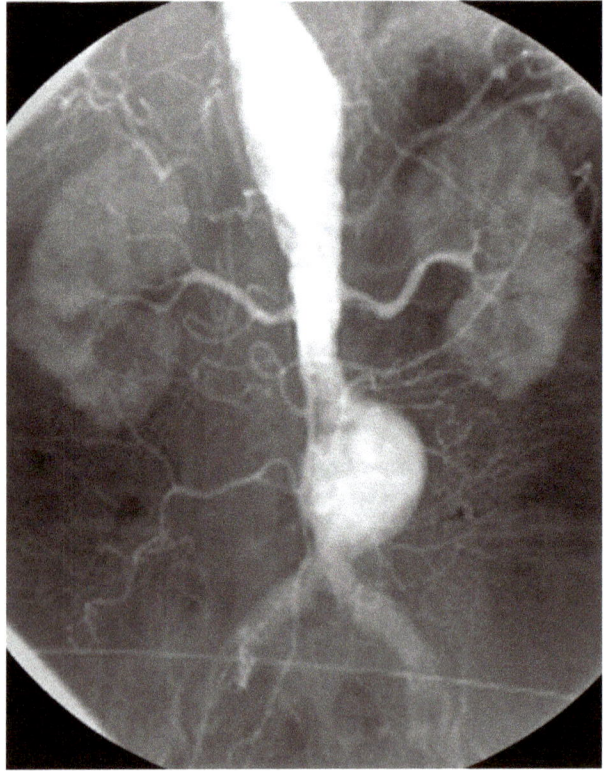

**Fig. 6:** Angiography is used to diagnose the renal area. In this instance, an endoleak represented continued pressurization of the sac.

is recommended. This is the generally accepted point where risk of rupture outweighs the risk of surgery. Long-term medical management should include smoking cessation and aggressive BP control with beta blockers.

Several repair mechanisms may be used and are to be decided by the vascular surgeon and the patient. Open repair and endovascular repair are the main differences. Endovascular repair has lower morbidity and mortality but is limited to certain types of aneurysms. Historical case: Albert Einstein died of severe bleeding from ruptured aortic aneurysm.

## AORTA SCAN

This has been represented with a portable 3D ultrasound device which helps the physicians to measure the abdominal aortic diameter quickly and accurately (Figs. 7A and B).

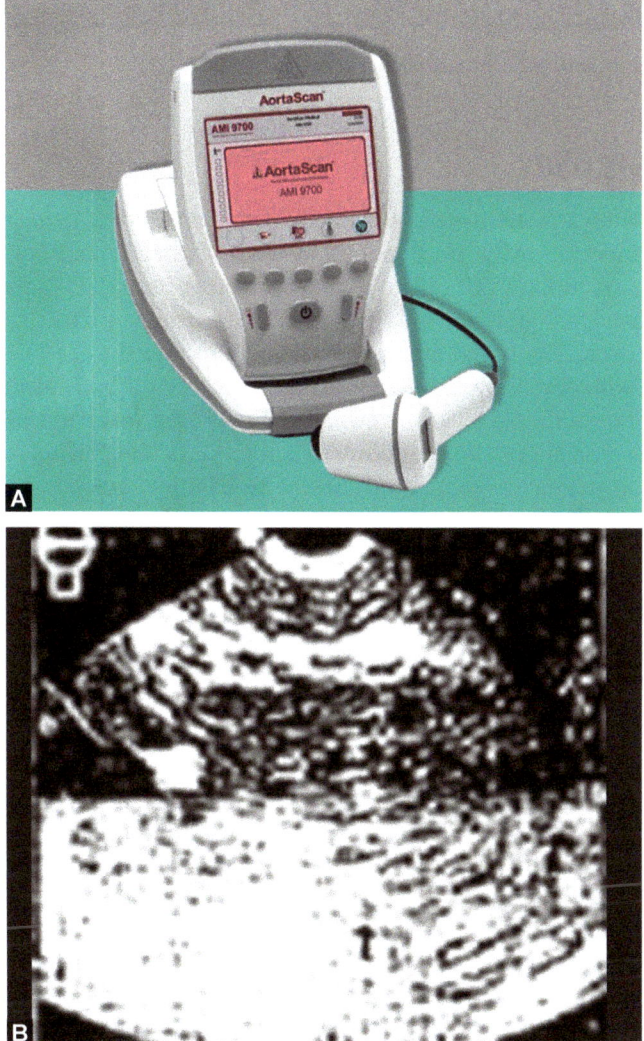

**Figs. 7A and B:** Aorta scan AMI 9700. Available online from http://www.verathon.com/Products/AortaScan/AMI9700.aspx. [Accessed June, 2012]
*Source:* With permission from Verathon, Bothell, Washington, USA.

## REFERENCE

1. O'Connor RE. Emergent management of abdominal aortic aneurysm rupture. [Online]. Available online from emedicine.medscape.com/article/756735; 2011 [accessed June, 2012].

## CASE STUDY 21: HEMORRHAGIC SHOCK

*"None of our patients should code in the CT scanner."*
—Badar M Zaheer

## CASE HISTORY

After a heated argument with his wife and two daughters, a 45-year-old male began drinking heavily. He punched through a window and cut his wrists with the glass "hoping to die." The patient then drove himself to the emergency department (ED) and stood in the parking lot drinking hard liquor, while bleeding profusely. Initial attempts to bring him into the ED for treatment were met with physical resistance. The patient agreed to come inside for treatment but he continued to curse and yell at the staff the entire time. He continued to become angry and more unintelligible. Once the patient's arms were secured, normal saline was started and the bleeding at his wrists was stopped. The patient became increasingly lethargic and O+ blood was ordered.

## USE OF BEDSIDE ULTRASOUND

Nowadays, ER physicians are being trained to preform bedside ultrasounds. Special training and workshops are available for ER Physicians to learn the skills necessary to perform the ultrasound. Many ER residencies are incorporating bedside ultrasound training as part of their curriculum. There are a number of conditions we should be looking for in the setting of shock. A bedside ultrasound scan can help you narrow down your differential: pericardial tamponade, pulmonary embolism (PE), myocardial infarction (MI), hypovolemia, aortic dissection, and rupture of abdominal aortic aneurysm (AAA) are some at the top of the list. Since there is no room to show all of these here, you may want to check out the free ultrasound image library at www.erpocketbooks.com as you read on. With cardiomegaly on the chest X-ray, especially if you do not know that it is chronic, your first consideration should be cardiac tamponade from a large pericardial effusion. A bedside echo should be able to rule this out quite easily. On a quick look, your patient does not have any signs of an effusion, so you move on. Given the heart murmur, your next consideration should probably be cardiogenic shock, and if this were the case, you would expect to see a dilated, hypokinetic left ventricle (LV). However, the LV is actually small and it is the right ventricle (RV) that appears enlarged. This should make you suspect a PE; however, this was eventually ruled out with a pulmonary angiogram. As it turned out, this patient was eventually diagnosed with acute pulmonary hypertension, possibly due to a combination or cirrhosis and methamphetamine abuse (see above for facts on pulmonary hypertension). Other conditions that the ultrasound machine could be helpful with include hypovolemic shock, where you would expect to see a small rapidly beating heart and a shrunken or flat inferior vena cava (IVC). If you look carefully in the right patient, it is possible to pick up an intimal flap from an acute aortic dissection. Imaging the belly for an AAA or free fluid from a ruptured spleen or hemorrhagic pancreatitis might also be helpful in narrowing down the cause of shock in a sick patient. In the setting of a new murmur, valvular pathology or an acute MI should also be considerations. Imaging for these conditions, however, is beyond the scope of most emergency physicians; so when you are worried about these, a formal echocardiogram is desirable.

## PEARLS AND PITFALLS OF DIAGNOSTIC/ THERAPEUTIC ULTRASOUND USE IN HYPOTENSIVE PATIENTS

- Start with the heart. Parasternal images tend to give the most information, but the subxiphoid view may be easier in some patients. Look for effusions, chamber dilation, and wall motion abnormalities (advanced).
- Use the curvilinear probe or the phased array transducer. Start in the fourth intercostal space and position the probe between the ribs. If you do not get a good image, try moving up or down one rib space and redirecting the angle of your probe. Remember to direct the beams of your probe through the long axis of the heart. If you need to decrease the distance between the patient's heart and the ultrasound beams, have the patient rolled over onto his left side and bring his heart closer to his chest wall.
- Take the time to adjust your depth and gain to maximize image quality. Make sure you have enough depth to look behind the heart for a pericardial effusion. You should always try to see the cross-sectional descending aorta coursing behind the LV.
- In the setting of hypotension, pericardial fluid, especially when accompanied by right ventricular collapse, may signify tamponade, a condition which is best treated by immediate pericardiocentesis. Pleural effusions may mimic pericardial effusions in certain instances. If you are unsure, find the retrocardiac aorta. If the fluid is between the heart and aorta, it is pericardial. If it is on the opposite side of the aorta from the heart, it is pleural.
- A hyperdynamic rapidly beating heart usually signifies hypovolemia. Look at the IVC to assess if the patient is indeed intravascularly depleted. Many studies have correlated IVC diameter to Swan Ganz RA pressures. If the heart is hyperdynamic and the IVC is compressed, the aggressive administration of fluids or blood products may be life-saving. Consider a search for the source of bleeding. Look for melena, hemoperitoneum, or an aortic aneurysm.

- A dilated RV should raise your suspicion for a massive PE. In such cases, tissue plasminogen activator (tPA) should be considered. Remember that congestive heart failure (CHF) or pulmonary hypertension can also cause a dilated RV, although these chronic conditions will show a dilated RV with hypertrophy of the RV walls. A dilated RV with thin walls prompts consideration of the diagnosis of an acute massive PE.
- Scanning further south may also help to find the cause. Image the abdomen for evidence of retroperitoneal bleeding from a ruptured AAA, or intraperitoneal bleeding from occult trauma, or ruptured ectopic pregnancy or spleen. Ultrasound of the legs may show deep vein thrombosis (DVT).
- Ultrasound may be useful for more than just establishing a diagnosis. It can also help with procedures such as central line placement and pericardiocentesis during the resuscitation.
- Consider the concentrated overview of resuscitative efforts (CORE) scan in all undifferentiated hypotensive patients. For more information, visit apps.acep.org/WorkArea/DownloadAsset.aspx?id=42470.

Brady Pregerson manages a free online EM ultrasound image library and is the author of the *Tarascon Emergency Department Quick Reference Guide*. For more information, visit EMResource.org.

Teresa S Wu is the Associate Residency Director and Director of Ultrasound and Simulation Based Training for the Maricopa EM Program in Phoenix.

## PHYSICAL EXAMINATION

- *Vital signs*: BP—could not be measured, *heart rate*—163 bpm, *respiratory rate*—35 breaths/min, *body temperature*—95.6°F
- *Skin/mucous membranes*: Pale, cold, clammy sweat
- *Cardiac activity*: Tachycardia.

## DIFFERENTIAL DIAGNOSIS

It includes shock (cardiogenic, toxic, hemorrhagic, obstructive shock, distributive shock, and neurogenic shock).

### Hypovolemic Shock

- *Loss of blood*
  - *External hemorrhage*: Trauma or gastrointestinal (GI) bleed
  - *Internal hemorrhage*: Hematoma, hemothorax, hemoperitoneum
- *Loss of plasma*: Burns, exfoliative dermatitis
- *Loss of fluid and electrolytes*
  - *External*: Vomiting, diarrhea, excessive sweating, hyperosmolar states *diabetic ketoacidosis* (DKA)
  - *Internal (third spacing)*: Pancreatitis, ascites, and bowel obstruction.

## Cardiogenic Shock
- *Dysrhythmia*: Tachyarrhythmia, bradyarrhythmia
- *Pump failure*: MI, cardiomyopathy
- *Acute valvular dysfunction*: Regurgitant lesions more common
- Rupture of ventricular septum or free ventricular wall.

## Obstructive Shock
- Tension pneumothorax
- *Pericardial disease*: Tamponade, constriction
- Pulmonary vasculature disease: PE, pulmonary hypertension
- *Cardiac tumor*: Atrial myxoma
- Left atrial mural thrombus
- *Obstructive valvular disease*: Aortic or mitral stenosis.

## Distributive Shock
Septic shock, anaphylactic shock, neurogenic shock, vasodilator drugs, and acute adrenal insufficiency.

# DIAGNOSIS
Considering the patient's obvious signs of trauma and excessive binge drinking, a hypovolemic and hemorrhagic shock is the most likely diagnosis. Refer to Table 1 for hemorrhagic shock according to the amount of blood loss.

## Workup for Shock
### Identifying Source of Bleeding
External bleeding (lacerations), pleural cavity (hemothorax), peritoneal cavity (bleeding from intra-abdominal injuries), pelvic girdle (pelvic fracture), and soft-tissue compartments (long-bone fractures).

## Imaging
Computerized tomography can be used for unclear bleeding sources in head, abdomen, and pelvis. Plain film can be used for extremities to show potential fractures (Fig. 1).

## Laboratory
During an acute hemorrhage, there is not much use for a complete blood count (CBC). The hemoglobin and hematocrit results will be normal initially because the body is losing equal normotonic fluid. Decrease in these results will show up after crystalloid fluid replacement has been initiated and the red blood cell (RBC) is essentially diluted.

**Table 1:** Clinical diagnosis of hemorrhagic shock using advanced trauma life support (ATLS) classification of hypovolemic/hemorrhagic shock.

| Class | Blood loss (mL) | Pulse | Blood pressure | Capillary blanch test | Respiratory rate (breaths/min) | Urine output (mL/h) | Psychology |
|---|---|---|---|---|---|---|---|
| Class I | 750 (15%) | <100 | Normal with normal or increased pulse pressure | Normal | 14–20 | >30 | Slightly anxious |
| Class II | 750–1,500 (15–30%) | >100 | Normal with decreased pulse pressure | Positive | 20–30 | 20–30 | Mildly anxious |
| Class III | 1,500–2,000 (30–40%) | >120 | Decreased with decreased pulse pressure | Positive | 30–40 | 5–15 | Anxious and confused |
| Class IV | >2,000 (>40%) | >140 | Decreased with decreased pulse pressure | Positive | >35 | Negligible | Lethargic |

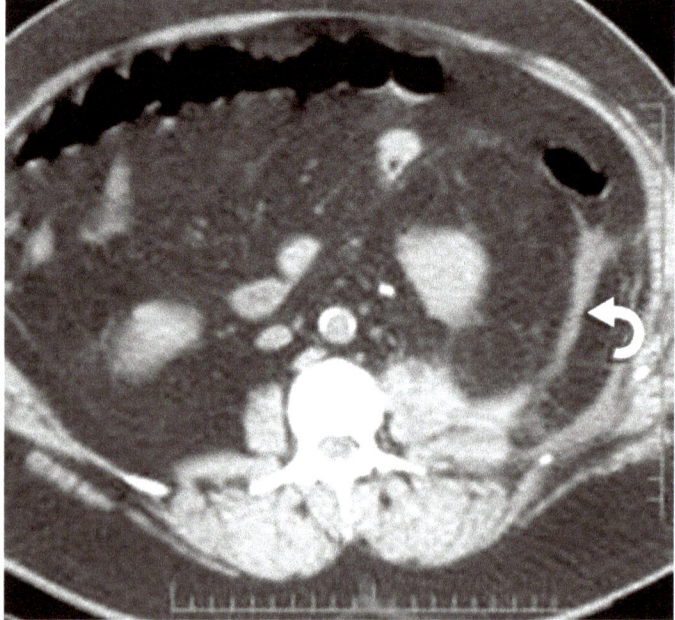

**Fig. 1:** Computed tomography scan shows hemorrhage into left retroperitoneum (arrow) and along iliopsoas compartment.

# MANAGEMENT

## Fluid Loss

*Initial Step*

Isotonic crystalloid fluid (isotonic saline or lactated Ringer solution) is given as the initial fluid. For each liter given, 300 mL stays in intravascular space meaning 3 mL of fluid = 1 mL of blood loss.
- Colloid (albumin, hetastarch, dextran) versus crystalloid—no clinical difference.

*Blood Transfusion*

If 2–3 L of crystalloid solution is not enough to increase the patient's saturation and cardiovascular collapse is imminent, blood transfusion is the next step. Ideally, cross-typed blood is the best option. However, in an emergency setting, O− blood is given to women and O+ blood is given to men.

## Hemorrhage

- Pressure, tourniquet, dressing and tamponade can be tried for external wounds
- Surgical consult needed for intra-abdominal injuries
- Interventional radiology-guided embolization can be used for advanced pelvic injuries.

## FURTHER READING

1. Beatrice Hoffman, MD, PhD, RDMS, John Hopkins http://www.sonoguide.com/introduction.html.
2. *Hemorrhagic shock* visit www.ncbi.nlm.nih.gov/pmc/articles/PMC 1065003.

# CASE STUDY 22: PERICARDITIS

## CASE HISTORY

The patient is a 45-year-old male who presents with acute sharp retrosternal pain that radiates to the shoulder. The pain is worse with inspiration and better when leaning forward. The patient has been experiencing a racing heart. He has been having a fever for the last 2–3 days. The fever has stayed consistent and his breathing has quickened. He noticed that his breathing has become more difficult. He says that the pain has been constant for the last 6 h. He has a history of gastroesophageal reflux disease (GERD) and esophageal spasm. Patient says that he has felt pain similar to this before but it would go away within a few minutes.

## PHYSICAL EXAMINATION

### Cardiovascular System

Tachycardic, regular, pericardial friction rub heard [coarse, high pitched, better in expiration at lower left sternal border (LLSB) with patient leaning forward (specifically, not sensitive)], new S3 present.

### Respiratory System

Patient develops hypotension, elevated *jugular venous pressure* (JVP), and blood pressure falls 10 mm Hg with inspiration.

### Laboratory Tests

- Complete blood count (CBC) of 12,000/µL with no shift
- Erythrocyte sedimentation rate (ESR) elevated
- Elevated C-reactive protein (CRP)
- Elevated cardiac enzymes include elevated creatine kinase-muscle and brain (CK-MB), and troponins
  *Note*: In young males, troponin levels are more like to be elevated.
- Electrocardiogram (ECG) shows ST-segment elevation that does not come back down to baseline.

## DIFFERENTIAL DIAGNOSIS

- *Cardiovascular system*: Aortic dissection, aortic stenosis, coronary artery vasospasm, myocardial infarction
- *Respiratory system*: Pulmonary embolism
- *Gastrointestinal system*: Esophageal rupture, esophageal spasm, esophagitis, gastritis, GERD, and peptic ulcer disease.

## PHYSICAL FINDINGS

- Increased heart rate out of proportion to fever
- S1, S4 faint on auscultation
- Mitral regurgitation murmur
- Pericardial friction rub
- The most frequent presentation is dyspnea (72% of all patients) followed by chest pain (32%) and then arrhythmias (18%)
- Signs of right heart failure (hepatomegaly, edema, distention in neck veins, and loud S3)
- Fever, malaise, and arthralgias. Difficulty in breathing may be the most common presentation in children
- Sudden cardiac death.

## WORKUP

- *Medical history*: The clinical presentation of pericarditis and myocarditis are both nonspecific and can consist of fatigue, palpitations, dyspnea, precordial discomfort, and myalgias.
- Diagnostic workup includes chest X-ray (CXR) examination, ECG, laboratory evaluation, echocardiogram, cardiac catheterization, and endomyocardial biopsy (in selected patients on the basis of the likelihood of finding specific treatable disorders such as giant cell myocarditis).

## Laboratory Studies

- Elevated cardiac troponin T is suggestive of pericarditis in patients with clinically suspected myocarditis. Troponin I specificity is 89%; sensitivity is 34%. A normal level does not rule out the diagnosis.
- Increased creatine kinase (with elevated MB fraction, lactate dehydrogenase) and aspartate aminotransferase from myocardial necrosis.
- Increased ESR (nonspecific but may be of value in following the progress of the disease and the response to therapy).
- Increased white blood cell count (increased eosinophils in case of if parasitic infection).
- Viral titers (acute and convalescent)
- Cold agglutinin titer, antistreptolysin O titer
- Blood cultures
- Lyme disease antibody titer.

### *Imaging*

- *Chest radiograph*: Enlargement of cardiac silhouette
- *ECG*: Sinus tachycardia with nonspecific ST-T-wave changes; intraventricular conduction defects and bundle branch block may be present
  - Lyme disease and diphtheria cause all degrees of heart block
  - Changes of acute myocardial infarction can occur with focal necrosis.
- *Echocardiogram*
  - Dilated and hypokinetic chambers
  - Segmental wall motion abnormalities
- *Cardiac catheterization and angiography*
  - To rule out coronary artery disease and valvular disease
- A right ventricular endomyocardial biopsy can confirm the diagnosis, although a negative biopsy result does not exclude myocarditis. Recent studies have shown that myocardial biopsy may be unnecessary because immunosuppression therapy based on biopsy results is generally ineffective.

## PERICARDITIS STAGING (FIGS. 1 TO 5)

Stage 1 = Diffuse ST elevation, PR-segment depression.
Stage 2 = Normalization of ST and PR segments.
Stage 3 = Widespread T-wave inversion.
Stage 4 = Normalization of T-waves, persistent inversion if chronic.

- ECG may show electrical alternans with tamponade
- CXR shows enlarged cardiac silhouette with large pericardial effusion of ≥200 mL (Fig. 2)
- Evaluating the presence of pericardial effusion tamponade of pericardial disease by transthoracic echo (Fig. 5)
- Computed tomography/magnetic resonance imaging (CT/MRI) is done if initial workup is inconclusive

## DIAGNOSIS

- Pericardiocentesis (Fig. 3) is indicated for cardiac tamponade, high suspicion of tuberculous, purulent, or neoplastic pericarditis
  - Purulence with neutrophil shows bacterial pericarditis
  - Purulence with lymphocytes shows neoplastic pericarditis
- Diagnosis of different types of pericarditis
  - Constrictive pericarditis
  - Restrictive pericarditis

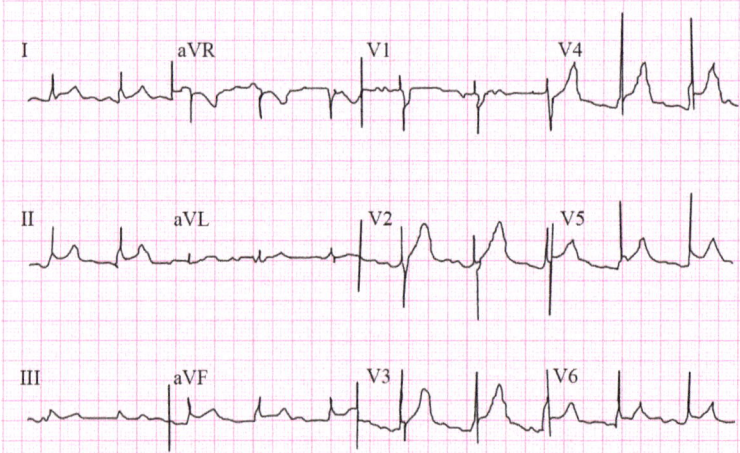

**Fig. 1:** Electrocardiogram in acute pericarditis showing diffuse upstaging ST-segment elevations seen best here in leads II, III, aVF, and V5–V6. There is also subtle PR-segment deviation (positive in aVR, negative in most other leads). ST-segment elevation is due to a ventricular current of injury associated with epicardial inflammation; similarly, the PR-segment changes are due to an atrial current of injury which is pericarditis, typically displaces the PR-segment upright in lead aVR and downward in most other leads.
*Courtesy*: Ary Goldberger, MD.

## DIFFERENTIAL DIAGNOSIS

- *Cardiac*: Congestive heart failure
- *Infection*: Tuberculosis (TB), pneumonia
- Neoplasm.

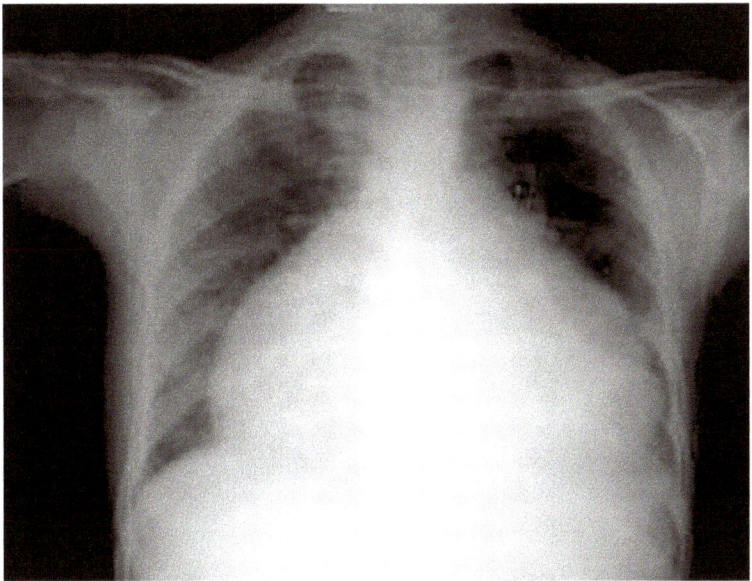

**Fig. 2:** Chest X-ray showing pericardial effusion.

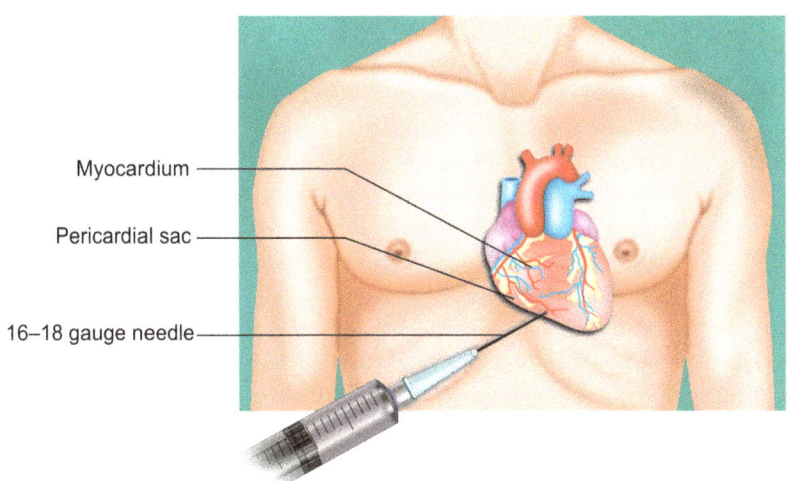

**Fig. 3:** Pericardiocentesis.
When the needle tip enters the pericardial sac, withdraw nonclotted blood as much as possible under ECG guidance.

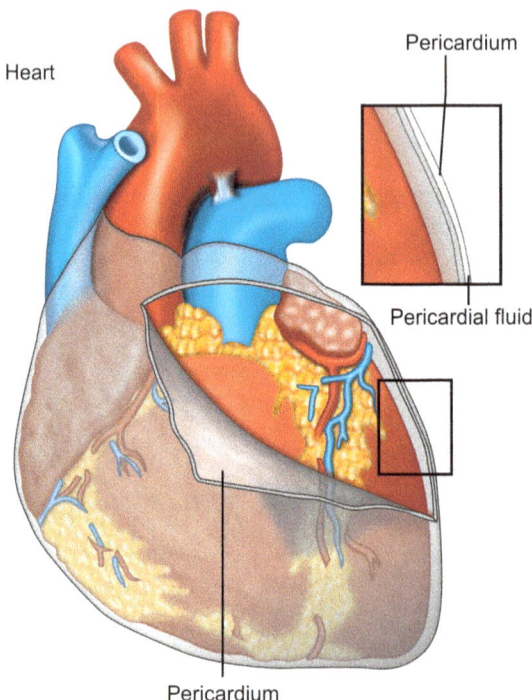

**Fig. 4:** Pericardium.
*Source:* Available online from http://www.medic2010.webs.com/pericardium_580x.jpg.

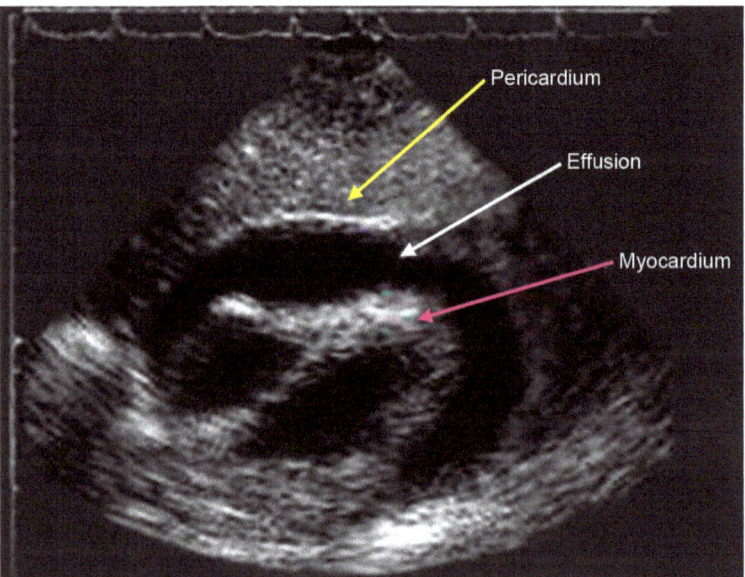

**Fig. 5:** Echopericardial effusion.

## TREATMENT

- Depends on the underlying cause and may include NSAIDs, steroids, antibiotics, etc.
- In severe situations, pericardiocentesis or surgery may be needed.

## CASE STUDY 23: CARDIAC ARREST

*"Saving a life is like saving a whole nation."*

—**Al Quran**

*"In Cardiac Arrest your priority is CAB, not ABC; compression first please."*

## CASE HISTORY

A 64-year-old female was traveling from Minnesota to Chicago in a blizzard weather in December. During the boarding process, it appeared that the passenger was having seizures and was approached by the pilot. The patient was not breathing and a call for assistance was made. A fellow passenger, who is an emergency room (ER) MD, offered to assist the pilot. Patient was pulseless and not breathing; one-person's cardiopulmonary resuscitation (CPR) was initiated until paramedics arrived on the scene with *automated external defibrillator* (AED) (Fig. 1).

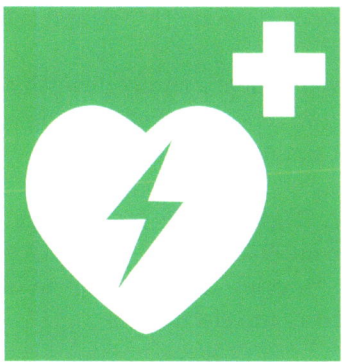

**Fig. 1:** Universal sign for AED. (AED: automated external defibrillator).

Weak and thready pulse was palpated after 30 min of resuscitation. Patient was transported to the nearest hospital for evaluation. After a successful resuscitation, the pilot moved the author to the first class cabin and offered his own dinner. Later, the pilot wrote a letter to the medical director of the author's hospital praising his heroism.

## TREATMENT (FIG. 2)

It involves the role of the following.
*Doctor*: Intubating and running the code.

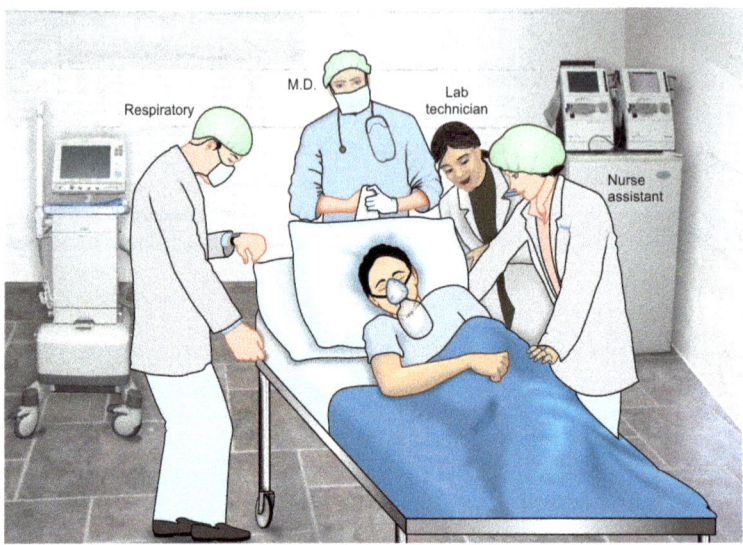

**Fig. 2:** A cardiac arrest patient's treatment.

*Nurse*: Monitors vital signs and IV access, reads crash cart, places transcutaneous pacer pads (Fig. 3) on patient, administers drugs (epi/atropine boluses), calls for electrocardiogram (ECG), and asks the charting nurse to time drugs.

*Nurse assistant*: Calls the patient's family, takes history, calls the patient's private doctor, and throws noncontributory people out of the room, "ALL CLEAR!" (If you're not against the wall or out of the room, you might get shocked.)

*Respiratory equipment*: Bagging with 100% oxygen, arterial blood gases (ABGs), and assisting in intubation.

*Laboratory technician*: Drawing blood, complete blood count (CBC), calcium, magnesium, glucose, and electrolytes.

## Initial Survey as Per the Latest American Heart Association Protocol (2010) (Fig. 4).

- Assess responsiveness (speak loudly, gently shake patient if no trauma—"Annie, Annie, are you OK?").
- Call for help or crash cart if unresponsive
- Compression, airway, breathing, and defibrillation (CABD)
    - Compression
        - Compressions of ≥100 per minute at a depth of 5 cm
        - Rotate the person doing the compressions every 2 min
        - See Figures 4 and 5 for 2010 AHA revised guidelines for CPR.

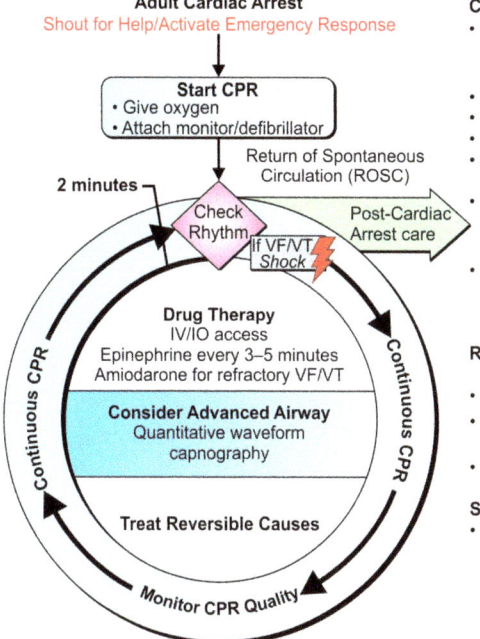

- **Monophasic:** 360 J
**Drug Therapy**
- **Epinephrine IV/IO Dose:** 1 mg every 3–5 minutes
- **Vasopressin IV/IO Dose:** 40 units can replace first or second dose of epinephrine
- **Amiodarone IV/IO Dose:** First dose: 300 mg bolus. Second dose: 150 mg.

**Advanced Airway**
- Supraglottic advanced airway or endotracheal intubation
- Waveform capnography to confirm and monitor ET tube placement

**Reversible Causes**
- Hypovolemia
- Hypoxia
- Hydrogen ion (acidosis)
- Hypo-/hyperkalemia
- Hypothermia
- Tension pneumothorax
- Tamponade, cardiac
- Toxins
- Thrombosis, pulmonary
- Thrombosis, coronary

**Fig. 3:** Flowchart of an adult's cardiac arrest.

- Airway
    - Head-tilt chin-lift (if provider suspects trauma: jaw thrust).
- Breath—Ventilations (Fig. 5).
    - Give ventilations at a ratio of 2 ventilations every 30 compressions for 1 healthcare provider
    - A ratio of 15:2 (compressions to ventilations) if two healthcare providers are present
    - If an advanced airway is in place
        - Give ventilations every 6–8 s
        - Asynchronous with chest compressions
        - About 1 s per breath
        - Visible chest rise.

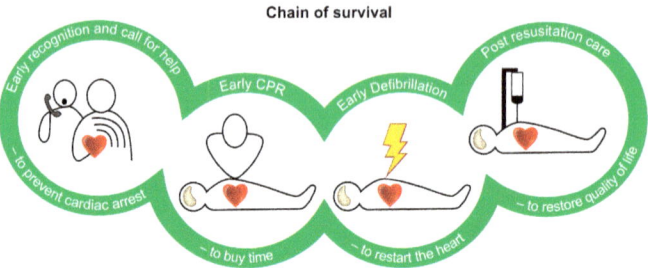

**Fig. 4:** Acute cardiac arrest.
*Source*: By Terezza89—Own work, CC BY-SA 4.0, https://commons.wikimedia.org/w/index.php?curid=45056808.

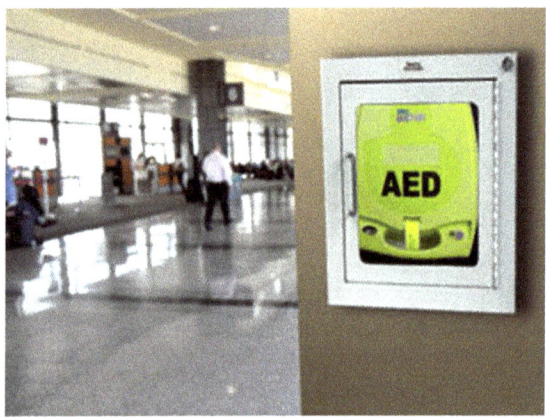

**Fig. 5:** AED in airport. (AED: automated external defibrillator).
*Source:* http://www.zoll.com/zoll-news/2010/07/15/sheriffs-save-airport-passenger-aed-cpr-automated-external-defibrillator/.

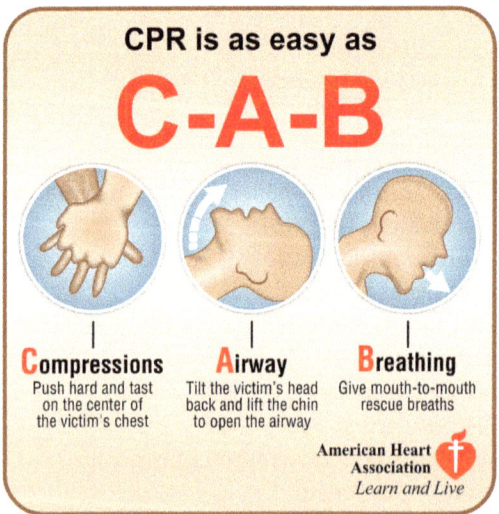

**Fig. 6:** A new order for CPR, spelled CAB.[2] (CPR: cardiopulmonary resuscitation).

- Defibrillation
  - Attach and use AED as soon as available. Minimize chest compressions before and after shock; resume chest compressions immediately after shock
  - Shock energy
    - Biphasic
      - Initial dose of 120–200 J (if unknown, use maximum).
      - Second and subsequent doses same as first
      - Higher doses may be considered after second dose
    - Monophasic
      - One dose of 360 J
- Repeat the cycle.

Lastly, in the developing countries, there is a misconception about the use of intraosseous lines in cases where no peripheral access is available–this procedure is confined to be used only in the pediatric population, but it is wide and clear that this is the method of choice for adults as well. Using a tibial intraosseous line is found to be the most preferable life-saving intervention in the out-of-hospital cardiac arrest setting. Research done by Reades et al. states that the tibial intraosseous access had the highest first-attempt success for vascular access.[1] It also had the most rapid time to vascular access during out-of-hospital cardiac arrest when tested against peripheral intravenous and humeral intraosseous access. Box 1 lists factors associated with better outcomes in cardiac arrest.

**Everybody should know how to use an AED.**
1. Power on the AED
2. Make sure the chest wall is dry
3. Follow the pictures on the pads and place the pads in their appropriate location
4. Clear the area of any bystanders
5. The machine will automatically analyze the heart rhythm and prompt you when to shock
6. Say "all clear" loudly before delivering the shock
7. Continue CPR.

**Box 1:** Factors associated with improved outcomes in cardiac arrest.

- Presenting rhythm of VT/VF
- Early/bystander CPR
- Early defibrillation
- CPR prior to defibrillation in the circulatory phase of cardiac arrest
- Minimal interruptions to chest compressions
- In-hospital and out-of-hospital use of AEDs
- Amiodarone use in shock-resistant VT/VF
- Therapeutic hypothermia in comatose cardiac arrest victims

*Source*: Available online from http://www.ebmedicine.net.

## REFERENCE

1. Reades R, Studnek J, Vandeventer S, et al. Intraosseous versus intravenous vascular access during out-of-hospital cardiac arrest: a randomized controlled trial. Ann Emerg Med. 2011;58(6):509-16.

## CASE STUDY 24: CARDIAC ARREST OUTSIDE HOSPITAL: USE OF INTRAOSSEOUS LINE

## CASE HISTORY

A 55-year-old man and his wife are on vacation in Seattle. While returning home, they stop for a slice of pizza at the airport when suddenly the man passed out and is unresponsive. His wife calls for help, and shortly after, paramedics arrived. Upon arrival, the paramedics determined that the man is in full cardiac arrest so one of the paramedics started cardiopulmonary resuscitation (CPR) while the other one started an intraosseous line (IOL). The patient is successfully resuscitated and brought to the emergency room for further treatment. Upon arrival to the emergency department (ED), the man's wife states that the patient was diagnosed with coronary artery disease 4 years ago by his physician.

## DISCUSSION

Within the past 5 years, emergency medical training companies have changed protocols to include IOLs as part of treatment for cardiac arrest with adults as well as children. When setting up an IOL on a patient, there are three preferred sites: (1) sternal, (2) tibial, and (3) humeral. The sternal site makes it difficult to perform CPR at the same time and is hardly used. Until recently, there is little evidence either way as to whether the humeral or tibial site is better. Current research has shown that IOL access to the tibia has a 40% greater initial success rate than humeral IOL or peripheral intravenous sites.[1] Also, the tibial site has a lower time to needle placement and provides less needle dislodgments. Although the peripheral intravenous site is the most common site used in health care, it is slower to place than IOLs and still has the same issues with dislodging. Though slower and less effective, intravenous access is still by far the cheapest access method used.

## INTRAOSSEOUS LINE PLACEMENT

### Treatment

When treating for cardiac arrest, time is of the essence because the lack of blood circulation means that no oxygen is perfusing to the cardiac tissue.

As little as 2 min of hypoxic conditions can cause tissue death. Immediately when paramedics arrive on the scene and suspect cardiac arrest, one paramedic should start doing CPR while the other paramedic inserts an IOL in the tibia (Figs. 1A to C). There are three important rules to remember when inserting a tibial IOL. The first is that the trapdoor effect is not seen when using the drill; the second is that the medical professional should estimate the depth needed prior to drilling. Lastly, the expert should stop sooner than they think, as you can always go back and drill deeper, if necessary.[1] Defibrillation is the next step in the treatment of this patient. Paramedics should focus on the airway, breathing, and circulation (ABC) till they get to the hospital where the ED physician will order drug therapy, and more cardioversion or surgery, if necessary.

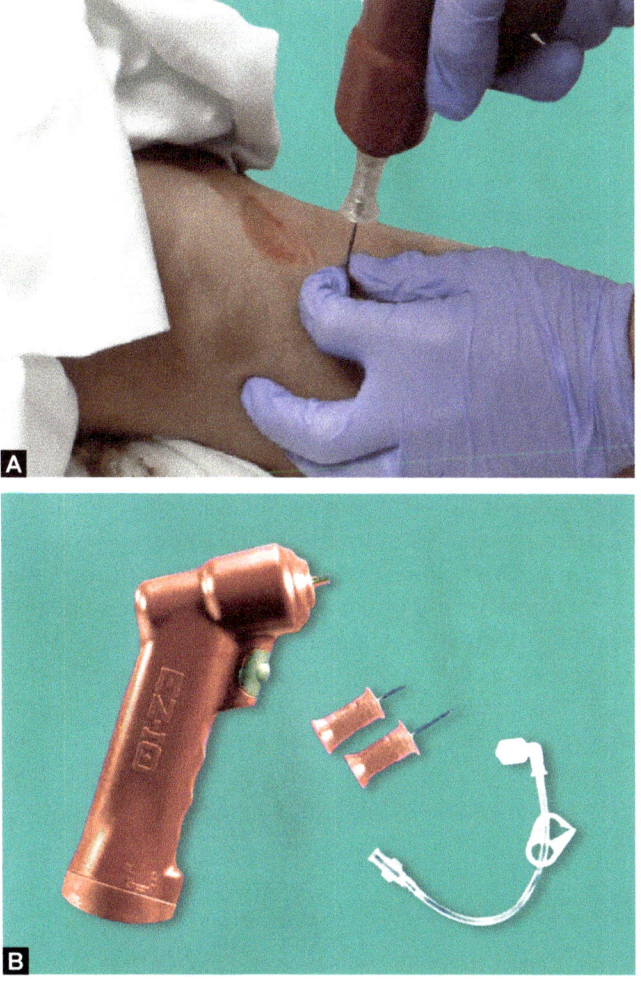

**Figs. 1A and B:** (A) Technique for IOL; (B) EZ IO (power driver drill, needle sets, IV catheter).

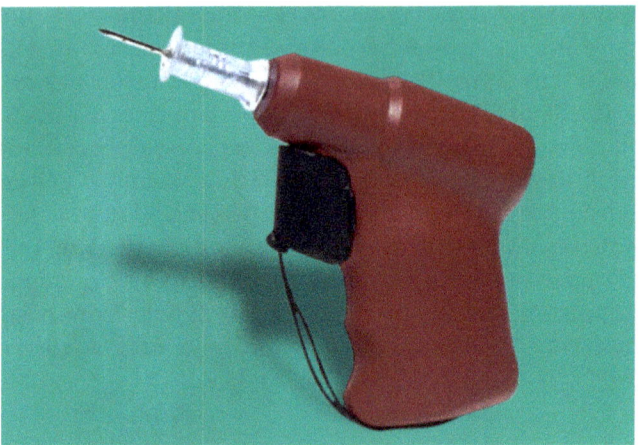

**Fig. 1C:** EZ IO power drill. (IOL: intraosseous line).

## REFERENCE

1. Reades R, Studnek JR, Vandeventer S, et al. Intraosseous versus intravenous vascular access during out-of-hospital cardiac arrest: a randomized controlled trial. Ann Emerg Mee 2011;58(6):509-16.

## CASE STUDY 25: CONGESTIVE HEART FAILURE

### CASE HISTORY

A 32-year-old certified nursing assistant (CNA) with a history of depression had stopped taking her medication. Recent social history included divorce and a family of five children to care for. She was presented to the emergency room (ER) with complaints of trouble in breathing and was brought to the examination room immediately. When transferred to the bed, the patient had completely stopped breathing and was intubated. Frothy and pink secretions were assessed with the endotracheal (ET) tube. This patient was presenting with congestive heart failure (CHF) exacerbation, a portable chest X-ray was ordered, and fulminant pulmonary edema was evident. An intravenous (IV) furosemide 80 mg was started and also an IV antibiotic was administered, and Foley catheter was inserted with 2 L of urine draining. Repeated chest X-ray showed improvement after 4 h and patient was admitted to intensive care unit.

### TREATMENT APPROACH

The primary goal of treatment in acute cases of CHF is to provide symptomatic relief. Initial management options include a combination of oxygen, morphine, diuretics, vasodilators, inotropes, and ultrafiltration therapy as a last resort. Morphine results in mild vasodilatation and slows the heart rate. Morphine can be particularly useful if the patient is restless and significantly dyspneic.[1] All patients should be admitted to the hospital. If the patient responds adequately to initial treatment, telemetry monitoring is acceptable. Those who are hypotensive or fail to respond to initial therapy require admission to the intensive care unit and may need invasive monitoring if tissue perfusion is compromised.[2] If cardiogenic shock is present, invasive evaluation is required.

## Maintenance of Oxygen Saturation

Oxygen therapy should be given to all patients to maintain oxygen saturation between 95% and 98% and to maximize tissue oxygenation. Ventilation with noninvasive positive pressure ventilation (NIPPV) or continuous positive airway pressure (CPAP) may be required if oxygen saturation cannot be maintained by oxygenation alone and is associated with a decreased requirement for intubation and mechanical ventilation. Mechanical ventilation is only used when other treatments, including noninvasive ventilation methods, fail.

## Hemodynamically Stable

### Diuretics and Vasodilators

- Loop diuretics are the mainstay of treatment and are effective in relieving symptoms. Non-loop diuretics, such as spironolactone and metolazone, may be added if there is an inadequate response to loop diuretics alone. Intravenous diuretics are indicated in patients with a systolic blood pressure (BP) higher than 85 mm Hg.
- Vasodilators (glyceryl trinitrate, nitroprusside, and nesiritide) are indicated in patients with pulmonary congestion/edema and a systolic BP higher than 90 mm Hg. Glyceryl trinitrate is the first-line agent with nesiritide-considered second line.
- Although there are no large-scale studies comparing diuretics alone with glyceryl trinitrate in patients with acute CHF, some have suggested that nitrates alone may be a better alternative in patients with acute CHF. In clinical practice, both these agents are used in combination [Level B Evidence].

In patients who do not respond to initial therapy, extracorporeal ultrafiltration is used to reduce volume overload [Level A evidence].

## Hemodynamically Unstable

Patients with hypotension or hypoperfusion (i.e., cold and dry, cold and wet profiles) should be commenced on inotropic support as this may improve hemodynamics [B evidence]. However, positive inotropes should be used with caution because there is evidence that they result in increased mortality and can cause arrhythmias and worsening of coronary ischemia [B evidence]. The occurrence of sustained arrhythmias should lead to their discontinuation. Concomitant use of amiodarone may be advisable, although there are no large-scale data on the use of antiarrhythmics in this setting. If the patient has symptomatic coronary ischemia, inotropes should be discontinued.

Patients with a systolic BP below 90 mm Hg or a drop of mean arterial pressure of >30 mm Hg with a pulse rate above 60 bpm and/or low urine output (<0.5 mL/kg/h) are defined as being in cardiogenic shock. Insertion of an intra-aortic balloon pump is indicated in patients with persistent cardiogenic shock, despite inotropic therapy. However, patients with significant aortic regurgitation or aortic dissection are not candidates.

Choice of inotrope depends on clinical findings.[2] Dobutamine or milrinone is recommended for patients with a systolic BP of 85–100 mm Hg and no clear clinical evidence of shock, such as cold extremities and low urine output. Levosimendan, a calcium sensitizer, may be used as an alternative to dobutamine or milrinone. It may not be available in some countries. Dopamine is recommended for patients with systolic BP below 85 mm Hg with clinical evidence of shock.[2] Norepinephrine (noradrenaline) is recommended for patients with systolic BP below 85 mm Hg and persistent signs of shock.

## Specific Treatment of Underlying Cause

### Coronary Artery Disease

- Intravenous glyceryl trinitrate (nitroglycerin) is first-line treatment.
- The common adverse effect of glyceryl trinitrate is headache and hypotension. The dose of nitrates should be reduced if systolic BP decreases below 90–100 mm Hg and discontinued permanently if BP drops further. From a practical point of view, a reduction of 10 mm Hg in mean arterial BP should be achieved.
- In cases of significant coronary artery disease (CAD) causing acute CHF, percutaneous revascularization or coronary artery bypass should be carried out. Aspirin is given to all patients with coronary ischemia and those undergoing revascularization.
- In the case of cardiogenic shock with acute myocardial infarction (AMI), revascularization is recommended. Thrombolysis in this setting is not effective.

### Hypertensive Emergency

- Use of IV beta blockers and glyceryl trinitrate is recommended.
- If additional medicines are needed, nitroprusside is recommended in addition to other choices.

## Valvular Heart Disease
- In cases of severe aortic stenosis with heart failure, nitroprusside can be used provided the patient is not hypotensive.
- The definitive treatment for aortic stenosis is transcatheter aortic valve implantation (TAVI) if the patient is not a suitable candidate for conventional surgery. Mitral stenosis, if severe, needs a valve replacement, but in resistant heart failure, a percutaneous valvotomy may be used as temporary measure until definitive valve replacement is carried out. In mitral stenosis, percutaneous valvuloplasty may be done if no thrombus is present on transesophageal echocardiogram (TOE).
- Similarly in heart failure associated with mitral regurgitation or aortic regurgitation, a vasodilating drug such as nitroprusside should be used. A decrease in the peripheral arterial resistance results in an increase in the cardiac output and a decrease in regurgitant volume which in turn is associated with a reduction in left ventricular end-diastolic volume and an augmentation of the ejection fraction.

## Acute Right Heart Failure
- Treatment is focused on the underlying pathology, for example, pulmonary embolism (anticoagulation, thrombolytics, catheterization, or surgically directed thrombectomy), right ventricular infarction [percutaneous coronary intervention (PCI) or thrombolytics], and chronic thromboembolic pulmonary hypertension (thromboendarterectomy).

## Acute Myocarditis
- Giant cell myocarditis is treated with single or combination of immunosuppressant therapy including corticosteroids, azathioprine, cyclosporine, and muromonab-CD3 (OKT3).
- Treatment of other forms of myocarditis is limited to supportive care.

# Resistance to Maximal Medical Therapy

In cases of resistance to maximal medical therapy, a left ventricular assist device (LVAD) should be inserted. In some cases of nonischemic cardiomyopathy, sustained reversal of severe heart failure is seen with implantation of an LVAD. The use of LVADs has evolved significantly over the past 25 years and various types of LVAD now exist. Extracorporeal devices, the most common of which are the extracorporeal membrane oxygenators (ECMOs), require full heparinization and are typically used for days or weeks as a bridge for patients who are expected to recover within days. Percutaneous short-term devices (e.g., Tandem Heart) are inserted through the femoral artery and advanced into the left ventricle. Longer term assist devices are divided into first-generation (e.g., Heart Mate I), second-generation (e.g., Heart Mate II), and third-generation (e.g., HVAD and Dura Heart) devices. The third-generation pumps are thought to last as long as 5–10 years and are currently being evaluated in several phase 1 studies.[2]

An intra-aortic balloon pump (IABP) is a catheter with a balloon on it that is pushed through the femoral artery and placed in the aorta. This device increases the cardiac output by 40% and decreases the left ventricular stroke work and myocardial oxygen demand.

## Ongoing Therapy (Flowchart 1)

Once the patient is stabilized, definitive medical therapy for heart failure should be commenced. Usually, an angiotensin-converting enzyme (ACE) inhibitor [A evidence] (or an angiotensin-II receptor antagonist if ACE inhibitors are not tolerated [B evidence]) is started first, followed by the addition of beta-blockers [A evidence]. The dose of ACE inhibitors and beta-blockers

**Flowchart 1:** Drugs used in the treatment of congestive heart failure.

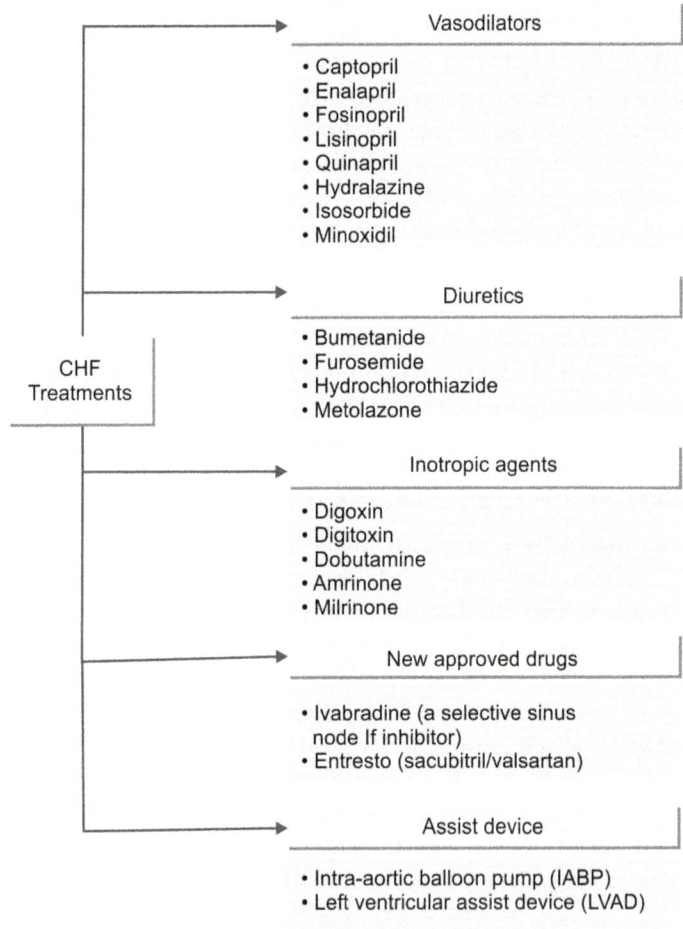

should be increased to the maximum tolerated dose depending upon BP and heart rate. Patients who have persistent signs of fluid overload will need ongoing diuretics. Patients with ongoing symptoms, despite this therapy, should be treated as having chronic CHF. Probability of CHF within 4 years for women aged 45–94 years with coronary disease, hypertension, or valvular disease.

## REFERENCES

1. books.mcgraw-hill.com
2. bestpractice.bmj.com

## CASE STUDY 26: BRUGADA SYNDROME

## CASE HISTORY

A 35-year-old male who has no history of cardiac risk factors is brought to the emergency room unresponsive. When hooked to the cardiac monitor, ventricular fibrillation (V-fib) is present. After 3–4 shocks at 360 J, his rhythm is restored.

## DISCUSSION

Brugada syndrome is a life-threatening heart rhythm disorder characterized by sudden death. It is a genetic disease causing abnormal heart rhythm due to the heart receiving excess electrical current. It was first identified by the Brugada brothers in a young child with abnormal electrocardiogram (ECG). It is a major contributor to causes of death in children. In fact, it may explain some cases of sudden infant death syndrome (SIDS). This syndrome may be present at any age from infancy to adulthood. It is inherited in an autosomal dominant manner. Patients inherit an abnormal *SCN5A* gene which alters $Na^+$ channel production and function. Because of this mutation, $Na^+$ channel function is altered which leads to decreased flow of $Na^+$ ions and therefore an irregular rhythm. Early repolarization occurs. This early repolarization may lead to malignant ventricular tachycardia which leads to ventricular fibrillation and possible sudden cardiac death (SCD). Symptoms may include syncope, shortness of breath, and SCD. Diagnosis is made by ECG and echocardiography (ECHO). ECG may show elevated ST segments and inverted T waves. The current treatment is *implantable cardiac defibrillator* (ICD) placement to prevent SCD.

There are three types of Brugada syndrome. Type 1 has ≥2 mm ST-segment elevation either spontaneously or induced with ajmaline/flecainide (a diagnostic test). Type 2 has a saddle back pattern with ≥2 mm J-point elevation and ST elevation. This type also shows a positive or biphasic T-wave.

Type 3 resembles either the shape of Type 1 or Type 2, except the elevation of the J-point is <2 mm, also with <1 mm ST elevation. Types 2 and 3 can be seen in healthy subjects (Flowchart 1 and Fig. 1).

**Flowchart 1:** Types of Brugada syndrome.

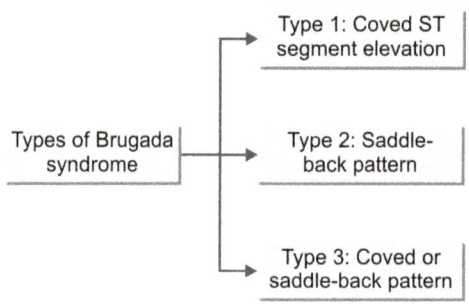

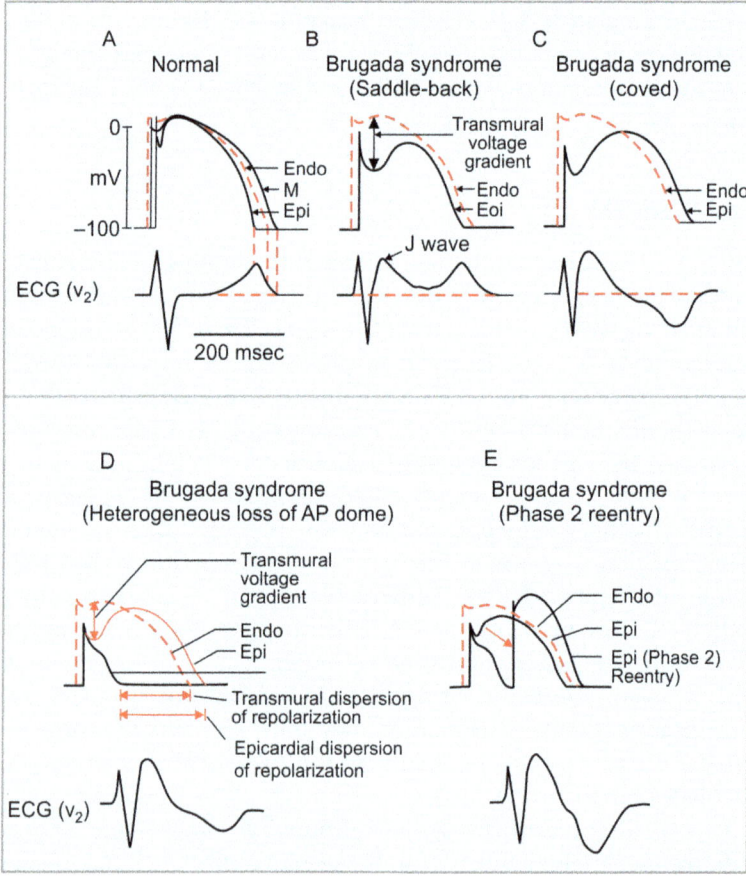

**Fig. 1:** Transmembrane action potentials.

Brugada syndrome is the most common cause of death in young men with no known underlying risk factors in Cambodia and Laos.

## CASE STUDY 27: HYPERTENSIVE URGENCY VERSUS EMERGENCY

*"... I will keep them from harm and injustice."*
—Hippocratic Oath

### CASE 1: HYPERTENSIVE URGENCY

A 60-year-old diabetic male presents to the emergency room with a chief complaint of headache. The patient was alarmed, when taking his blood pressure at home, that the reading was 200/110 mm Hg. His past medical history is significant for diabetes, hypertension, and chronic kidney disease (CKD) stage 3, with a *glomerular filtration rate* (GFR) between 30 and 59 mL/min for the past 6 months. He was diagnosed to have nephrosclerosis. The patient has been hypertensive for the past 20 years, but recently he has been having difficulty controlling his blood pressure. Presently, he is on three different medications: lisinopril 20 mg, amlodipine 10 mg, *hydrochlorothiazide* (HCTZ) 25 mg. His laboratory tests show protein uria and a spot protein-urine sample shows urine protein excretion is <500 mg/day. Physical examination shows body mass index (BMI) of 32 but does not reveal any evidence of abdominal bruit. Also, there is no mental status change and no significant neurological deficits. Funduscopic examination of the eye shows no diabetic retinopathy and no hypertensive retinopathy. Ultrasound examination shows bilateral renal disease without obstruction. Kidney size is 9.1 cm right and 9.6 cm left. This case represents hypertensive urgency (Flowchart 1).

### Patient's Management

Cautious reduction of blood pressure within 24–48 h with oral medications can be achieved. You can do more harm to a patient with hypertensive urgency by aggressively reducing the blood pressure. You may complete angina to full-blown acute myocardial infarction (AMI), or you may complete a partial stroke/stroke in evolution to complete stroke.

### CASE 2: HYPERTENSIVE EMERGENCY

A 77-year-old male is brought to the emergency department by the paramedics after a sudden onset of right-sided weakness associated with difficulty of speaking. His wife called the ambulance when she observed him returning from the washroom with right-sided weakness and he was slurring his speech. Past medical history is significant for poorly controlled hypertension and diabetes secondary to poor compliance, and there is no history of atrial fibrillation (Flowchart 2). He had a hemoglobin A1c drawn last week which

**Flowchart 1:** Hypertensive crisis.

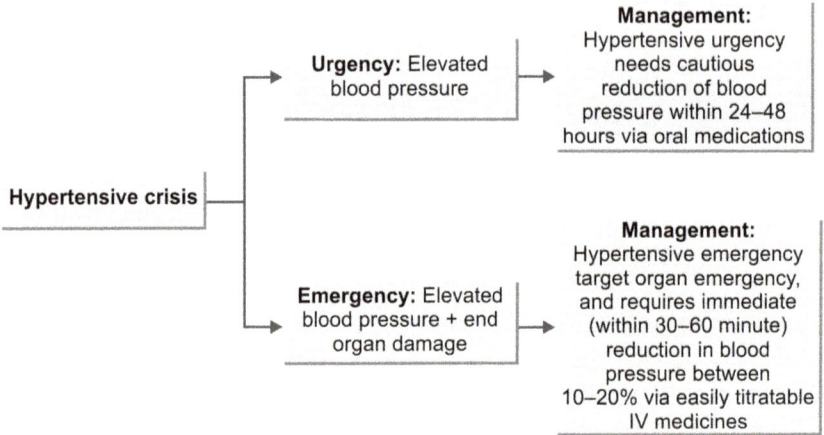

showed 8%. diagnostic tests; computed tomography (CT) head (noncontrast) shows multiple old lacunar infarcts and parietal ischemic stroke. On arrival to the emergency department, his vitals are blood pressure of 200/110 mm Hg, pulse rate 100 bpm, temperature 36.9°C, and complete blood count (CBC) and chemistry profile within normal limits (WNL).

## Patient's Management

This is a true hypertensive emergency where elevated blood pressure has caused end-organ damage/dysfunction (Figs. 1A to D). In this scenario, the ischemic injury needs to be treated very cautiously and slowly. Since this is a target organ injury to the brain, hence, cerebral autoregulatory ability is disrupted. In this situation, there are two causes of injury to the patient, ischemia and decrease in cerebral blood flow. A variety of studies have shown a relationship between systolic BP reductions and stroke outcomes. The higher the blood pressure, the better the outcome. Another study has shown that a poor outcome was independently associated with the degree of systolic blood pressure reduction. As a result of varied data from different studies, a scientific statement from the stroke council of the American Stroke Association has recommended that blood pressure, generally, not be lowered in patients suffering from acute ischemic strokes who are not otherwise candidates for thrombolysis. Mainly treating the cause of hypertension is very helpful.

Chest

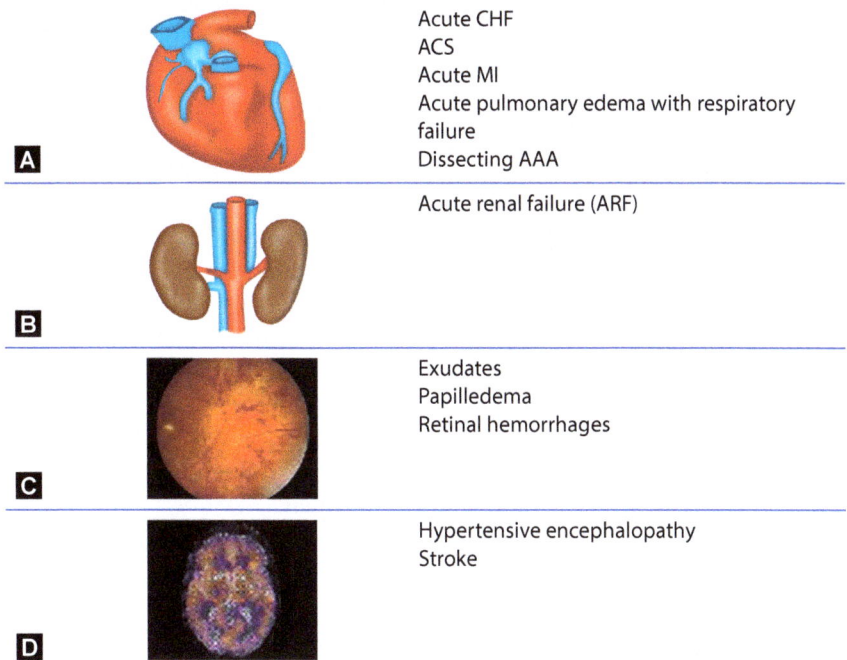

Figs. 1A to D: End-organ damage in hypertensive emergency.

## DISCUSSION

Flowchart 2: Causes and treatment of hypertensive emergency.

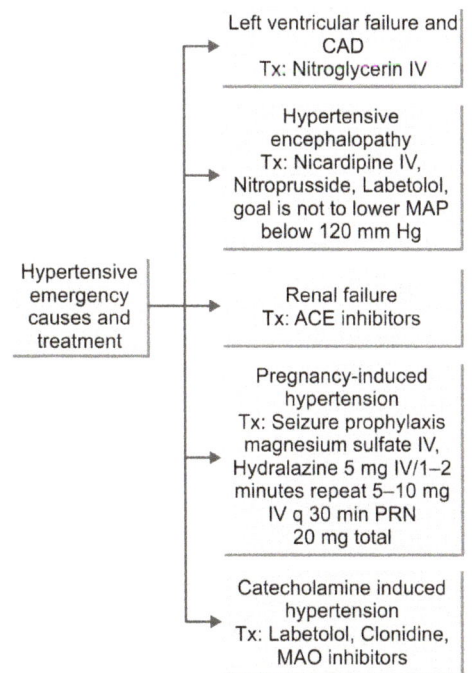

## CASE STUDY 28: LEFT VENTRICULAR ASSIST DEVICE

*"Except for the occasional heart attack, I never felt better."*

—Dick Cheney

## CASE HISTORY

A 55-year-old man is on a business trip from Seattle to a rural area in Southern Illinois. He is out to dinner and starts experiencing chest pain and throws up bright red blood, so his co-workers call the ambulance. While riding in the ambulance, he insists that he did not receive cardiopulmonary resuscitation (CPR) and gives a card to the paramedics about a left ventricular assist device (LVAD) and a doctor's name. While talking to the patient, the paramedics cannot find a pulse on the patient's body. By the time they get to the hospital, the patient is unconscious but his orders are transferred from the paramedics to the emergency department (ED) doctor. None of the ED doctors has heard of an LVAD, so the patient's cardiologist on the card is called.

## DISCUSSION

LVADs have been around for almost 20 years but are not widely used since heart transplant is still the gold standard. The first-generation devices used a pulsating flow to push the blood in waves out of the ventricle into the aorta. Current devices (second generation) use a continuous flow to keep blood moving but can also cause more alarm to an ED doctor as a patient may present without a pulse but still able to talk! To qualify for an assistive device [right ventricular assistive device (RVAD) and both ventricular assistive device (BiVAD) also exist], the patient must have Stage IV New York classification heart failure and an ejection fraction of ≤25%.[1] Most of the time, these devices are used to keep a person alive until a transplantation can be found. In some cases, they are used as a destination treatment for heart disease, because most patients do not fit the specific criteria for transplantation.

Patients with heart failure are often limited in what they can do and often not able to accomplish many activities of daily living. After having a LVAD inserted, most patients go from Stage IV heart failure to Stage I or II and regain much functioning (with the exception of swimming). The longest lasting second-generation device to date has been 6 years, but there is no reason they cannot last longer. In addition, if problems with the pump happen, the device should be able to be replaced as many times as necessary limited only by patient healing (Fig. 1).

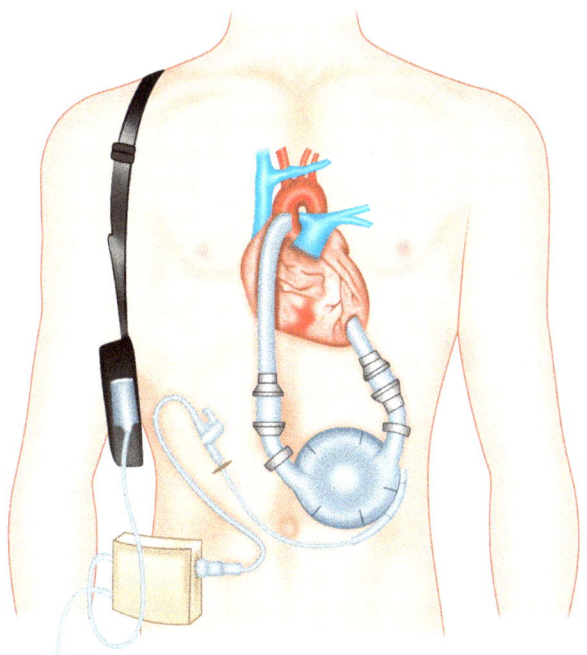

**Fig. 1:** A LVAD pumping blood from the left ventricle to the aorta, connected to an externally worn control unit and battery pack. (LVAD: left ventricular assist device).

## TREATMENT

Until recently, we have only seen people coming for dobutamine IV weekly for treatment of congestive heart failure (CHF), since the advance of modern medicine LVADs have replaced such treatments (Table 1). There are four very distinct reasons why medicine is moving toward LVAD implantations which include limited need for medication, less follow-up, fewer invasive procedures, and they still have the option for transplant. Former Vice President of America, Dick Cheney, had an LVAD implanted.

**Table 1:** Complications from left ventricular assistive device and its treatment.

| Complications from left ventricular assistive device | Treatment |
| --- | --- |
| Infection/cellulitis | Hospitalize and give IV antibiotics |
| Bleeding | Look and treat for coagulopathy |
| Pulselessness/no heart sounds | Listen to precordium for humming sound of the device |
|  | Examine power supply and battery, change if necessary and call the control center. Place the patient on cardiac monitor and obtain Doppler blood pressure |

*(Contd...)*

*(Contd...)*

| Complications from left ventricular assistive device | Treatment |
|---|---|
| Ventricular dysrhythmias | Defibrillate |
| Hypoxia/acidosis | Intubation and administer $NaHCO_3$ IV |
| Right ventricular failure from thrombosis in left used for non-bleeding patients | Anticoagulation (heparin) therapy ventricular assist device or pulmonary embolism |

## REFERENCE

1. Swadron S. The LVAD: walking, talking and pulseless. Emerg Physicians Mon 2012;19(7):12.

## FURTHER READING

1. The Nebraska Medical Center. Left ventricular assist device (LVAD) as destination therapy—the nebraska medical center. [Online]. Available from www.youtube.com/watch?v=ggtAJHVYifc; 2011 [accessed August, 2012].

# CHAPTER 3

# Abdomen

## CASE STUDY 29: UPPER GASTROINTESTINAL BLEED

### CASE HISTORY

A 45-year-old investment banker presents with an episode of black vomit. He has been experiencing stomach pains for weeks, often after he finishes a meal. He wakes up at night with burning chest pain and describes a foul taste in the morning. The patient also complains of bloating and fullness. His job has been stressful, as the economy has been taking massive downturns. He describes himself as an easily stressed person. The patient has had tension headaches for many years that he usually responded by using a few capsules of Advil. The patient also admits that he has been feeling weak and a reduced sex drive.

### PHYSICAL EXAMINATION

Patient is tachycardic. Abdomen examination shows tenderness in the epigastrium.

### Laboratory Tests

Low hematocrit. Hypochromic anemia.

### Imaging

*Endoscopy*: Gastric ulcer.

### DIAGNOSIS

The patient is suffering from upper gastrointestinal (GI) bleeding secondary to nonsteroidal anti-inflammatory drug (NSAID) overuse.

## DISCUSSION

Before the details of the case are discussed, it is helpful to define a number of terms:
- *Hematemesis*: Vomiting of blood
- *Coffee ground emesis*: Vomiting of blood that has been broken down by stomach acid, which shows the color of oxidized heme
- *Hematochezia*: Presence of fresh blood in stool
- *Melena*: Presence of digested blood in stool.

This is a case of upper GI bleeding. The presence of "coffee ground" emesis, epigastric discomfort, and history of stress and NSAID use highly suggest an upper GI bleed before endoscopic confirmation of a gastric ulcer. Upper GI bleed refers to any bleeding above the ligament of Treitz of the duodenum. The form of blood in either emesis or stool can give clinicians clues as to where the location of bleeding may be, even within the scope of upper GI bleeding. In the case of "coffee ground" emesis, an upper GI bleed is most likely. The bleed is unlikely to be in the esophagus due to its oxidized nature. If it is a gastric bleed, the bleeding may be low-grade, which allows blood the time to be oxidized. In contrast, the presence of hematemesis suggests bleeding in the esophagus or heavy bleeding in the lower upper GI tract.

The forms of blood in stool are also helpful in diagnosing GI bleeds. In the case of melena, the bleeding location is likely to be upper GI due to the fact that the blood had the time to pass through the GI system to be digested. If hematochezia is present, the bleeding is likely to be in the lower GI due to its proximity to the anus. Hematochezia may also occur with severe upper GI bleeding, in which the volume of blood overcomes the digestive capacity of the system. In such cases, the patients are likely to exhibit signs of hypovolemia, anemia, and even shock.

There are many causes of upper GI bleeding. Gastric ulcer secondary to NSAID use is a prevalent problem. NSAIDs inhibit cyclooxygenases, which are responsible for producing prostaglandins that protect the gastric mucosa. Another common cause of gastric ulcer is *Helicobacter pylori (H. pylori)* infection. The bacterium erodes the mucosa, allowing gastric acid to further damage the underlying gastric and duodenal tissues. Ulcers may also result from heavy alcohol consumption, in which the alcohol irritates the gastric mucosal lining and causes acid damage. Other causes of upper GI bleeding include Mallory–Weiss syndrome, cancer, and esophageal/gastric varices.

The diagnosis of GI bleeding is through upper endoscopy. Endoscopy can verify the presence and site of the bleed and perform coagulation therapy (Fig. 1). Nasogastric tube may also be used to aspirate gastric content to determine if blood is present (to differentiate between lower GI bleeding). Other diagnostic tests, such as hemoglobin, hematocrit, colonoscopy, and stool occult blood, are also helpful in differentiating upper GI bleed from other diagnoses.

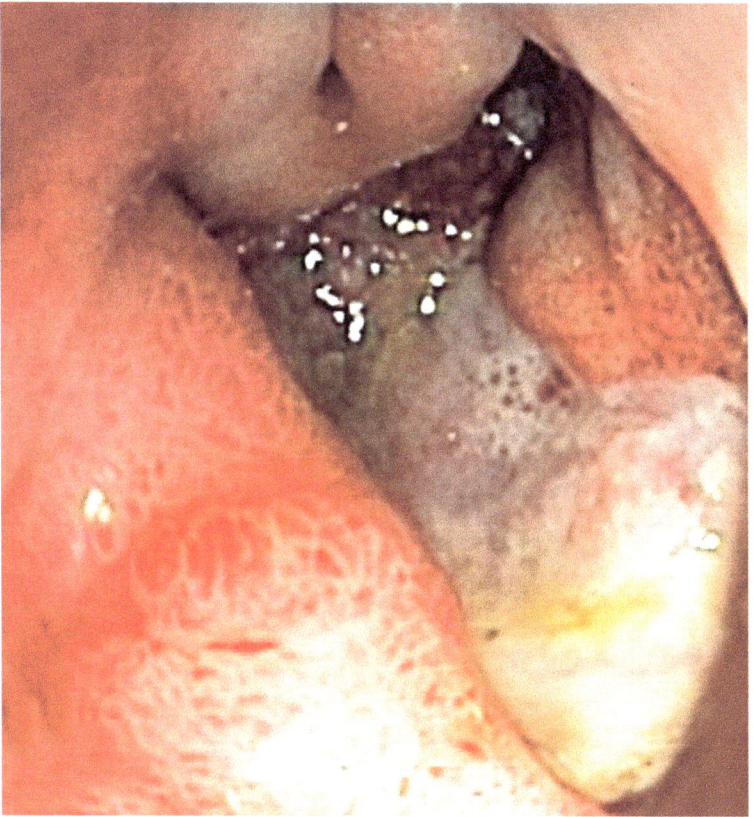

**Fig. 1:** Endoscopy showing deep gastric ulcer.
*Source:* http://www.cleanandsoberlive.com/stomach-pain-after-drinking-its-probably-gastritis/.

The first priority of treatment of an upper GI bleed is resuscitation and stabilization if the patient is hemodynamically compromised. The subsequent management depends on the severity and the underlying cause of bleeding. Active bleeding is treated with endoscopy with coagulation to stop the bleed. If the bleeding cannot be stopped with endoscopic procedures, surgery would be the next step (Flowchart 1). Pharmacological interventions may follow to treat the underlying cause of the bleed. In the case of *H. pylori* infection, a proton pump inhibitor and combinations of antibiotics are necessary. Octreotide is used to treat esophageal or gastric varices.

Depending on the comorbidities and rate of blood loss, transfusions are almost necessary if the hemoglobin (Hgb) is <7 g/dL (Fig. 2).

1. Sometimes when Hgb <10, patient may require transfusions.
2. If patient is thrombocytopenic, they may require platelet transfusion.
3. If patient has international normalized ratio (INR) >1.5, you should administer fresh frozen plasma.

**Flowchart 1:** Lower gastrointestinal bleeding management.

```
Resuscitate and stabilize
            ↓
Endoscopy (to exclude upper GI bleeding)
            ↓
Colonoscopy (to identify the source and
cause of bleeding and to control the
bleeding via ligation, diathermy, clipping,
injection, etc.)
            ↓
           If
       ↙       ↘
CT angiogram    Mesenteric angiogram
                (for embolization)
       ↘       ↙
         Surgery
```

*Modified from:* http://www.slideshare.net/sirajshiferaw/agi-bleedingseminar.

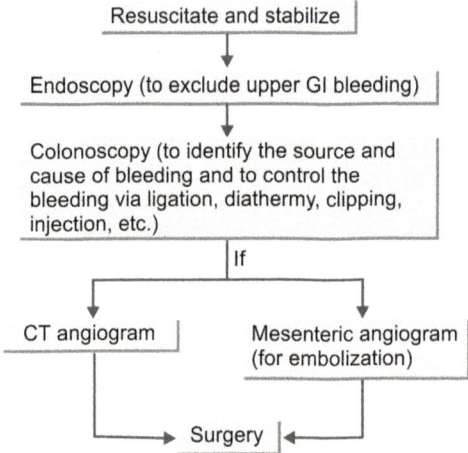

**Transfusion**
- Almost always for Hgb <7
- Sometimes for Hgb <10
- Depends on comorbidities and rate of blood loss
- If patient is thrombocytopenic (platelets less than 50,000), transfuse platelets
- If patient has INR >1.5, administer fresh frozen plasma
- Follow labs every 2–6 hours

**Fig. 2:** Criteria for transfusion of blood.
*Source:* Gastrointestinal emergencies. 2nd edn. ISBN: 978-1-405-14634-0.

4. Continue to follow laboratories ever 2–6 h.

For very severe hemorrhage, prophylactic antibiotics can be administered to reduce the morality.

## FURTHER READING

1. Gastrointestinal emergencies. 2nd ed. ISBN: 978-1-405-14634-0.
2. http://www.slideshare.net/sirajshiferaw/agi-bleedingseminar.

## CASE STUDY 30: DIVERTICULITIS

*"If you believe the patient has appendicitis on the left side, you are most likely dealing with diverticulitis"*

—Badar M Zaheer

## CHIEF COMPLAINT

An 84-year-old postmenopausal white female with abdominal and flank pain.

## CASE HISTORY

An 84-year-old lady with a history of smoking presents to the emergency room (ER) early in the morning with sudden constant left lower quadrant (LLQ) pain that radiates to the groin with an onset of 3 h. Current pain level is 2–3/10 and maximum was 10/10. Last bowel movement was 20–25 min prior to arrival which was normal but thinner. She presents with a mild fever, but no chills, sweating, chest pain, nausea, and vomiting. No diarrhea or constipation was noticed. Nothing seems to exacerbate or relieve her symptoms.

## PAST SURGICAL HISTORY

Right hip surgery.

## DIAGNOSTIC TESTS

- CBC—Patient has 16,000 white blood cell (WBC) count with shift to the left.
- Abdominal X-rays—Not useful
- Barium enema—Outdated and not useful
- Computed tomography (CT) abdomen—Preferred choice. Highly sensitive and specific (Figs. 1 and 2)
- Ultrasound—Safe, less invasive, low cost, but operator dependent and not as accurate as CT. Not a useful tool for surgical planning.

## DISCUSSION

Many people have small pouches in the lining of the large intestine that bulge outward through weak spots. The small pouches are called diverticula, and the condition of having diverticula is called diverticulosis. As we age, this condition becomes more prominent.[1]

In 10–25% of people with diverticulosis, the pouches become inflamed. Acute diverticulitis is the most common complication of diverticular disease,

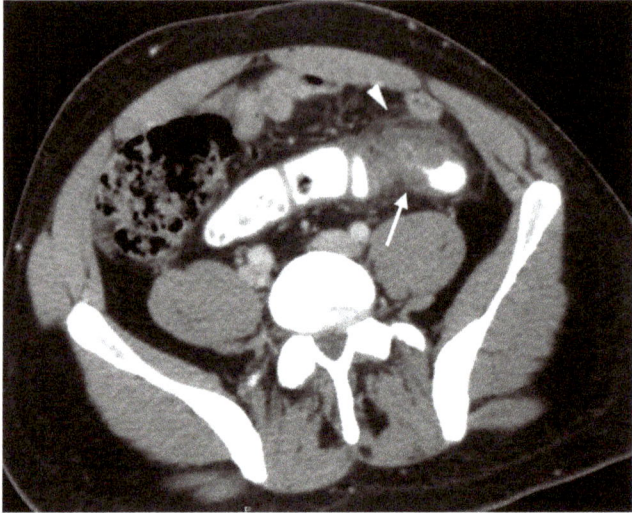

**Fig. 1:** Computed tomography scan shows abdomen with sigmoid wall thickening and adjacent fat stranding.
*Courtesy:* Badar M Zaheer, MD, Chicago, USA.

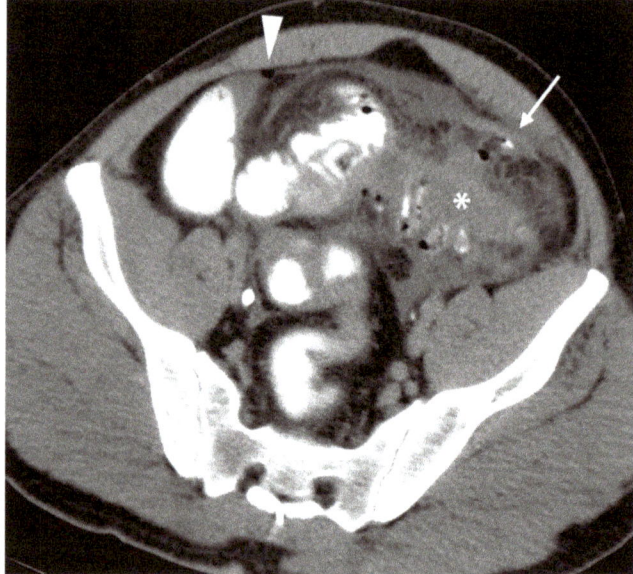

**Fig. 2:** Computed tomography scan shows severe diverticulitis with perforation. This patient presented with abdominal pain, fever, and rebound tenderness.
*Courtesy:* Badar M Zaheer, MD, Chicago, USA.

but 20% of the patients with diverticular disease may also develop other complications, such as infection, abscess, fistula, obstruction, perforation, or even diverticular bleeding. Patients usually present with visceral abdominal pain and tenderness localized to the area of maximal inflammation.

Nausea, vomiting, and altered bowel habits often occur. There may also be rectal tenderness, fever, and leukocytosis.

## MANAGEMENT

In mild cases, where the patient has the ability to tolerate oral intake, he or she can be treated as an outpatient. Put the patient on clear liquid diet and a broad spectrum antibiotic for 7–10 days (amoxicillin–clavulanate, trimethoprim–sulfamethoxazole, or fluorquinolone and metronidazole), and discharge home for a close follow-up.

Patients suffering from a severe attack of diverticulitis may require hospitalization. The patient must be put on analgesia, bowel rest, intravenous fluid, and a broad-spectrum antibiotic for anaerobes and gram-negative rods for 7–10 days. Anaerobes are treated with metronidazole or clindamycin. Gram-negative rods are treated with aminoglycoside, monobactam, or third-generation cephalosporins (Tables 1 and 2).

Pericolic abscesses are drained under CT or US guidance. The patient may also be treated with conservative methods, as those stated above.[2]

Treatment focuses on clearing up the inflammation and infection, resting the colon, and preventing or minimizing complications. Gradually increasing the amount of high-fiber foods in the diet will help in recovery.

**Table 1:** Medications.

| Time | Medication | Dose (mg) | Route | Site |
| --- | --- | --- | --- | --- |
| 08:07 | Zofran | 4 | IV | LW |
| 08:13 | Morphine sulfate | 2 | IV | LW |
| 08:45 | Nitro patch | 0.4 | TOP | Left Chest |
| 09:45 | Ativan | 0.3 | IV | LW |
| 10:06 | Zofran | 4 | IV | LW |
| 10:20 | Compazine | 5 | IV | LW |
| 11:25 | Tylenol | 650 | PR | |
| 12:05 | Motrin | 400 | PO | |

**Table 2:** IV medication infusion.

| Time | Solution/Medicine Type | Rate (mL/h) | Stop time | Amount infused |
| --- | --- | --- | --- | --- |
| 10:20 | 0.97 NS1 Med. | 200 | | |
| 10:25 | Rocephin, 1 GM 1 Med. | 200 | 10:50 | 100 |
| 10:51 | Gentamicin, 125 mg 1 Med. | 300 | 11.20 | 100 |
| 11:20 | 0.9% NS Pump | 999 | 11:45 | 300 |
| 11:46 | 0.9% NS Pump | 999 | 11:59 | 300 |

## PHYSICAL EXAMINATION

### General Appearance
The patient is alert, oriented and not in acute distress.

### Head, Eyes, Ears, Nose and Throat (HEENT)
There is no evidence of trauma, tumors, facial edema, goiter, or thyroid nodules. Pupils are equal, round, reactive to light, and accommodation (PERRLA) and sclera icterus. Ear, nose, throat (ENT) inspection is normal. Pharynx is normal. The neck is supple.

### Cardiovascular System
Regular rate and rhythm. S1 and S2 are normal.

### Respiration
Breath sounds are normal.

### Abdominal
- Soft, tenderness in LLQ
- Normal bowel sounds. No abdominal bruit. No pulsatile mass. No hepatosplenomegaly.

### Skin
Color is normal. No rash. Warm and dry.

### Extremities
Nontender, normal range of motion (ROM), no pedal edema, no joint effusions, rashes, or cyanosis.

### Laboratory
Complete blood count (CBC), comprehensive metabolic panel (CMP), amylase, lipase, blood culture and sensitivity (C&S) × 2 sites, urinalysis (UA), blood culture × 2.

### Results
*White blood cell (WBC): 15.5.*
*Platelets (PLT): 265.*

Normal chemistry.
Lipase and amylase are normal.
*UA*: WBC: 10–25, UA: Bacteria + 1.

## Procedures

- *Portable chest X-ray (CXR)*: Normal; normal bowel gas
- Flat and upright abdominal X-ray
- *CT*: Abdomen and pelvis, oral and IV contrast (*see* Figs. 1 and 2).

## DISPOSITION

## Discharge Vitals

*BP*: 109/70 mm Hg, HR: 123 bpm, RR: 24 breaths/min, *T*: 102°F, and $SaO_2$: 96%. Pain: 4/10.

## Impression

*Diverticulitis*: LLQ (radiates to groin), leukocytosis, and fever.
*For most definitive diagnosis:* CT.

### Computerized Tomography

- Diverticula, thickened colonic wall >4 mm
- Inflammation within pericolic fat more or less
- Collection of contrast material or fluid.

## Differential Diagnosis

- *Sepsis*: Fever, leukocytosis, HR >90 bpm, RR >20 breaths/minute, WBC count <4,000 or >12,000 is a sign of sepsis
- *Acute urinary tract infection*: Dysuria, urinary frequency, pyuria, hematuria, bacteriuria, foul, and cloudy urine
- *Acute pyelonephritis*: Fever, dysuria, vomiting, flank pain, U/A: WBC, white cell casts
- *Inflammatory bowel syndrome*: Abdominal pain, vomiting and diarrhea, rectal bleeding, internal cramps/muscle spasms in pelvic region, weight loss, arthritis, pyoderma gangrenosum, and primary sclerosing cholangitis
- *Acute appendicitis*
- *Sigmoid malignancy*
- *Ovarian cyst*
- *Endometriosis*
- *Pelvic inflammatory disease.*

## Treatment

One of the following course of treatment is followed.
- *Antibiotics*: Ciprofloxacin and metronidazole
- Ampicillin or sulbactam and piperacillin or tazobactam
- Gentamicin and cefotetan or cefoxitin.

*Mild Disease*

*Oral antibiotics*: Amoxicillin/clavulanic acid (Augmentin)

## DISCUSSION

### True Diverticulum

Sac-like herniation of entire bowel wall.

### Pseudodiverticulum

- Mucosa protrusion through muscularis propria of colon is the most common.
- *Protrusion point*: Nutrient artery (vasa recti) penetrates through muscularis propria
- Break in integrity of colonic wall
- *Common site*: Sigmoid colon, 1/20: pancolonic diverticula
- *Cause*: The main cause is higher amplitude contractions and constipated, high-fat content stool within sigmoid lumen.

## DIVERTICULITIS

- Inflammation of diverticulum
- Retention of particulate material within diverticular sac and fecalith formation
- Compression or erosion of vasa recti causes bleeding indicates perforation.

### Acute Uncomplicated Diverticulitis

*Presentation*: Fever, LLQ abdominal pain, anorexia/obstipation, generalized peritonitis (diverticular perforation)
*Examination*: Abdominal distension and signs of localized or generalized peritonitis
*Laboratory*: Leukocytosis.

## Diagnosis

*Computerized tomography*
- Sigmoid diverticula, thickened colonic wall is >4 mm
- Inflammation is within pericolic fat.

### Contraindications for Testing in Acute Diverticulitis
- Barium enema or colonoscopy in acute setting for fear of perforation and pertonitis
- Perform 6 weeks after diverticular disease to rule out sigmoid malignancy.

## Complicated Diverticulitis
- *Presentation*: Abscess > perforation > stricture > fistula
- *Perforation staging*: Hinchey classification system, predict outcome of postoperative management
- *Fistula formation*: Cutaneous, vaginal, vesicle fistulae, stool passage through skin or vagina, air in urinary stream (pneumaturia)
- *Colovaginal fistulae*: More common in women with history of hysterectomy.

## MANAGEMENT
- Radiographic and hematologic confirmation of inflammation or infection within the colon
- Initially with antibiotic and bowel rest
- Three-fourth of hospitalized acute diverticulitis patients respond to antimicrobial regimen
- Trimethoprim/sulfamethoxazole or ciprofloxacin
    - + Metronidazole: Aerobic gram-negative rods + anaerobic bacteria
    - + Ampicillin: If not responding
- *Single agent*: 3G penicillin, IV piperacillin, oral penicillin/clavulanic acid
- *Duration*: 7–10 days.

## REFERENCES
1. Destigter KK, Keating DP. Imaging update: acute colonic diverticulitis. Clin Colon Rectal Surg. 2009;3:147-55.
2. Kaltenback T, Soetikno R. Diverticular disease. In: Gastrointestinal Emergencies. 2nd ed. Hoboken, New Jersey: Blackwell Publishing Ltd. 2009.

## CASE STUDY 31: ACUTE PANCREATITIS

### CASE HISTORY

A 45-year-old female patient presents with pain that started suddenly in the epigastric region while she was sitting at work. Pain is sharp 8/10 and radiates to the back. Since the onset of the pain, patient has had three episodes of non-bloody, non-bilious vomiting. Patient has never had pain quite like this before, although she states that she has had several episodes of right upper quadrant (RUQ) pain for which she was told that she should eventually have her gallbladder taken out. Past medical history is significant for gastroesophageal reflux disease (GERD) for which she takes omeprazole. Her only past surgery was a tubal ligation after her third pregnancy. She does not smoke, drink alcohol, or use any other recreational drugs. On physical examination, patient is afebrile with a blood pressure of 156/95 mm Hg, heart rate 108 bpm, respiratory rate 18 breaths/min, and oxygen ($O_2$) saturation of 100% on room air. What is the most likely diagnosis? What testing would help confirm your suspicion?

### DISCUSSION

The most likely diagnosis is gallstone pancreatitis. The patient's epigastric abdominal pain radiating to the back is characteristic of pancreatitis. The patient's history of biliary colic suggests gallstones are the cause. Lipase or computed tomography (CT) of abdomen could confirm pancreatitis. Aspartate aminotransferase/alanine aminotransferase (AST/ALT), alkaline phosphatase, electrolytes, complete blood count (CBC), and urinalysis (UA) should also be obtained. Urine pregnancy test in women of child-bearing age should be obtained. Other causes of the patient's abdominal pain that should be considered are biliary colic, cholecystitis, cholangitis, peptic ulcer disease, and ulcer perforation.

Acute pancreatitis is an inflammatory disease of the pancreas that is associated with little or no fibrosis of the gland. It has high morbidity and mortality rates contributing to 300,000 hospital admits per year as well as 20,000 deaths. The exact mechanism is unknown and varies with a specific cause. In general, it is thought that there is an activation of digestive zymogens inside acinar cells that leads to injury. In addition, there is activation of inflammatory mediators. If severe, this can lead to systemic inflammatory response syndrome (SIRS) and multiorgan failure or local necrosis of the pancreas.

Typical presentation includes abdominal pain in 95% of cases. The pain is most likely to have a sudden severe onset that is either located in the epigastric region, RUQ, or less commonly the left upper quadrant (LUQ). The pain has a tendency to radiate toward the back due to the retroperitoneal positioning of the pancreas. The quality is usually boring and deep, alleviated by resting in the fetal position and exacerbated by eating and drinking alcohol. In 90% of cases, there are associated symptoms of nausea and vomiting. Often patients feel restless and agitated. In the cases of biliary pancreatitis, the exception is that the pain may come on more gradually and be more localized to the RUQ.

The physical examination depends on the severity of the attack. Mild disease will cause mild abdominal tenderness, whereas severe disease will cause severe tenderness and guarding in the upper abdomen. Generally, no rebound tenderness is present. In terms of vitals, patients are usually tachycardic. Mild hypotension may be present due to sequestration of fluid in the pancreatic bed. Low-grade fevers are present without evidence of infection in 60% of cases. Respirations are generally rapid and shallow. Signs suggestive of severe disease include Grey Turner sign and Cullen sign. Grey Turner sign consists of ecchymoses in the flanks that are indicative of hemorrhage from hemorrhagic pancreatitis. Cullen sign is ecchymoses in the periumbilical region that is similarly suggestive of intra-abdominal hemorrhage. Other associated findings that are suggestive of peripancreatic spread of inflammation include generalized ileus, signs of pleural effusion, subcutaneous fat necrosis, and jaundice.

Expected laboratory findings include leukocytosis, mild hyperglycemia, mild increase in AST/ALT from alcoholic pancreatitis, large increase in AST/ALT from biliary causes. More importantly, serum lipase has a high sensitivity of 90% and high specificity when elevated up to two times normal. Serum amylase is sensitive but not specific for pancreatitis unless three times normal. Other pancreatic enzymes can be measured but generally not done clinically.

Abdominal CT is the most accurate for diagnosing pancreatitis and identifying its localized effects. CT abdomen should be done when you are uncertain or the diagnosis, suspect complications, or in cases of mild-to-moderate disease that do not improve over several days. Intravenous (IV) and oral contrast should be used. Findings on imaging will include pancreatomegaly, peripancreatic streakiness, or "dirty fat," necrotic areas that fail to enhance. CT severity index may be used as an aid in prognosis. Other methods of imaging that may be used are abdominal X-ray, ultrasound, and magnetic resonance cholangiopancreatography (MRCP). Abdominal X-ray is often used to rule out perforation. Findings include dilated loops or air-fluid levels secondary to paralytic ileus, sentinel loop, colon cut-off sign, widening of the C-loop, and calcifications of the gallbladder. Ultrasound may provide evidence of the cause of pancreatitis and may aid in ruling out gallstones. It is often difficult to identify the pancreas due to overlying intestinal gas or fat. If able to visualize, a hypoechoic and enlarged pancreas may be present. MRCP is useful for the select patient populations: pregnancy, contrast allergy, and renal insufficiency. It is most accurate for visualizing bile and pancreatic ducts and pancreatic fluid collections. This test may be most useful while awaiting endoscopic retrograde cholangiopancreatography (ERCP) for definitive management.

There are many causes of pancreatitis. Remember the mnemonic "**GET SMASHED.**"
**G**allstones
**E**thanol
**T**rauma
**S**teroids
**M**umps
**A**utoimmune
**S**corpion
**H**yperlipidemia
**E**RCP
**D**rugs.

It is important to identify the cause in order to direct the present therapy and prevent future recurrences. The most common cause overall is gallstones making up to 40%. Combined, gallstones and alcoholism can cause 75% of cases. In 15% of cases, the cause can never be identified. For alcoholic pancreatitis, it requires more than eight alcoholic drinks per day for >5 years. Smoking is an important cofactor. Frequently, alcoholics develop chronic pancreatitis. Hypertriglyceridemia accounts for 2% of the cases. Triglyceride levels >1,000% are suggestive, but levels >2,000% are diagnostic. Levels should be measured early. If found to be >10,000%, plasmapheresis may be required. It has been suggested that mumps, coxsackie, and *Mycoplasma* infections may cause pancreatitis because titers have been shown to be elevated during an attack, but none have been isolated in the pancreas. ERCP causes 2% of cases. Mild-to-moderate elevations in amylase and lipase occur after ERCP regardless, so it is unnecessary to measure levels immediately after the procedure.

Patients with pancreatitis are most likely going to be admitted except in some cases of chronic pancreatitis. However, a decision has to be made on whether to admit these patients to the intensive care unit. This is where the severity of the criteria can be useful. Ranson's CT severity index, acute physiology and chronic health evaluation II (APACHE II) are the most commonly used. APACHE II generally has the best predictive value, but the criteria involves more testing. Please see Box 1 and Table 1 for these criteria. Any signs of organ failure warrant admission to the intensive care unit. For this to happen, coordination must take place between the intensive care unit team, gastrointestinal (GI) team, surgery, and infectious disease. First line therapy is supportive. Aggressive fluid hydration is required to prevent acute tubular necrosis (ATN) and lessen pancreatic necrosis for 48 h. Glucose should be monitored because elevations may occur even without history of diabetes. Analgesia is essential for patient comfort. Historically, meperidine 50–100 mg q 6 h has been used, but long-term build-up of toxic metabolites has caused this drug to fall out of favor. It was once thought that morphine use would worsen pancreatitis due to sphincter of Oddi contraction, but this

> **Box 1:** Ranson's criteria.
>
> *Ranson criteria on admission:*
> - Age over 55 years
> - A white blood cell count of >16,000/μL
> - Blood glucose >11 mmol/L (>200 mg/dL)
> - Serum LDH >350 IU/L
> - Serum AST >250 IU/L
>
> *Ranson criteria 48 h of admission*:
> - Fall in hematocrit by >10%
> - Fluid sequestration of >6 L
> - Hypocalcemia [serum calcium <2.0 mmol/L (<8.0 mg/L)]
> - Hypoxemia ($PO_2$ <60 mm Hg)
> - Increase in BUN to >1.98 mmol/L (>5 mg/dL) after IV fluid hydration
> - Base deficit of >4 mmol/L
>
> *The prognostic implications of Ranson criteria are as follows*:
> - Score 0–2: 2% mortality
> - Score 3–4: 15% mortality
> - Score 5–6: 40% mortality
> - Score 7–8: 100% mortality

**Table 1:** CT severity index.

| Prognostic indicator | Points |
| --- | --- |
| Pancreatic inflammation | |
| Normal pancreas | 0 |
| Focal or diffuse enlargement of the pancreas | 1 |
| Intrinsic pancreatic abnormalities with inflammatory changes in peripancreatic fat | 2 |
| Single, ill-defined fluid collection of phlegmon | 3 |
| Two or more poorly defined collections or presence of gas in or adjacent to the pancreas | 4 |
| Pancreatic necrosis | |
| None | 0 |
| ≤30% | 2 |
| >30–50% | 4 |
| >50% | 6 |

is now thought to be more theoretical. Morphine is frequently used for pain control. Patients should be nil per os (NPO) for bowel and pancreatic rest. Diet should be advanced slowly when there is no longer pain, nausea, vomiting, or distention. If patient is expected to be NPO for more than a few days, then parenteral nutrition should be considered with total parenteral nutrition (TPN) or nasojejunal (NJ) tube. Nasogastric tubes are no longer used because randomized trials did not show faster times to per os (PO) intake. Vitals should be frequently monitored.

Directed therapy depends on the cause of pancreatitis. For patients with gallstone pancreatitis, ERCP and sphincterotomy may be considered in conjunction with GI consult. This should be urgently done if cholangitis is suspected. Cholecystectomy should be done at some point during the hospitalization. Timing is controversial but typically done between 48 and 72 h or after 72 h. Intraoperative cholangiogram should be done to rule out the presence of stones in the common bile duct if ERCP has not already been done.

Many complications can occur as a result of pancreatitis. It is important to be aware of these in order to both prevent and rapidly treat them. The most common complication, which occurs in 10% of patients, is a pancreatic pseudocyst, which is defined as a collection of pancreatic fluid surrounded by a nonepithelialized wall of granulation tissue. Typical presentation includes a history of pancreatitis with now worsening pain, distention, and difficulty eating. Drainage is required whether it is done by CT-guided endoscopy or surgery. Regardless of the mode of procedure, the treatment involves making a connection between the cyst and one of three places: stomach, duodenum, or jejunum. Surgical intervention is done when the cyst lasts >6 weeks and/or is >5 cm. A severe complication is pancreatic abscess. This typically occurs 2–6 weeks after the initial attack. Patients will become septic. CT scan is necessary to diagnose and treatment is drainage. Mortality rate is high. Other complications include hypocalcemia, disseminated fat necrosis, *acute respiratory distress syndrome* (ARDS), renal insufficiency, sterile pancreatic necrosis, infected pancreatic necrosis in the first few hours or days, ascending cholangitis, pancreatic abscess, abdominal compartment syndrome, splenic artery or gastroduodenal artery pseudoaneurysm, pancreatic fistula, pancreatic ascites, splenic vein thrombosis, cardiovascular shock with hypovolemia, and hemorrhagic pancreatitis.

In summary, the most common symptoms are abdominal pain, nausea, and vomiting. Lipase has the highest sensitivity and specificity. CT is the most sensitive imaging, but it is not always needed for diagnosis. The most common causes are gallstones and alcoholism. It is important to assess the need for intensive care unit admission. The mainstay of treatment is supportive therapy with aggressive fluid resuscitation, NPO, and analgesia.

## FURTHER READING

1. Cappell MS. Acute pancreatitis: etiology, clinical presentation, diagnosis, and therapy. Med Clin North Am. 2008;92:889-923.
2. Haney JC, Pappas TN. Necrotizing pancreatitis: diagnosis and management. Surg Clin North Am. 2007;87:1431-46.
3. Howell DA, Shah RJ. Endoscopic management of pseudocysts of the pancreas: efficacy and complications. Up-To-Date Wolters Kluwer Health; 2010.
4. Sielaff TD, Curley SA. Liver. In: Brunicardi FC, Andersen DK, Billiar TR, editors. Schwartz's principles of surgery. 8th ed. New York: McGraw-Hill; 2005. p. 1163.

5. Tenner S, Steinberg WM. Acute pancreatitis. In: Feldman M, Friedman LS, Brandt LJ, editors. Sleisenger and Fordtran's gastrointestinal and liver disease. 9th ed. Philadelphia, PA: Saunders Elsevier; 2010.
6. Vege SS. Clinical manifestations and diagnosis of acute pancreatitis. Up-To-Date Wolters Kluwer Health; 2010.
7. Vege SS. Treatment of acute pancreatitis. Up-To-Date Wolters Kluwer Health; 2012.

## CASE STUDY 32: ACUTE CHOLECYSTITIS

## CASE HISTORY

A 26-year-old Caucasian female is presented to the emergency department with a chief complaint of right upper quadrant pain, associated with nausea and vomiting, after a night at the pizza parlor with her friends. She is obese with a body mass index (BMI) of 35 kg/m$^2$. Her vital signs are temperature 37.7°C, pulse rate 120 bpm, and score on pain scale is 9/10. On examination, there is tenderness in the right upper quadrant. Murphy sign cannot be elicited because of severe pain in that area. After conducting a complete blood count (CBC), white blood cell (WBC) count is 12,000/μL with no shift, serum lipase is within normal limits and liver enzymes are slightly elevated. A gallbladder ultrasound done by the doctor, which is shown in Figure 1, shows two gallstones and thickening of the wall to the gallbladder. Upon seeing the ultrasound image, the nurse exclaimed, "That's where I left my marbles!"

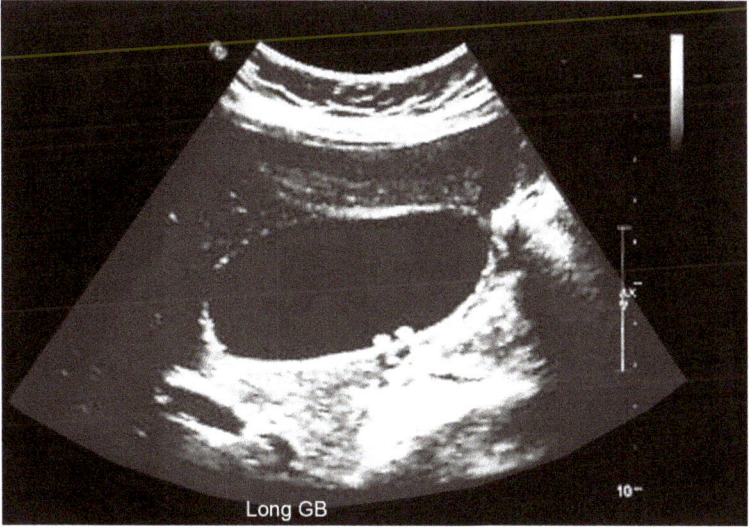

**Fig. 1:** Bedside ultrasound in the ER done by the author showing gallstones.

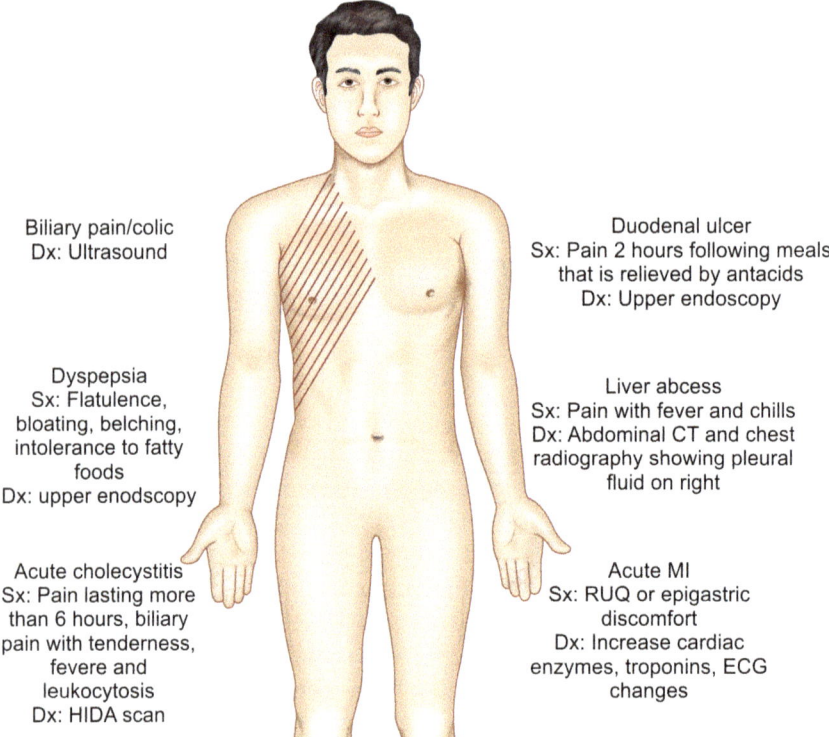

**Fig. 2:** Differential diagnosis of acute cholecystitis (by symptoms and diagnostic tests).
*Source:* Modified from Diverticular disease. In: Gastrointestinal emergencies. 2nd ed. Blackwell Publishing Ltd; 2009.

## DIFFERENTIAL DIAGNOSES

Differential diagnoses of cholecystitis are shown in Figure 2.

## DIAGNOSIS AND TREATMENT

Patients who develop symptoms/complications related to gallstones (biliary colic, acute cholecystitis, cholangitis, and/or pancreatitis), definitive therapy (cholecystectomy, cholecystostomy, endoscopic sphincterotomy, medical gallstone dissolution) is recommended.[1] Watchful waiting is the best treatment option for most patients with asymptomatic gallstones. Patients with cholecystitis should have a laparoscopic cholecystectomy in the early course of treatment. According to Bellows et al.,[2] gallstone pancreatitis requires a laparoscopic cholecystectomy (Fig. 3).[2] Oral dissolution therapy is appropriate for those who are not fit for surgery [elderly, at risk, heart conditions, past medical history (PMH) including stroke]. Selection criteria are based on three main characteristics: age of patient, condition of gallbladder, and characteristics of the stone.[3]

Abdomen

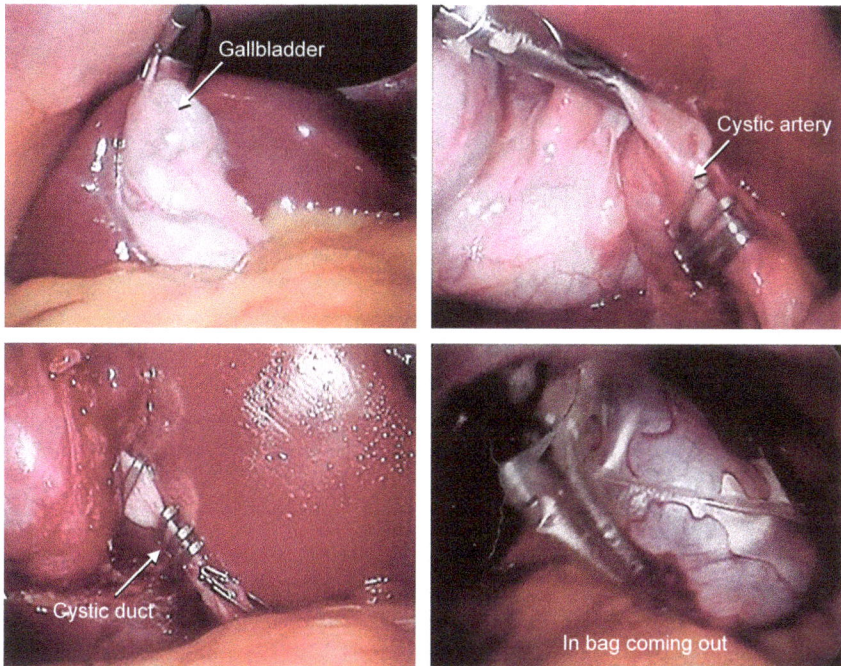

**Fig. 3:** Laparoscopic cholecystectomy.
*Source:* By User:Pschemp–User:Pschemp, CC BY-SA 3.0, https://commons.wikimedia.org/w/index.php?curid=1192663

## REFERENCES

1. https://www.uptodate.com/contents/treatment-of-acute-calculous-cholecystitis#H1053804.
2. Bellows C, Berger D, Crass R. Management of gallstones. Am Fam Physician. 2005;72(4):637-42.
3. Konikoff FM. Gallstones—approach to medical management. Med Gen Med. 2003;5(4). http://www.medscape.com/view article/460309.

# CHAPTER 4

# Pelvic and Urogenital

## CASE STUDY 33: TESTICULAR TORSION

### CASE HISTORY

Patient is a 14-year-old male who is presented to emergency department (ED) with a chief complaint of pain in the right testis since yesterday which continues to worsen. The patient is now experiencing difficulty in walking. He reports that he had similar pain in the past, but this time, it is more severe. He denies any history of trauma but states that he was exercising strenuously in the gym a few nights ago. Patient denies fever and history of sexually transmitted infections (STIs). His vital signs are temperature 97.4°F, pulse rate 90 bpm, blood pressure 100/62 mm Hg, and pulse oximetry 98% on room air. Physical examination reveals an enlarged, erythematous, edematous, and extremely tender scrotum on the right side. The cremasteric reflex is absent. Doppler ultrasound is ordered immediately, and it reveals swelling and lack of flow. Radionuclide testicular scan with technetium-99 pertechnetate (also known as Tc-99m) demonstrates decreased vascularity, venous thrombosis, and tissue edema. Patient has a presumed testicular torsion, and an immediate urologic consultation is obtained for definitive management.[1]

### DISCUSSION

Each year, testicular torsion affects 1 in 4,000 males younger than 25 years. All prepubertal and young adult males with acute scrotal pain should be considered to have testicular torsion until proven otherwise.

Based on the presentation, the patient likely has a testicular torsion. Given the presence of right testicular pain, several other diagnostic considerations may be made, but torsion is a "do not miss" diagnosis because over time, the testis will no longer be viable due to a disruption in blood flow.[2] The differential includes epididymo-orchitis, incarcerated inguinal hernia, hematoma either traumatic or idiopathic, acute hydrocele, testicular tumor, epididymitis, orchitis, spermatocele, hydrocele, varicocele, or torsion of the appendix testis.

Testicular torsion is defined as twisting of testis and spermatic cord causing acute ischemia (Fig. 1). The most common anomaly is high insertion of tunica vaginalis on the spermatic cord causing increased testicular motility bilateral in 80% of patients (Flowchart 1). Presentation includes pain, swelling, and absence of cremasteric reflex.[3] Absence of ipsilateral cremasteric reflex is the most accurate sign of testicular torsion. Blue dot sign (a tender nodule with blue discoloration located at the upper pole of the testis) may also be seen and used for diagnosis. One testis may appear less descended than the other (Fig. 1) Ultrasound with Doppler flow may confirm diagnosis (Fig. 2).

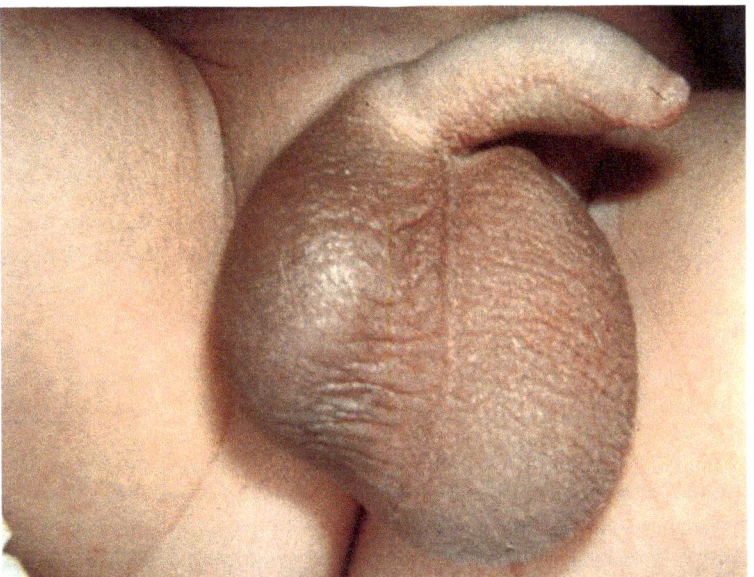

**Fig. 1:** Torsion of testicle—one testis is appearing less descended than the other.
*Source:* http://www.sciencephoto.com/media/146577/view.

**Flowchart 1:** Types of testicular torsion.

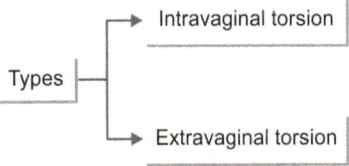

*Courtesy:* Badar M Zaheer, MD, Chicago, IL USA.

Testicular torsion is a true urologic emergency (Flowchart 2). If the physical examination is imperfect or inconclusive, quick imaging studies like ultrasonography and nuclear scans are very useful when the testicular torsion has to be ruled out or ruled in.

## TREATMENT

Very early urology consult is mandatory for detorsion and orchipexy or possible orchiectomy. If urology consult in the ER is unavailable, a quick transfer to urologists with sufficient analgesic medication (Figs. 3 and 4).

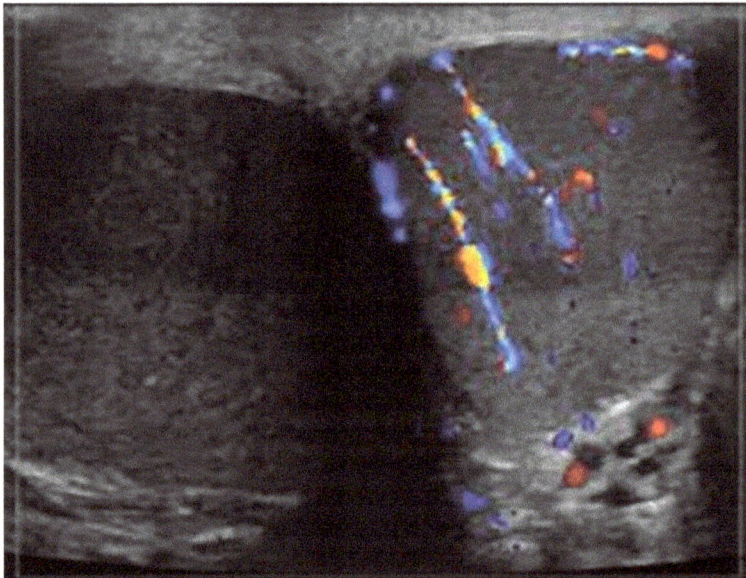

**Fig. 2:** Ultrasound with Doppler flow showing testicular torsion.
*Source:* 19-year-old male presented with acute onset right scrotal pain. (2016). In B. Khurana, J. Mandell, A. Sarma, & S. Ledbetter (Eds.), Emergency Radiology COFFEE Case Book: Case-Oriented Fast Focused Effective Education (pp. 204-210). Cambridge: Cambridge University Press. doi:10.1017/CBO9781139237185.030

**Flowchart 2:** Treatment of testicular torsion.

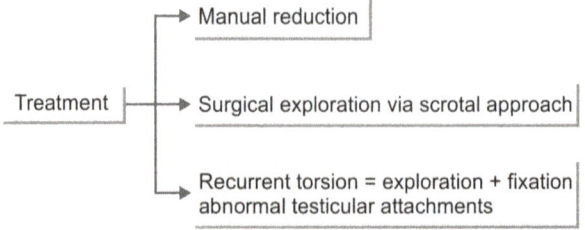

*Courtesy:* Badar M Zaheer, MD, Chicago, IL USA.

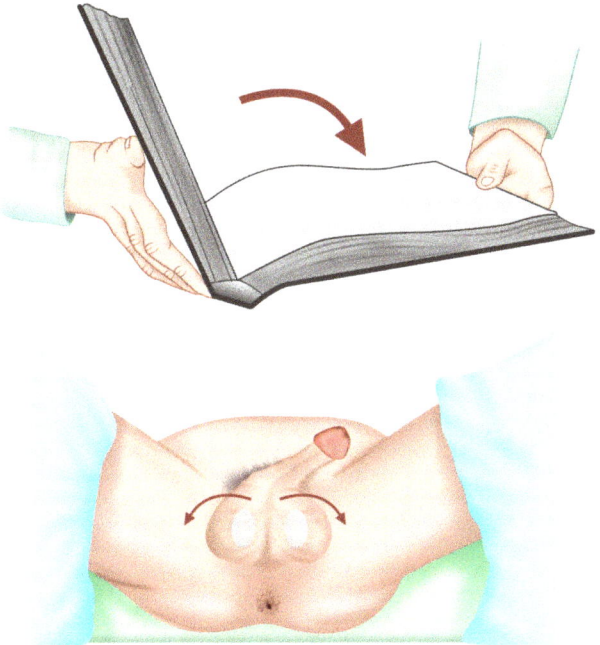

**Fig. 3:** Direction of rotation for testicular detorsion.
*Source:* https://www.barnardhealth.us/emergency-medicine/testes-and-epididymis.html.

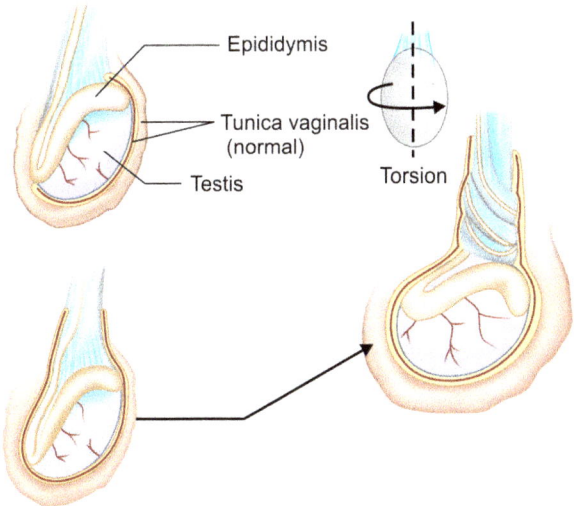

**Fig. 4:** Testicular detorsion.
*Source:* http://clinicalgate.com/urologic-procedures/.

## REFERENCES

1. Available from https://www.google.com/images/cleardot.gif.
2. Black TL. The 5 minute clinical consult. 20th ed. Phliadelphia, PA: Lippincott Williams and Wilkins; 2012. p. 1296
3. Ringdahl E, Teague L. Testicular torsion. Am Fam Physician. 2006;74(10):1739-43. Available from: http://www.aafp.org/afp/2006/1115/p1739/html.

# CHAPTER 5

# Musculoskeletal

## CASE STUDY 34: SEPTIC ARTHRITIS

### CASE HISTORY

A 40-year-old female is presented to the emergency department (ED) with left knee pain for the last 3 days. Patient noticed the pain when she woke up 3 days ago. Pain has been worsening since then. She is having difficulty in ambulating due to excruciating pain. She was having no fever at home. No history of sexually transmitted infections is present. No history of gout or arthritis is there. Patient is afebrile with unremarkable vitals. Physical examination reveals a tender, erythematous, warm joint on the left knee. Ambulation is extremely limited due to pain. Due to concern for septic arthritis, the joint is tapped. Results of the tap include approximately 5 cm$^3$ of yellow-green fluid. White blood cell (WBC) count is >100,000/µL with initial gram stain inconclusive. Fluid is sent for culture, and blood cultures are also drawn at this time. Intravenous (IV) antibiotics are started. Orthopedic consult is obtained for possible arthroscopy.

### DISCUSSION

Septic arthritis is a form of infectious arthritis in which various microorganisms invade the joint.[1] Risk increases with prosthetic joints as well as rheumatoid arthritis (RA) and *systemic lupus erythematosus* (SLE). Classification is either gonococcal or nongonococcal. The most common pathogen is *Neisseria gonorrhoeae* among young, sexually active individuals. However, overall the most common cause is *Staphylococcus aureus*. The knee is the most commonly involved joint.

Septic arthritis is a medical emergency because bacterial invasion can lead to destruction of the joint (Fig. 1).[2] The destruction results from initial damage to articular cartilage. The pathophysiology starts with destruction, followed by pannus formation and subsequently cartilage erosion. Severe damage may

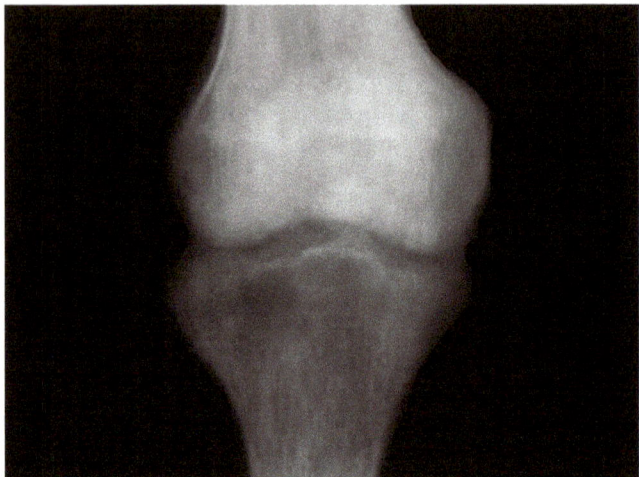

**Fig. 1:** X-ray shows septic arthritis.[2]
*Source:* http://emedicine.medscape.com/article/395381-overview.

occur in a little as 3 days. Morbidity from dysfunction of the joint can manifest as decreased range of motion or chronic pain. Other complications include dysfunctional joints, osteomyelitis, and sepsis. Prognostic signs for poor outcomes include age >60 years, infection in hip or shoulder joints, underlying RA, positive synovial fluid cultures after 7 days of appropriate antibiotics, and delay of 7 days in starting therapy. Mortality rate is low for *N. gonorrhoeae* but may be as high as 50% in cases where *S. aureus* is the causative agent.

History should determine acute onset of joint pain, or superimposed acute on chronic symptoms, history of trauma, which joints are involved, presence of extra-articular symptoms, and use of IV drugs. Patients should be questioned regarding exposure to sexually transmitted infections, exposure to ticks, and immunocompromised risk factors. Physical examination should assess for signs of erythema, swelling, warmth, and tenderness. Effusions are generally present when the joint is infected. Assess active and passive range of motion which will usually be markedly limited. Differential includes Lyme disease, prosthetic joint infection as well as reactive and tuberculous arthritis.

Synovial fluid should be obtained in all suspect cases. Even patients with a history of gout warrant synovial fluid analysis. Septic joints will generally have a lack of crystals, pus like synovial fluid, Gram's stain may be positive, WBC will exceed 50,000/μL with the majority of polymorphonuclear leukocytes. Polymerase chain reaction (PCR) may further assess for specific viral or bacterial causes. PCR is especially helpful in the setting of patients who have recently been given antibiotics that would otherwise influence the culture. Blood cultures should also be obtained to look for bacteremic origin, like swabbing, rectum, cervix, urethra, or pharynx of confirm possible gonococcal infection X-ray may assess for osteomyelitis. Ultrasound may confirm effusions in distorted joints.

## DIAGNOSTIC CRITERIA[3] (FIGS. 2 AND 3)

- General variables
  - Fever (>38.3°C)
  - Hypothermia (core temperature <36°C)
  - Heart rate >90/min or more than two SD above the normal value for age
  - Tachypnea
  - Altered mental status
  - Significant edema or positive fluid balance (>20 mL/kg over 24 h)
  - Hyperglycemia (plasma glucose >140 mg/dL or 7.7 mmol/L) in the absence of diabetes.
- Inflammatory variables
  - Leukocytosis (WBC count >12,000/µL)
  - Leukopenia (WBC count <4,000/µL)
  - Normal WBC count with >10% immature forms
  - Plasma C-reactive protein more than two SD above the normal value
  - Serum lactate >2 mmol/L (>18 mg/dL)
  - Plasma procalcitonin more than two SD above the normal value (more sensitive marker).
- Hemodynamic variables
  - Arterial hypotension (SBP <90 mm Hg, MAP <70 mm Hg, or an SBP decrease >40 mm Hg in adults or less than two SD below normal for age).

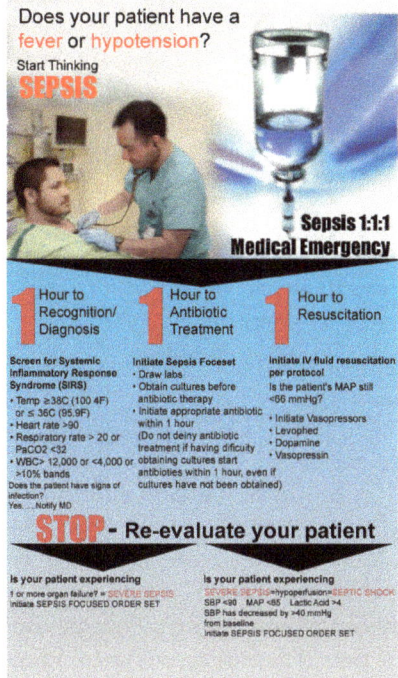

**Fig. 2:** Think SERIOUSLY of SEPSIS if your patient has fever/hypotension or both.
*Source:* OSF St. Francis Medical Center in Peoria, Illinois.

> **Surviving Sepsis**
>
> **SEPSIS** is an infection causing a systemic inflammatory repsonse (SIRS). SIRS can also be due to trauma, inflammation, or ischemia. But think **SEPSIS** and assess and respond!
>
> Patient presents with 2 or more of the following criteria:
> - Temp >100.4 or <96.8
> - HR >90
> - Respiratory rate >20 or ↑ $O_2$ requirements
> - SBC <90 after 30 cc/kg fluid bolus or lactate >4
> - WBC >12,000 or <4000 or bandemia
> - Blood glucose >140 in non-diabetic patients
>
> **CONSIDER SEPSIS**
> - Insert 2 large bore needle IVs 18 g or larger
> - Fluid bolus 2L.9NaCl with MD order RAPIDLY
> - Will need CBC, CMP, Lactate, PT/PTT, ABG, blood cultures × 2
> - After blood cultures drawn start broad spectrum antibiotic within 1 hour of screening positive for sepsis
> - CXR and EKG
> - Place Foley; send UA and culture; maintain accurate I & O
> - Cardiac monitor, frequent vitals, 5–15 minutes
> - May need vasopressor therapy: Norepinephrine 5–20 mcg/min IV

**Fig. 3:** Diagnostic management of sepsis.

- Organ dysfunction variables
  - Arterial hypoxemia ($PaO_2/FiO_2$ <300)
  - Acute oliguria (urine output <0.5 mL/kg/h for ≥2 h despite adequate fluid resuscitation)
  - Creatinine increase >0.5 mg/dL or 44.2 μmol/L
  - Coagulation abnormalities (INR >1.5 or a PTT >60 s)
  - Ileus (absent bowel sounds)
  - Thrombocytopenia (platelet count <100,000/μL)
  - Hyperbilirubinemia (plasma total bilirubin >4 mg/dL or 70 μmol/L).
- Tissue perfusion variables
  - Hyperlactatemia (>1 mmol/L)
  - Decreased capillary refill or mottling.

## TREATMENT

Treatment should include admission, pain control, consultation, and antibiotic therapy. Length of antibiotic course depends on the pathogen. In general, ≥2 weeks will be required. Some cases with complications, such as osteomyelitis, will require PORT-A-CATH placement and several months of antibiotics. Start empirically and tailor to both the hospital resistance patterns and the cultures. Consider starting with a combination of penicillin and gentamicin or a later generation cephalosporin (Fig. 4).

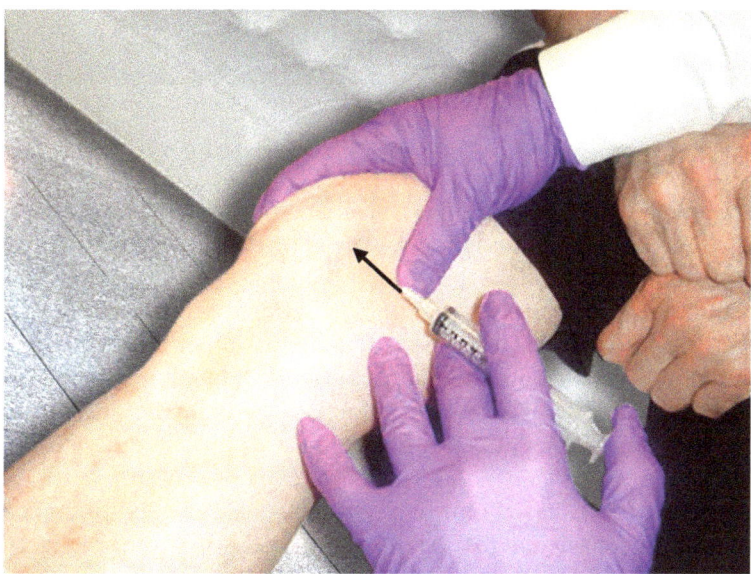

**Fig. 4:** Aspiration of keen joint for synovial fluid analysis.
*Source:* http://reference.medscape.com/features/slideshow/arthro-practice.

## PITFALLS OF MISSING SEPSIS

All patients with the signs and symptoms of sepsis as well as those who meet systemic inflammatory response syndrome (SIRS) criteria for sepsis are at a big risk for mismanagement or misdiagnosis for a potential lawsuit. Patients in sepsis are at an increased risk for mortality and morbidity as a result of organ hypoperfusion and failure.

All patients with a presentation of monoarticular joint pain should be assumed to have septic arthritis, until proven otherwise. Severe medical malpractice may result from a missed case. This is due to delays in treatment that can result in severe morbidity as well as mortality. Long-term disability is a strong motivator for taking legal action. Consider a young man with a missed diagnosis, the misery and long-term disability after knee surgery. Regardless of why the diagnosis was missed, the patient required a skin graft, and eventual above the knee amputation. This story emphasizes why it is always important to consider this diagnosis.

## REFERENCES

1. Brusch JL. Septic arthritis. Available from http://emedicine.medscape.com/article/236299-overview.
2. http://emedicine.medscape.com/article/1268369-overview.

## CASE STUDY 35: ACROMIOCLAVICULAR JOINT SEPARATION

### ACROMIOCLAVICULAR JOINT INJURIES

A 23-year-old man is presented to the emergency room with shoulder pain after falling on his left shoulder (Fig. 1). On physical examination, his vital signs are temperature 98.5°F, pulse rate 84 bpm, respiratory rate 16 breaths/min, and blood pressure 120/80 mm Hg. Examination shows tenderness of the left lateral clavicular area. He is unable to abduct his shoulder, internal rotation is restricted and painful, but he can touch his right shoulder with his left hand. Radial and brachial pulses are palpable, and there is no evidence of neurovascular compromise. X-ray of the shoulder is shown in Figure 2.

The diagnosis is based on the physical examination and findings of an X-ray of acromioclavicular (AC) joint separation due to a torn coracoclavicular ligament.

### FEATURES OF ACROMIOCLAVICULAR JOINT INJURIES

Acromioclavicular joint injuries are classified as type 1, type 2, or type 3 based on the severity of the injury and the X-ray findings (Flowchart 1). Type 1 injury is a strain or partial tear, which will have normal X-ray findings. Type 2 injuries

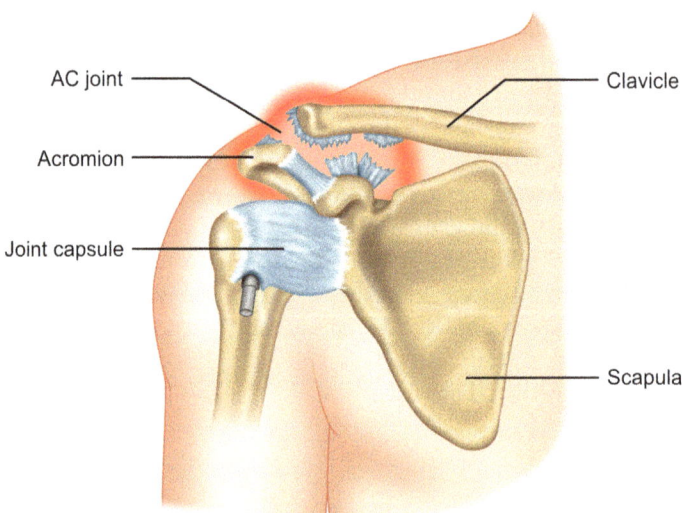

**Fig. 1:** Anatomy of acromioclavicular joint.

Musculoskeletal

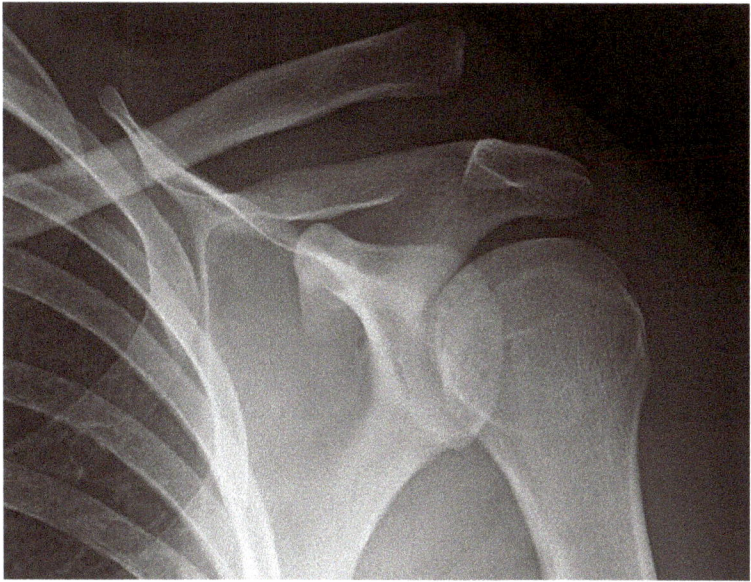

**Fig. 2:** X-ray of the shoulder showing acromioclavicular joint separation.

**Flowchart 1:** Acromioclavicular (AC) joint separation types.

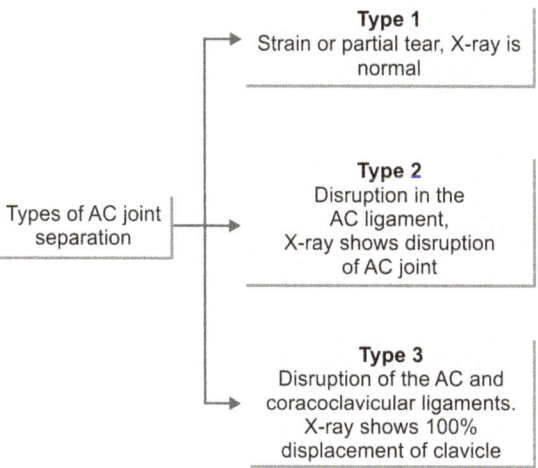

result in a disruption in the AC ligament. If X-ray shows 25–50% elevation of the clavicle above the acromial process, then types 1 and 2 will have a widening of the coracoclavicular space between 1.1 and 1.3 mm. Type 3 injuries are associated with a complete disruption of the AC and coracoclavicular ligaments and are identified on X-ray by a 100% superior displacement of the clavicle and a widening of the coracoclavicular space of >5 mm.

## TREATMENT

Treatment of type 1 and 2 injuries is done conservatively with rest, ice, analgesics, and arm immobilization with a sling for 1–3 weeks. Range of motion and strengthening exercises are started once the patient gets better and is pain free. For type 3 injuries, treatment approach is controversial. Many prefer conservative treatments similar to that of types 1 and 2, although some physicians opt for surgical repair. More severe injuries are managed surgically.

## CASE STUDY 36: GLENOHUMERAL JOINT DISLOCATION

### CASE HISTORY

A 19-year-old baseball player is presented to the emergency department complaining of right shoulder pain. The injury occurred during a baseball game when he slid headfirst into second base with his arms outstretched.

On physical examination, his vital signs are stable with a temperature of 98.7°F, pulse rate 74 bpm, respiratory rate 16 breaths/min, and blood pressure 116/70 mm Hg. He holds his arm in a slightly flexed position, supported by the left hand. The shoulder has a "squared off" appearance and he complains of severe pain on examination. He refuses to move the extremity. X-ray of the shoulder is shown in Figure 1.

### CLINICAL FEATURES

Glenohumeral joint dislocation is the most common type of joint dislocation (Flowchart 1). About 95–97% of these injuries are anterior dislocations caused by indirect force on the joint capsule with the arm abducted, extended, and externally rotated. The patient is presented with severe pain and holds the joint in a slightly abducted and externally rotated position, supported by the other arm. On visual inspection, the shoulder appears "squared off" and shortened. The most common complication is axillary nerve injury. Function can be assessed by pinprick sensation over the skin of the lateral shoulder.

### DIAGNOSIS

Diagnosis is made by physical examination combined with anteroposterior (AP) and lateral scapular "Y" or axillary X-ray views. The X-ray can also often identify concomitant fractures, although these require no additional treatment. Common associated injuries include compression fractures of the

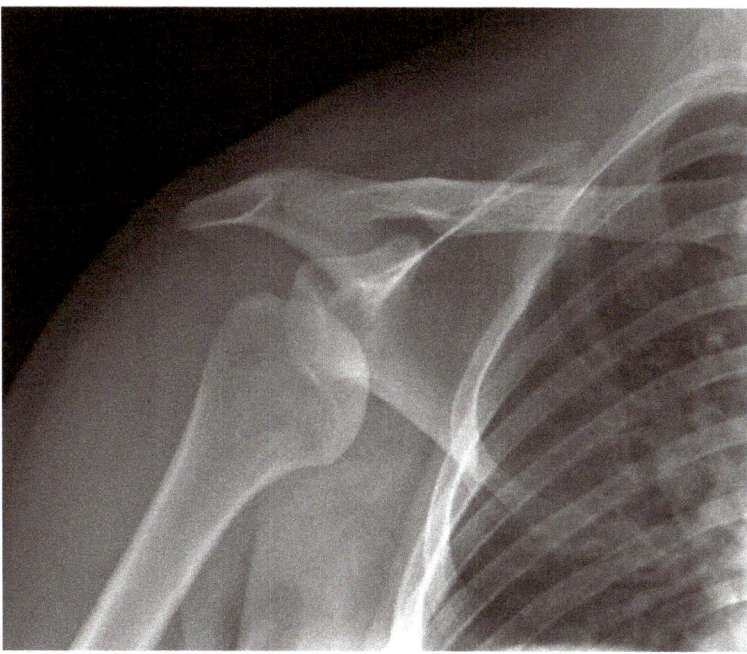

**Fig. 1:** Shoulder X-ray.
*Courtesy:* Badar M Zaheer, MD, Chicago, USA.

**Flowchart 1:** Types of shoulder dislocation.

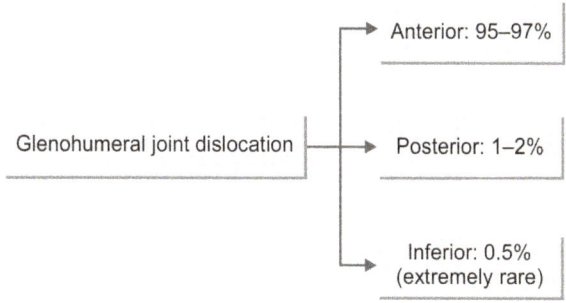

*Courtesy:* Badar M Zaheer, MD.

humeral head, anterior glenoid rim fractures, greater tuberosity avulsion fracture, and rotator cuff tears.

## TREATMENT

Anterior glenohumeral joint dislocations are treated with reduction followed by immobilization of the joint. There are a number of techniques that can be used to reduce the dislocation, the most common of which is the modified Hippocratic technique (Fig. 2).

Closed reduction with intravenous (IV) sedation and muscle relaxation.
1. Modified Hippocratic technique.
2. *Stimson technique*: While patient lies prone with arm hanging over the edge of the table, hang a 5-lb weight on wrist for 15–20 min applied.
3. *Traction–counter-traction technique*: An assistant stabilizes the torso with a folded sheet wrapped around the patient's chest while the physician applies gentle steady traction (Fig. 3).

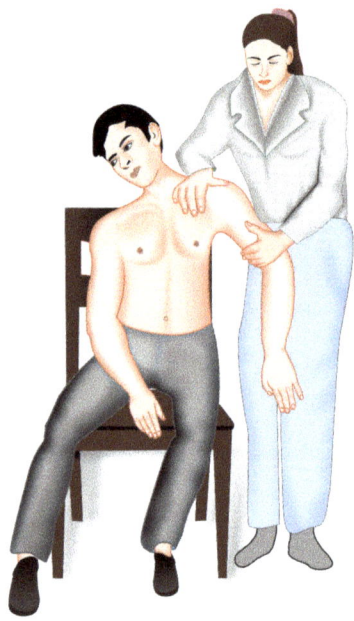

**Fig. 2:** Patient's treatment with Hippocratic technique.

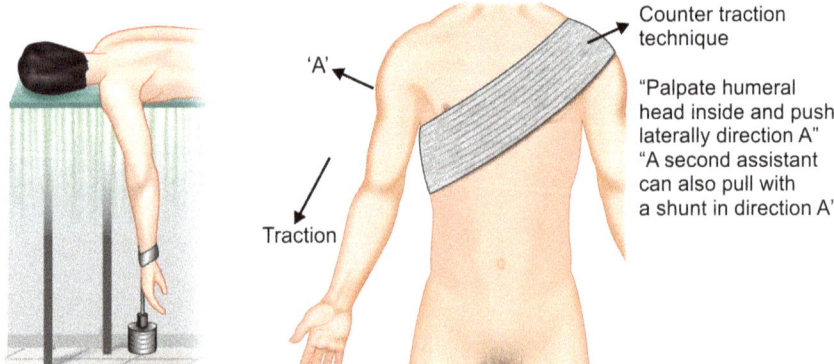

**Fig. 3:** Reduction of anterior dislocation. Traction and counter-traction technique. Assistant stabilizes the torso with a folded sheet wrapped across the chest while the physicians apply gentle steady traction.

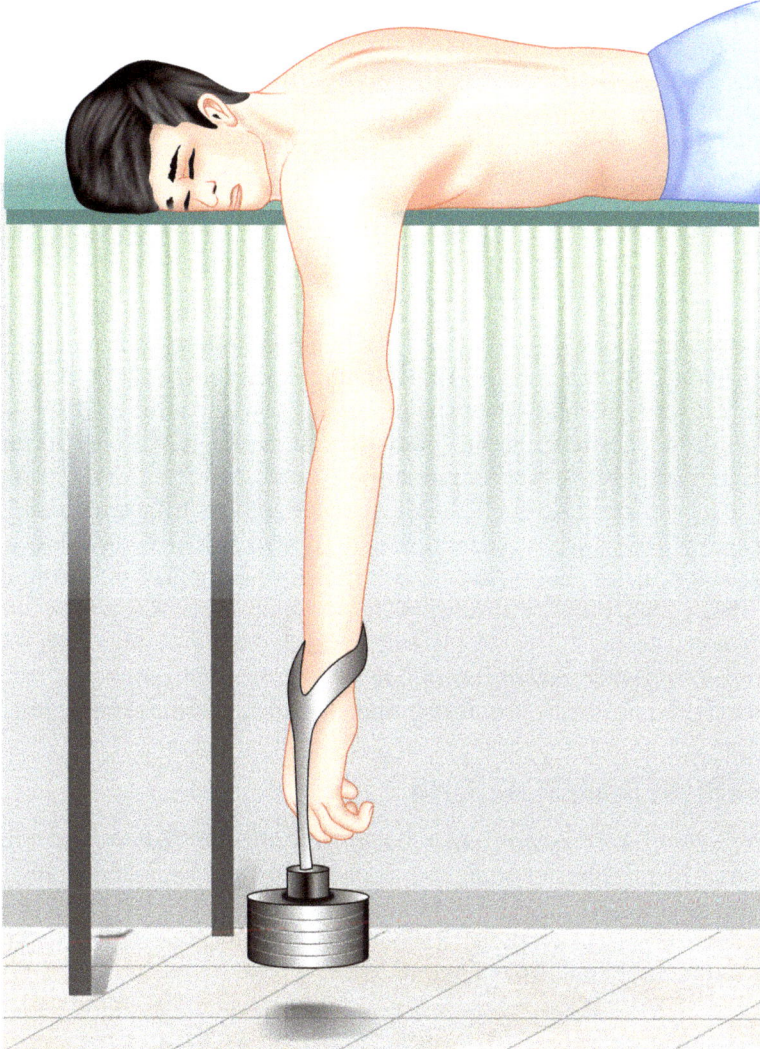

**Fig. 4:** Patient's treatment with Stimson's technique.
*Source:* Available online from http://www.eorthopod.com/sites/default/files/images/shoulder_dislocation_treatment01.jpg.

Obtain postreduction X-rays and check for neurovascular status. Put shoulder in sling for 3 weeks followed by physical therapy. Immediate orthopedic referral for failed/unstable closed reductions.

## Other Common Treatment Techniques

In the Stimson's technique, the patient is placed prone on a gurney with the dislocated shoulder hanging off the side. A 10-lb weight is hung off the wrist (Fig. 4) If muscle relaxation is obtained, reduction can occur in 30 min.

Aronen technique is used for recurrent dislocations. This technique is useful because it can be taught to the patients for self-reduction of an injury. In this method, the patient is seated on a gurney with the ipsilateral leg and knee in flexion. The patient is then told to clasp his hands behind the knee and relax the shoulder muscles. Countertraction is applied by the patient's own body weight and his own paraspinous muscles. Taping the patient's hands together can help reduction.

## POSTERIOR DISLOCATIONS

These account for approximately 1–2% of glenohumeral dislocations. They occur with convulsive seizures, direct trauma to the anterior shoulder, or falls on an outstretched arm. The patient presents with the arms held across the chest in adduction and internal rotation. On active range of motion examination, abduction is severely compromised and external rotation is completely blocked. On inspection, the anterior shoulder appears flat with a prominent coracoid process and the posterior aspect appears full. AP X-ray shows a loss of the elliptical half-moon-shaped overlap seen on normal films. The humeral head has a "light bulb" or "drumstick" appearance. The diagnosis can be confirmed with scapular Y-view of lateral views. Reduction is done on a supine patient by applying axial traction along the long axis of the humerus, anterior directed pressure on the posterior humeral head, and some external rotation.

## INFERIOR DISLOCATIONS

These injuries are very rare and make up only about 0.5% of shoulder dislocations. The mechanism of injury is usually a forceful hyperabduction or an inferior directed axial load on the abducted shoulder. The patient will present with the arm-locked overhead. Reduction is completed with an upward and outward force in line with the humerus.

## FURTHER READING

1. Cutts S, Prempeh M, Drew S. Anterior shoulder dislocation. Ann R Coll Surg Engl. 2009;91:2-7.

## CASE STUDY 37: LOW-BACK PAIN

## CASE HISTORY

A 52-year-old male presents with low back pain of 4 months. Patient reports that he has had low-back pain problems for "years," but over the last 4 months, it has been worsening and now includes left-sided weakness. It is now to the point where the patient is having difficulty staying still for any amount of time; only standing in certain positions alleviates the pain. Patient has been taking over-the-counter (OTC) nonsteroidal anti-inflammatory drug (NSAIDs) without relief. He occasionally has shooting and tingling pain down to his foot. He decided to come in today because he just cannot take the pain anymore. He has a 54-pack-year history of smoking, drinks 6-12 beers per day, and denies use of recreational drugs. Patient is afebrile and normotensive. On physical examination, he does not have spinal tenderness but is positive for paraspinal tenderness. Cranial nerves are intact. Strength is 5/5 in upper extremity flexors and extensors, but it is difficult to assess strength in the lower extremities due to pain. He has a loss of muscle bulk in the left anterior thigh. The sensation to pinprick is intact throughout. Reflexes are symmetrical. He has no cerebellar signs. Gait is difficult to assess due to pain. Straight leg raise test is positive on the left. Toes are downgoing. Rectal tone is intact. What should be taken into consideration when deciding if this patient should have imaging? What should be done and how quickly?

## Should Imaging be Done for this Patient?
- Usually conservative management for the first 4-6 weeks is sufficient
- *Acute concerns*: Epidural abscess, epidural compression syndrome, malignancy, spinal stenosis, and back pain in children. Always think of *abdominal aortic aneurysm* (AAA) in hypotensive and elderly patients.

## Indications for Plain Films
- Patient's age should be <18 or >50 years
- Any history of malignancy or unexplained weight loss
- Any history of fever, immunocompromised status, or intravenous (IV) drug use
- Recent trauma other than simple lifting
- Progressive neurologic deficits or other findings consistent with cauda equina syndrome
- Prolonged duration of symptoms beyond 4-6 weeks.
  Additional views are given if spondylolysis or spondylolisthesis suspected.

## Look for Red Flag Signs
### History
Patient should be in age group of under 18 years or over 50 years, with pain lasting for >6 weeks, history of cardiac arrest, fevers or/chills, night sweats or unexplained weight loss, recurrent bacterial infection, unremitting pain, night pain, IV drug users, major trauma, and minor trauma in the elderly patients.

*Physical Examination*

Below mentioned points should be checked during physical examination: fever, writhing in pain, bowel or bladder incontinence, saddle anesthesia, decreased or absent anal sphincter tone, perianal sensory loss, severe or progressive neurological defect, and major motor weakness.

*Computed Tomography versus Magnetic Resonance Imaging*

Computed tomography (CT) scan is done for evaluating the spinal canal and risk for impingement. For cauda equina, spinal infection, and malignancy, magnetic resonance imaging (MRI) scan is useful. MRI has to be emergently done if neurologic findings are acute or progressive.

**If you have clinical suspicion for any compromise of the spinal canal and spinal cord, it is indicated to consult a neurosurgeon and order an MRI without delay.**

## FOLLOW-UP CASE OUTCOME

Given patient's age, recent weight loss, and history of smoking, a lumbosacral X-ray was ordered but found to be inconclusive. CT scan of lumbosacral spine was ordered and showed evidence of multiple areas of disk bulging, but no fractures or signs of metastasis. Given history of acute and chronic weakness, emergent MRI was considered. However, the patient was reassessed after receiving pain medication, and it was determined that he did not have weakness on physical examination. Patient was instructed to follow-up with an MRI as an outpatient, as well as with neurosurgery for further evaluation.[1]

## ASSESSMENT OF BACK PAIN

It is important to do a thorough neurovascular examination including deep tendon reflexes, sensation, and muscle strength. It is also important to assess peripheral pulses and palpate the abdomen for masses or organomegaly. Lower extremities should also be assessed for flexibility and the spine should be examined for posture, stance, gait, and straight leg raise.

## MANAGEMENT

Non-surgical management is focused on pain control, bracing, and rehabilitation. This usually requires extensive inpatient physical therapy, occupational therapy, and recreational therapy.[2,3] Never miss a spinal epidural abscess for it can lead to a devastating and irreversible outcome. Always keep this diagnosis in mind for every backache complaint.

## PITFALLS OF MISDIAGNOSING LOWER-BACK PAIN

Although most cases of lower back pain are musculoskeletal in origin, keep in mind that serious syndromes that require immediate neurosurgical consult to avoid disability and medicolegal issues such cauda equina can present with initial symptoms, such as lower back pain. Therefore, a thorough history and physical exam is vital. Look for classic.

## REFERENCES

1. Marx JA. Rosen's emergency medicine: concepts and clinical practices. Mosby Elsevier; 7th ed. (2010); 2010. ISBN-10: 9996073521. Headquarters for the publishing company are located in Maryland Heights, Missouri.
2. Corwell BN. The emergency department evaluation, management, and treatment of back pain. Emerg Med Clin North Am 2010;28(4):811-39.
3. Sherman AL. Lumbar compression fracture treatment & management. [Online]. Available from http//emedicine.medscape.com/article/309615 treatment; 2012 [accessed July, 2012].

## CASE STUDY 38: HEADACHE

*"Holding on to anger, resentment and hurt only gives you tense muscles, a headache and a sore jaw from clenching your teeth. Forgiveness gives you back the laughter and the lightness in your life."*

—**John Lunden**

## CASE HISTORY

Patient is a 46-year-old female who presents with headache of 4 days. Patient states that she woke up in the morning with a headache 4 days ago. Since then the headache has been waxing and waning but has never been completely resolved. She has never had headaches in the past and describes this headache as the worst of her life. Ibuprofen which she also takes for her osteoarthritis has not been alleviating her pain. For the past week, the patient has generally been feeling unwell without specific symptoms. She does have associated photophobia and nausea but no vomiting. The patient states that her neck is stiff although she has full neck range of motion (ROM). She has no fevers or chills. No intravenous (IV) drug use, no history of immunocompromise, no loss of consciousness (LOC), no head trauma, and no numbness, tingling, or weakness were observed. Past history includes hypertension, diabetes type 2, and osteoarthritis for which the patient takes metformin, lisinopril, *hydrochlorothiazide* (HCTZ), and ibuprofen. Surgical history includes tubal ligation and family history of diabetes. Socially, the patient does not smoke, drink, or use other drugs. At baseline, the patient has difficulty getting around her house.

On physical examination, patient had temperature 36.8°C, blood pressure 160/94 mm Hg, pulse rate 76 bpm, respiratory rate 20 breaths/min, and oxygen ($O_2$) saturation 96%. Head, eyes, ears, nose, and throat (HEENT) and neck examination were significant for photophobia, but negative for meningeal signs and sinus tenderness. Neurologically, the patient did not have any deficits. Cranial nerves II–XII are intact. Strength is 5/5 in upper and lower extremity flexors and extensors. Sensation is intact to pinprick throughout. Reflexes are 2+ throughout. No cerebellar signs were noticed. She has normal gait.

## DISCUSSION

Differential for this patient includes migraine headache, *subarachnoid hemorrhage* (SAH), and viral meningitis. Patient has nausea and photophobia consistent with migraine, but no history of migraines in the past. The positive sudden severe onset warrants consideration of SAH. Viral meningitis is a possibility because the patient had generally been feeling unwell in addition to some subjective neck stiffness but did not have any fevers or toxic appearance that would suggest a bacterial meningitis. Computed tomography (CT) and lumbar puncture (LP) were done in a given time frame where CT scan would have a decreased sensitivity. CT scan was unremarkable. *Cerebral spinal fluid* (CSF) analysis is clear in appearance. Opening pressure was 24 cm $H_2O$. High lymphocyte count with elevated protein and normal glucose and clearing of red blood cells (RBCs) from tube 1 to tube 4. Patient was transferred to a university hospital for further treatment and specialty case.

### Headache

The initial differential is aimed at determining whether the cause of the headache is primary or secondary. Primary causes include migraine, tension-type headaches, cluster headache, chronic paroxysmal hemicrania, miscellaneous headaches unassociated with structural lesion (idiopathic stabbing, external compression, cold stimulus, benign cough, benign exertional, associated with sexual activity). Secondary causes include head trauma, vascular disorders [*cerebrovascular accident* (CVA), *arteriovenous malformation* (AVM), *cerebral venous thrombosis* (CVT), and SAH], nonvascular intracranial disorder (neoplasm), substance use or withdrawal, infection, metabolic disorders, craniofacial disorder (including cranium, neck, sinuses, etc.), and neuralgias.

Although the majority of headaches can be benign, always think about the possibility of a headache being the first presentation of a life threatening pathology, such as subarachnoid hemorrhage or brain tumor. If you have a patient with clinically suspicious signs and symptoms of a bleed or tumor, order a magnetic resonance imaging (MRI) or CT head.

Several clinical pearls can be used to determine a likely cause of the headache (Table 1).

**Table 1:** Findings and considerations of several clinical pearls.

| Finding | Consideration |
|---|---|
| Thunderclap headache | SAH |
| Worst headache | SAH, CVT |
| Use of space heater, gas leak, pets dying in household* | Carbon monoxide |
| Pregnancy | Eclampsia, CVT |
| Change in vision | Glaucoma, optic neuritis |
| Pain with eye movement | Optic neuritis |
| Fever | Infection (CNS vs systemic) |
| Double vision | Intracranial mass, idiopathic intracranial hypertension |
| Ptosis, miosis | Carotid artery dissection |
| Papilledema | Mass lesion, optic neuritis, pseudotumor |
| Dilated pupil | Aneurysm compressing third nerve |
| Age over 50 years | Temporal arteritis, mass lesion, glaucoma |

SAH: subarachnoid hemorrhage; CVT: cerebral venous thrombosis.
*This clinical pearl refers to the famous case of an elderly woman who left her gas on and presented with a headache with the incidental finding that her pet cat had just died unexpectedly.

# PEARLS

Studies show that onset/severity may be the most predictive of a SAH, meaning headaches that initiate suddenly with excruciating pain. According to Godwin and Villa,[2] "In one prospective study, 70% of patients (35/49) presenting with a thunderclap headache has an SAH. Another study prospectively examined all patients presenting with severe headache of sudden onset with no past history of the same. Of 27 patients enrolled, nine had SAH, one had intraventricular hemorrhage, and two had meningitis."[1-3]

Several danger signals may be used to identify the high-risk headaches. Historical danger signals include sudden onset of headache (thunderclap), worst headache of life, headache dramatically different from past headaches, immunocompromise, new onset of headache after the age of 50 years, headache that begins with exertion. Danger of physical findings includes altered mental status, meningeal signs, positive "jolt" test, focal neurologic signs, rash suspicious for spotted fever, and meningococcemia. In 2008, American College of Emergency Physicians (ACEP) created guidelines to better help and determine what evidence was in the literature on the management of headaches. Based on their guidelines, level A is generally accepted with strong evidence. Level B has moderate clinical certainty. Level C has preliminary, inconclusive, or conflicting evidence.

The guidelines argue that there is very little evidence that response to therapy can be used to diagnose the etiology of a headache. There is level B evidence to suggest that patients requiring an emergent CT are those with a headache and new neurologic findings, those with a new sudden onset of severe headache, and *human immunodeficiency virus* (HIV) positive patients with a new headache. There are level C recommendations that patients over the age of 50 years without Neurological findings may be able to have an urgent CT as an outpatient. Lumbar puncture is considered the gold standard for diagnosing SAH when xanthochromia is measured by spectrophotometry. CT and LP alone each has its limitations. CT often misses small bleeds or those disguised by bone. CT is unable to identify other etiologies. There is reader variability as well as decreased sensitivity in the setting of anemia and over time. LP can miss unruptured aneurysms, arterial dissections, CVT, or pituitary apoplexy. Some patients are difficult. One main advantage is the ability to measure the opening pressure. There is level B evidence that LP should be done even when CT is negative.

The data on when to perform a CT before LP is extremely limited by a lack of prospective randomized controlled trials (RCTs) so the recommendations are currently for level C. However, ACEP recommends CT first when there are signs of increased intracranial pressure (ICP). Finally, ACEP currently recommends with level B data that emergent angiography is not necessary when CT head and CSF analysis are negative. These patients may be discharged home with close follow-up.

## REFERENCES

1. Edlow JA, Panagos PD, Godwin SA, et al. Clinical policy: critical issues in the evaluation and management of adult patients presenting to the emergency department with acute headache. Ann Emerg Med. 2008;52(4):407-36.
2. Godwin SA, Villa J. Acute headache in the ED: Evidence-based evaluation and treatment options. Emerg Med Pract. 2001;3(6):1-32.
3. Sherman SC, Weber JM, editors. "Approach to headache" and "intracranial hemorrhage". For more information visit www.cdemcurriculum.org. Headache. In: USMLE road map: emergency medicine. 1st ed. New York: McGraw-Hill; 2007. p. 406-11.

## CASE STUDY 39: LUMBAR COMPRESSION FRACTURE

## CASE HISTORY

An 80-year-old female is presented to the emergency department with low back pain. The pain began suddenly when she bent over to pick up a book from the floor. On physical examination, she has vital signs of temperature 98.6°F, pulse rate 85 bpm, respiration rate 16 breaths/min, and blood pressure 140/80 mm Hg. She has point tenderness over the L5 vertebrae on palpation. Straight leg raise is negative bilaterally and neurovascular examination is intact. X-ray of the lumbar spine shows a compression fracture of the L5 vertebrae.

## DISCUSSION

The five lumbar vertebrae are very strong and therefore a fracture in one of these vertebrae is suggestive of severe trauma or pathology in the bone. Osteoporosis is a common cause of lumbar compression fractures in postmenopausal women, whereas violent trauma is the most common cause in younger patients.[1] In the absence of severe trauma, malignancy should be ruled out. Although mortality from these fractures is very rare, morbidity may be severe whether it is a complication from pain and bed rest or neurologic deficits.

The normal function of the lumbar spine is to provide stability and support while walking upright. Injuries will affect the lumbar curvature of the spine and subsequently the curvature of the thoracic and cervical spine. Fractures of the lumbar spine may cause significant disability whether it is through pain or the alterations of posture mechanics. Altering posture may cause secondary pain as well as increased risk for falls.

Different types of fractures may occur as a result of trauma. The Denis system of classification may be used to determine whether or not a fracture is stable. Wedge fractures generally result from malignancy or osteoporosis. These fractures are generally symmetric, but 8–14% of them are lateral wedge fractures. Lap belts in motor vehicles accidents (MVAs) may cause flexion and distraction forces, and therefore the posterior columns are injured. This most commonly occurs in children who remain neurologically intact. Finally, burst fractures can occur from axial loads to the spine. These are serious fractures that may lead to neurologic deficit.

In nontraumatic cases, the bone density is diminished to a point where minor accidents can cause a trauma. In this case, the fracture is generally wedge shaped and will increase kyphosis. In cases of malignancy, metastasis is usually the underlying cause. Other cases may include aneurysmal bone cysts, hemangiomas, and spinal infections resulting in osteomyelitis.

The typical presentation involves midline back pain that is axial, nonradiating, aching, or stabbing in quality. Signs or symptoms of neurologic injury should be elicited. Referred pain may also be present in ribs, hip, groin, or buttocks. Pain is not always present especially in cases involving osteoporosis. Neurological examination should include assessment of rectal tone. Spine curvature should be assessed and vertebrae should be palpated. Site of pain often correlates to the site of fracture. Hip flexor contractures should also be assessed. Differential diagnosis includes coccyx pain, lumbar degenerative disk disease, lumbar facet arthropathy, lumbar spondylolysis and spondylolisthesis, mechanical low back pain, and osteoporosis.

## WORKUP

Workup should include both blood tests and imaging. Blood tests should include complete blood count (CBC), prostate-specific antigen (PSA), and erythrocyte sedimentation rate (ESR). Urine may be tested for Bence Jones protein. Initially, plain films are the standard. Minimally anteroposterior and lateral views of the lumbar and thoracic spines should be obtained. If possible, lateral flexion and extension views with standing should be obtained to look for gross instability and burst fractures. CT scan may be further utilized to assess the severity of the fractures as well as rule out middle column and burst fractures that are not as easily seen on plain films. CT is also the best method for evaluations of fractures of posterior elements and laminae of the neural arch. When spinal cord injury is suspected, magnetic resonance imaging (MRI) must be done. MRI is also helpful for the evaluation of hemorrhage, tumor, and infection. Dual energy radiographic absorptiometry (DRA) and positron emission tomography (PET) scanning are also considering, but not likely to be done emergently.

## MANAGEMENT

Management may be either operative or nonoperative. Appropriate consults to either orthopedics and neurosurgery, or rheumatology should be made. Nonoperative patients require pain management, bracing, and physical therapy. One method of bracing is the thoracic–lumbar–sacral orthosis (TLSO). Physical therapy includes early mobilization and weight-bearing exercises. This usually begins on an inpatient basis and progresses to outpatient. Monitoring with plain films is required on a monthly basis to screen for fractures that worsen to the point where they require surgical intervention.

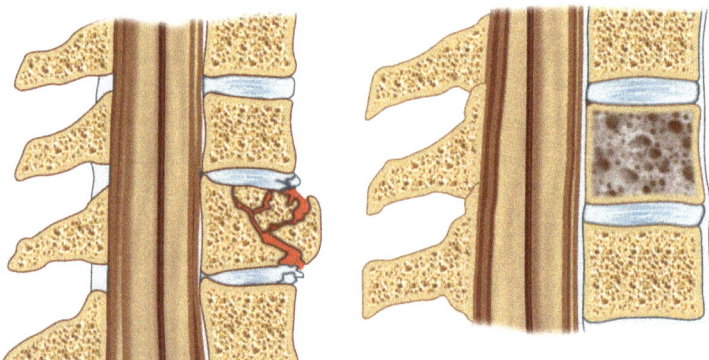

**Fig. 1:** Transcutaneous vertebroplasty.

Surgery is indicated when there is either neurological dysfunction or instability. Surgical technique depends upon the type of fracture and the overall health of the patient. If a patient continues to experience pain from a wedge fracture after conservation management, then a vertebroplasty may be considered (Fig. 1). This procedure involves injecting a cement polymer into the fractured vertebral body. This procedure has proven promising with the possibility of cement going to surrounding structures. A similar procedure called kyphoplasty involves injecting a balloon before cement, and, therefore, the cement is injected into a close balloon. Severe fractures will not permit the injection of the balloon. Despite the risks, these procedures have many benefits and are being used more frequently as well as earlier in the treatment process. A brace is generally used postoperatively with the time frame done on a patient-by-patient basis.

## REFERENCE

1. Sherman AL. Lumbar compression fracture. [Online]. Available from http://medicine.medscape.com/article/309615-clinical 2010; [accessed July, 2012].

CHAPTER 6

# Neurology

## CASE STUDY 40: MYASTHENIA GRAVIS

### CASE HISTORY

**History of Present Illness**

The patient is a 54-year-old female who presents to the emergency room (ER) complaining of increased difficulty in walking. She has weakness in her legs, requiring assistance from her family to walk. Upon further questioning, it is also found that she has difficulty chewing meat and other hard foods. Her eyelids are droopy and she has difficulty keeping them open, she has to lift them with her fingers in order to see. Family members state that over the years, she slowly became more fatigued, weak, leading to a decreased mood. She also reports that her symptoms seem to improve after a good night of sleep.

**Past Medical History**

Before the onset of ptosis, an initial onset of diplopia prompted an eye examination in early 2011. An ophthalmologist found no neurological or muscular abnormality. She was given a few trials of botox injections which did not resolve the ptosis and in fact made it worse. Since the patient was not able to pay her medical bills from the prior botox injection, the patient did not seek any further medical workup.

**Family History**

Negative.

### PHYSICAL EXAMINATION

**Neurologic Examination**

- *Mental status*: The patient is alert and oriented to time, place, and person. Cranial nerves II–XII are intact. When asked to smile, a snarling

appearance is noted. The patient has mushy speech (like she is talking with marbles in her mouth).
- Sensation and cerebellar function are intact.
- Deep tendon reflexes (DTR) are 2+ and intact.
- Weakness in extremities is noticed when asked to clench fist or when asked to resist pushing anterior region of calf.

## LABORATORY TEST RESULTS

- *Complete blood count (CBC)*: It showed no anemia, leukocytosis, or thrombocytopenia.
- *Basic metabolic panel*: Electrolyte, glucose, blood urea nitrogen (BUN), and creatinine are within normal limits.
- *Urinalysis*: Urine culture showed no hematuria, pyuria, and bacteriuria.
- *Liver function test*: Aspartate transaminase (AST), alanine transaminase (ALT), bilirubin, and alkaline phosphatase are within normal limits.
- Amylase and lipase are within normal limits.
- *Cardiac markers*: Creatine kinase-muscle and brain (CK-MB), troponin, and myoglobin are within normal limits.
- *Drugs*: Negative for illicit or over-the-counter (OTC) drugs.

## DIAGNOSTIC ADJUNCTS

### Computed Tomography

- *Brain*: Rules out intracranial mass, stroke, and skull fracture
- *Chest*: Rules out masses.

### X-ray

Search for a thymoma which is often associated with myasthenia gravis.

## DIFFERENTIAL DIAGNOSIS

- Senile ptosis
- Lambert–Eaton syndrome (increasing muscle strength on repetitive contraction, a paraneoplastic syndrome that may indicate the presence of small cell carcinoma—lung)
- Cerebral vascular disease/transient ischemic attack (TIA)/stroke
- Generalized fatigue
- amyotrophic lateral sclerosis
- Botulism (pupils dilated and repetitive nerve stimulation, incremental increase in muscular fiber contraction)
- Intracranial mass lesion
- Mitochondrial myopathy
  - Oculopharyngeal muscular dystrophy
  - Muscular dystrophies.

## DIAGNOSTIC TESTS

- *Preferred initial test*: Antiacetylcholine receptor (ACh-R) antibodies (Ab)
- *Edrophonium (Tensilon)*: Sensitive and easy to perform at the bedside but not specific
- *Side effects from edrophonium*: Nausea/diarrhea, fasciculation, bradycardia, and syncope
- *Imaging*: X-ray and computed tomography (CT) scan
  - *Thymoma*: Present in 10–15% of patients
  - *Thymic hyperplasia*: Present in up to 65% of patients
- *Accurate tests*: Definitive tests include electromyography (EMG) showing a decrease in muscular fiber contraction on repetitive nerve stimulation and serologic tests showing positivity for anti–acetylcholine receptor antibody (anti-AChR-ab). Both tests are accurate and reliable.
- Other tests you may order in order to rule out other processes that may cause gradual onset weakness include thyroid function tests, CBC, and chemistry panel.

## IMPRESSION

- *Myasthenia gravis*: Patient presents with muscle weakness and fatigue (Fig. 1)
- Initially she had diplopia and now prominent ptosis and difficulty in swallowing.
- Her speech is mushy with nasal voice.
- Facial weakness with snarling appearance is noted when smiling.

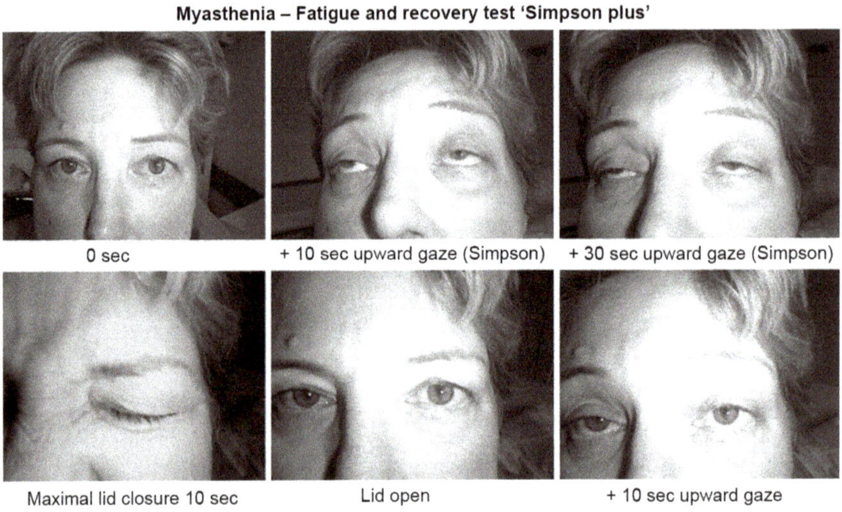

**Fig. 1:** Myasthenia gravis.
*Source:* Available online from http://www.neurology.org/content/67/8/1524.full.

- The disease progressed due to lack of a correct diagnosis and management, leading to generalized weakness involving proximal muscles in an asymmetric pattern.
- Sensation and DTR are intact.
- No evidence of respiratory muscle being affected
- After intravenous (IV) injection of 30 mg of physostigmine three times in 24 h, the patient shows a dramatic improvement of ptosis and motor activity.

## TREATMENT

- *Anticholinesterase drugs:* Pyridostigmine, neostigmine (used for symptomatic treatment)
  - Indicated in thymectomy
  - Used if thymoma present
  - Used before toxic immunosuppressive therapy
- *Immunosuppressive therapy*: Used if thymectomy not effective
  - *Glucocorticoids*: Improve weakness, 1-3 months to see effect
  - Steroids first, but if ineffective, consider
    - *Combination*: Azathioprine (3-6 months for effect) + steroid
    - *Cyclosporine and cyclophosphamide*: Alternative to azathioprine; more toxic
    - *Mycophenolate*: Newer immunosuppressive drug; less side effects than steroids or cyclophosphamide
    - *Plasmapheresis*: IV immunoglobulin (Ig), rapid improvement of weakness.

## ACUTE MYASTHENIC CRISIS

Respiratory involvement.

## AVOID

Aminoglycoside antibiotics may exacerbate Mysthenia gravis.

Glucocorticoids also have the potential to exacerbate symptoms, although they are sometimes a part of therapy for MG.

Beta-blockers, calcium channel blockers, some antiepileptics, phenothiazines, procainamide, magnesium, and opioids can also increase symptoms of weakness and although not contraindicated, it is preferable to avoid them in the setting of a patient recovering from myasthenic crisis with recent extubation.

## FOLLOW-UP

Ptosis and generalized muscle weakness improved with physostigmine injection. The patient is being treated daily with anticholinesterase and sustained-release tablets for symptom control.

## DISCUSSION

Although myasthenia gravis is a rare disorder affecting approximately only 7–23 out of every million people, it is important to recognize the condition and especially the emergencies that might present, such as respiratory muscle weakness that may lead to respiratory failure in myasthenic crisis. Symptoms may relapse and remit spontaneously for several weeks then reappear with worsening or new symptoms.

The most common presenting symptoms include ptosis, diplopia, and general weakness, especially of muscle groups that are used repetitively throughout the day such as with eye blinking and chewing. The pathophysiology stems from the development of auto-Ab to postsynaptic ACh-R. Classically, symptoms worsen towards the end of the day after repetitive muscle use. Treatment with acetycholinesterase (AChE) inhibitors increase the amount of acetylcholine available at the synaptic cleft and improve symptoms.

The most serious symptoms in myasthenia gravis involve the respiratory muscles. This potentially life threatening situation can be precipitated by interventions, such as surgery, infections, and certain medications or adjustments to immunosuppressant therapy. Respiratory involvement may warrant intubation and mechanical ventilation until the patient is able to ventilate on their own. Medications to be avoided in patients with myasthenia gravis, especially those with respiratory involvement, are listed in Box 1.

*Lambert–Eaton syndrome*: Auto-Ab to presynaptic $Ca^{2+}$ channel resulting in decreased ACh release. It causes proximal muscle weakness usually associated with paraneoplastic syndromes (small cell lung cancer). The symptoms improve with muscle use and there is no reversal with AChE inhibitors.

| **Box 1:** Drugs that may worsen myasthenia gravis. | |
|---|---|
| *Anesthetic drugs:* <br> Neuromuscular blocking agents <br> *Antibiotics:* <br> Aminoglycosides <br> Clindamycin <br> Fluoroquinolones <br> Ketolides <br> Vancomycin | *Cardiovascular drugs:* <br> Beta-blockers <br> Procainamide <br> Quinidine <br> *Others:* <br> Botulinum toxin <br> Chloroquine <br> Hydroxychloroquine <br> Penicillamine <br> Quinine <br> Anti-PD-1-monoclonal antibodies |

## PRACTICE PEARL

For rapid sequence intubation, the dose of succinylcholine for inducing anesthesia in patients with myasthenia gravis should be 2 mg/kg (verify with Train of Four (TOF) stimulator if available to prevent laryngospasm) versus 1.5 mg/kg in individuals without MG.

## FURTHER READING

1. Cogan DG. Myasthenia gravis: a review of the disease and a description of lid twitch as a characteristic sign. Arch Opthalmol. 1965;74:217-21.
2. Levitan R. Safety of succinylcholine in myasthenia gravis. Ann Emerg Med. 2005;45:225-6.
3. Oosterhuis H. Clinical aspects. In: DeBaets M, Oosterhuis H, editors. Myasthenia gravis. Boca Raton: CRC Press; 1993. p. 19.

## CASE STUDY 41: GUILLAIN–BARRÉ SYNDROME

## CASE HISTORY

*Chief complaint*: A 14-year-old Caucasian male presents with complaints of bilateral (BL) lower extremity weakness that started 3 h prior to admission.

### History of Present Illness

When the patient got out of bed this morning, he suddenly felt weak and was not able to walk. The patient started feeling BL lower leg weakness with intermittent tingling. He noticed weakness in both legs with loss of sensation on the right. The patient reported no recent trauma, injuries, pain, headache, or other complaints. The patient did not have any neurological symptoms previously and has not recently been seen or treated by a doctor or hospitalized. His parents state that the patient had four vaccinations 1 week ago.

### Past History

Past medical history is negative.

## PHYSICAL EXAMINATION

### General Appearance

Alert and anxious appearing 14-year-old white male who is not in acute distress and interacts very well with family members and staff. His growth and development are appropriate for his age. Vital signs and physical examination unremarkable except for neuromuscular examination.

## Musculoskeletal Examination

The patient's back is symmetrical, no masses found, and appears nontender.

## Neurologic Examination

- The patient is alert and oriented with good eye contact, and pupils are equal, round, reactive to light, and accommodation (PERRLA). Babinski sign is absent.
- Decreased BL lower extremity strength, reflexes, and proprioception
- Cerebellar function is normal.

## Extremities/Skin Examination

No joint effusions, tenderness, rashes, edema, or cyanosis found. Capillary refill rate is normal. The patient's skin is warm, dry, intact with no rash and good turgor.

## Laboratory Assessment

*Lumbar Puncture*: Increased protein, with fewer than 10 cells/mm$^3$.

# DIAGNOSTIC ADJUNCT

STAT computed tomography (CT) of lumbar spine was negative for acute pathology.

# IMPRESSION

*Guillain–Barré syndrome (GBS):* Patient presents with sudden and acute onset of BL lower extremity weakness which disables the patient from walking with decreased reflexes and proprioception. This patient's neurological examination is consistent with GBS as he feels weakness with absence of reflexes, fever, and constitutional symptoms (Fig. 1). Patients classically present with paresthesias of the toes and fingers followed by symmetric leg weakness and ascending involvement to the arms. Severe cases may ascend to affect the respiratory muscles.

# DIFFERENTIAL DIAGNOSIS

- *Basilar artery occlusion*: Asymmetric limb paresis
- *Botulism:* Descending paralysis
- *Spinal cord compression*
- Brainstem infection or stroke
- *Transverse myelitis:* Abrupt BL leg weakness and ascending sensory loss
- *Poliomyelitis:* Purely motor neuron destruction of the anterior horn cells
- *Polymyositis*: Chronic, affects proximal limb muscles.

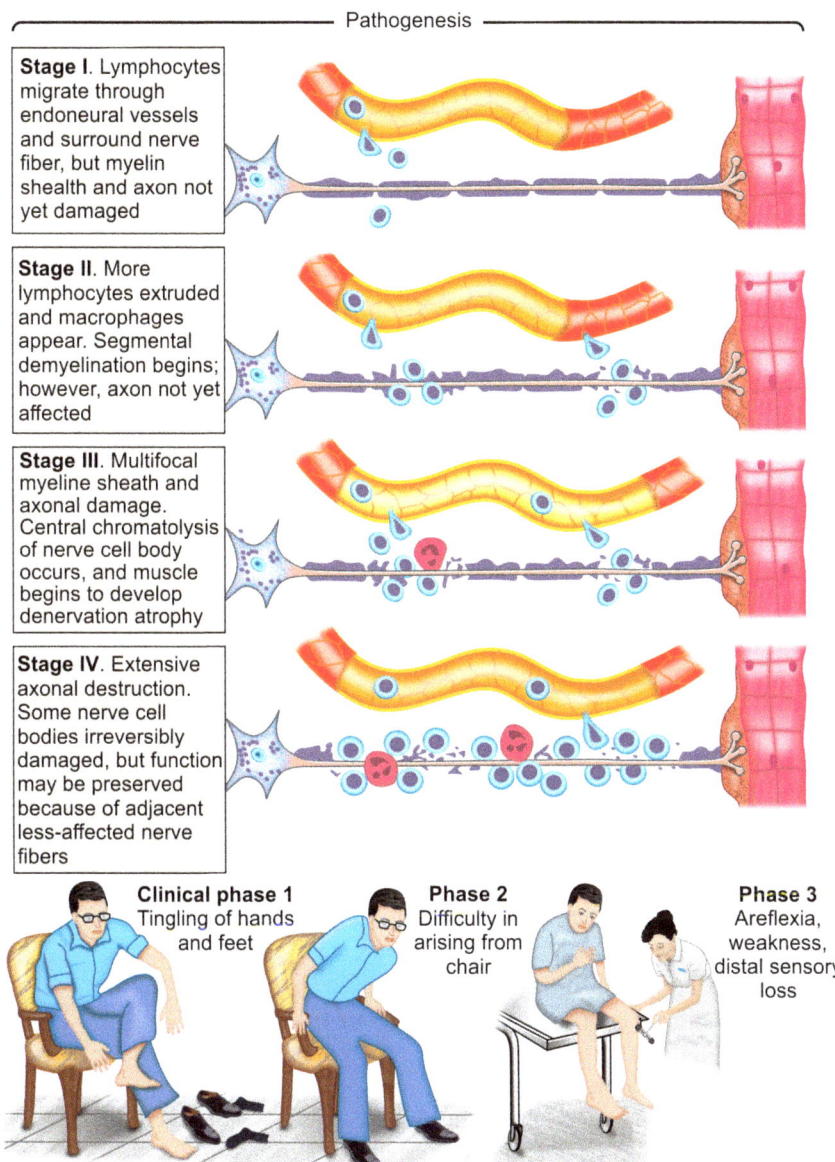

Fig. 1: Clinical stages/phases of Guillain–Barré syndrome.

- Toxic neuropathy
- Acute intermittent porphyria—abdominal weakness, psychosis, and abdominal pain
- Muscular conditions, such as periodic paralysis, rhabdomyolysis, or myopathy
- Metabolic abnormalities, such as hypokalemia, hypophosphatemia, uremia, or porphyria

- Recent diphtheria
- Myasthenia gravis
- Paraneoplastic disease
- Sarcoidosis
- Toxicity due to industrial chemicals
- *Vasculitic neuropathies:* In GBS, cerebrospinal fluid (CSF) protein levels elevate without elevating pleocytosis in about 80-90% of patients. CSF in Lyme or HIV disease may have pleocytosis demonstrating analogous meningeal reaction. If white blood cell count in CSF consists of elevated protein higher than 0.55 g/dL (5.5 g/L) that increases the possibility of Lyme disease, neoplasia, HIV, and sarcoid meningitis.

## DIAGNOSTIC TESTS

- There is no single diagnostic test that can confirm or rule out the diagnosis of GBS, a combination of clinical picture, CSF, electromyography (EMG), imaging, and serum immunoglobulin (Ig)G antibodies are taken into account
- *Best initial test:* Lumbar puncture for CSF protein and cell count
- *More than 48 h after onset of symptoms:* Elevated protein without rise in cell count
- *Most accurate test:* EMG which detects evidence of demyelination of peripheral nerves.

## DIAGNOSTIC CRITERIA

AAFP Diagnostic Criteria for typical GBS
*Features required for diagnosis:*
- Progressive weakness in both arms and legs
- Areflexia

*Features strongly supporting diagnosis:*
- Progression of symptoms over days, up to 4 weeks
- Relative symmetry of symptoms
- Mild sensory symptoms or signs
- Cranial nerve involvement, especially BL weakness of facial muscles
- Recovery beginning 2-4 weeks after progression ceases
- Autonomic dysfunction
- Absence of fever at onset
- High concentration of protein in CSF, with fewer than 10 cells/mm$^3$
- Typical electrodiagnostic features
- Features excluding diagnosis
- Diagnosis of botulism, myasthenia, poliomyelitis, or toxic neuropathy
- Abnormal porphyrin metabolism
- Recent diphtheria
- Purely sensory syndrome, without weakness.

## TREATMENT

Treatment is given as soon as possible because it becomes ineffective after 2 weeks from the onset of symptoms.
- Intravenous Ig or plasmapheresis is equally effective, no benefit to combination treatment
- *Glucocorticoids*: Not effective in treatment of acute GBS.

## MANAGEMENT

- Monitor vital capacity in patient with GBS
- Figure 1 shows the progression of the disease in different stages
- Initiate early respiratory support to prevent death from respiratory failure.

## Guillain–Barré Syndrome

GBS is an acute polyradiculopathy due to an autoimmune destruction of myelin (Fig. 2). There is misdirection of immune response due to molecular mimicry. Patient presents with rapidly developing weakness that begins in the lower extremities and moves upward. Patient lacks reflexes in affected muscle groups. Progression of symptoms develops over the course of hours to days. Legs are usually more affected than arms and face due to ascending nature of paralysis. Fever, constitutional symptoms, or bladder dysfunction are rare. Sensory disturbances can cause pain or tingling dysesthesia. Sensory changes are due to loss of large sensory fibers, resulting in reflex and proprioception loss. Autonomic instability occurs in severe GBS, requiring patient treatment in intensive care unit.

Seventy-five percent of patients with GBS have a history of infection 1–3 weeks prior to onset of symptoms. The infection is typically in the respiratory

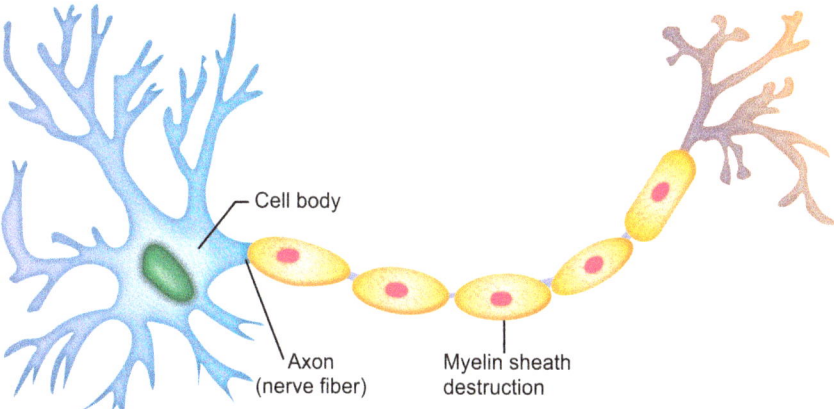

**Fig. 2:** Destruction of myelin sheath in Guillain–Barré syndrome.

or gastrointestinal system (*Campylobacter jejuni*, associated with up to 30% of cases). It may also be preceded by infections with human herpes virus, cytomegalovirus, and Epstein–Barr virus. Approximately one in every million person vaccinated for seasonal flue may develop GBS; however, the risk of developing GBS after a flu infection is substantially higher. Current available evidence suggests that the H1N1 vaccine is not associated with increased GBS risk in children. In addition, a very small percentage of GBS patients develop their symptoms following surgery, bone marrow transplant, or trauma.

*CSF findings:* CSF is often normal when symptoms have been present for <48 h, but by the end of the first week, CSF protein level is >5.5 g/L with no pleocytosis (<10 cells/cm).

## FURTHER READING

1. Asbury AK, Cornblath DR. Assessment of current diagnostic criteria for Guillain-Barré syndrome. Ann Neurol 1990;27(suppl):S21-4.
2. Berger AR. Guillain-Barré syndrome and its variants. [online]. Available at: www. HYPERLINK "http://neuropathy.org/site/DocServer/GBS-AlanBergerMD.pdf" neuropathy.org/site/DocServer/GBS-AlanBergerMD.pdf. [accessed May 9th, 2013].
3. Kimura J. Proximal versus distal slowing of motor nerve conduction velocity in the Guillain-Barré syndrome. Ann Neurol 1978;3;344-50.
4. Ropper AH. The Guillain-Barré syndrome. N Engl J Med 1992;326:1130-6.

## CASE STUDY 42: DELIRIUM TREMENS

## CASE HISTORY

A 67-year-old man was arrested on a Saturday night for drunk driving, this is his seventh driving under the influence (DUI) violation, and he was driving with a revoked license. He was taken to the local jail. The following afternoon (Sunday), he was noted to be acting restless, pacing around his jail cell. He later became agitated and tremulous. The following Monday afternoon, he became increasingly anxious and had several episodes of vomiting. Tuesday morning, he did not eat due to additional nausea and vomiting. In the early afternoon on Tuesday, he had a generalized seizure of approximately 45 s and was taken to the emergency room (ER). On the way to the hospital, he remained mildly confused about the situation but did not have any signs of head trauma. In the ER, he was initially found to be quite anxious with mild tachycardia and hypertension.

## EMERGENCY ROOM MANAGEMENT

Intravenous (IV) fluids like normal saline (NS) were started immediately upon arrival to the emergency department (ED), and he was given thiamine, naloxone, and glucose. Over the following hours while he was being assessed, he became progressively more agitated and confused about where he was, began having hallucinations of people telling him that he must get out of town, and he developed severely worsening tachycardia and hypertension.

He was given a bolus of diazepam and was transferred to the detox unit. There, he was monitored with the revised clinical institute withdrawal assessment for alcohol (CIWA-Ar) protocol using Ativan (lorazepam) for the following 4 days as he progressively returned to baseline and required decreasing amounts of Ativan. Upon discharge, he agreed to attend an alcoholic rehabilitation program.

## DISCUSSION

This patient is a chronic and heavy alcohol user, which is evidenced by his multiple DUIs with revoked driver's license and his progression to withdrawal symptoms. Although not usually the case, this patient demonstrated a progression through the various forms of alcohol withdrawal: minor withdrawal, major withdrawal, withdrawal seizure, and delirium tremens (DTs). Chronic alcohol use affects both the $\gamma$-aminobutyric acid (GABA) and *N*-methyl-D-aspartate (NMDA) receptors in the brain, with counter-effects occurring when alcohol is removed. This combination leads to the symptoms associated with alcohol withdrawal. Treatment is generally aimed at preventing adverse effects and additional withdrawal episodes. Progression to DTs is associated with high morbidity and mortality, so it is important to recognize and treat alcohol withdrawal quickly, while monitoring the patient through the withdrawal and detoxification stages. Finally, preventing future recurrences should be addressed by assessing willingness to change and providing information regarding rehabilitation opportunities. While the approach to quitting smoking and heroine encourages repeated attempts, data for alcoholics points to an association of decreased chances of successful rehabilitation with numerous failed or half-hearted attempts. Therefore, it is encouraged to only go forward with detoxing an alcoholic patient if they are serious about rehabilitation (vs trying to please you or simply looking for a bed to stay in).

## DELIRIUM TREMENS DISCUSSION

### General

Alcohol withdrawal syndrome can manifest with variable symptoms and occurs as a result of abrupt alcohol cessation in an alcohol-dependent individual. These include minor withdrawal, major withdrawal, withdrawal seizures, and DTs. These do not have to occur in any particular order, nor do they all even have to present at all. Minor withdrawal generally occurs within the first day after alcohol cessation and includes symptoms, such as tremor, anxiety, nausea, vomiting, and insomnia. Major withdrawal usually presents within 2–3 days of the last drink, exhibited by potential visual and auditory hallucinations, whole body tremor, vomiting, diaphoresis, and hypertension. Withdrawal seizures also may occur within the first 2–3 days. These tend to be brief, generalized, motor seizures in those who do not have a history of seizures. In some cases, this can be the initial and only symptoms during alcohol withdrawal. Without treatment, as many as 60% can have multiple seizures, but this rarely develops into status epilepticus. As many as 30–40% of people experiencing withdrawal seizures may progress to DTs. This is the most severe form of alcohol withdrawal, which tends to occur within the first week after alcohol cessation and can include symptoms such as agitation, global confusion, disorientation, hallucinations, fever, hypertension, diaphoresis, and autonomic hyperactivity. Risk factors for developing DTs include prior withdrawal seizures or DTs, concurrent illness, prolonged heavy daily alcohol consumption, current severe withdrawal symptoms, or prior detoxification. While <50% of alcohol-dependent people experience severe withdrawal needing pharmacological intervention, only about 3% will progress to DTs.

## Pathophysiology

Alcohol has effects on several receptors within the central nervous system. These include both the inhibitory GABA receptor and the excitatory NMDA receptor. Alcohol activates the GABA receptor and inhibits the NMDA receptor. With chronic alcohol use, this leads to downregulation of the GABA receptor and upregulation of the NMDA receptor. Upon removal of the alcohol stimulus, there will be less inhibitory GABA stimulation and more excitatory NMDA stimulation, which both lead to an increase in neuroexcitation. The combination of these effects leads to the mental confusion and autonomic hyperactivity associated with the various stages of alcohol withdrawal syndrome. The longer a person is exposed to chronic alcohol, more alterations occur with the GABA and NMDA receptors. This leads to increased frequency and severity of withdrawal episodes over time, which is a phenomenon known as kindling.

## Assessment

It is important to obtain a detailed history of the patient's situation. Remember that everything should not be blindly attributed to alcohol since people with alcohol dependence can also have other illness. Keep in mind the anecdote about the drunk patient who was left alone in the ER waiting room to sober up, but when finally examined, it was found that he had also suffered multiple trauma wounds due to being beat up while drunk.

With this in mind, be sure to determine the length of time and amount of regular alcohol intake, the time since the last drink, prior withdrawal episodes or detox admissions, past seizure history, additional medication or substance use or abuse, and any concurrent medical or psychiatric history. A detailed history alone can give you a very good idea of whether the symptoms are related to alcohol withdrawal syndrome.

The physical examination is nondiagnostic, so it should be used in conjunction with additional history and laboratory studies to obtain information regarding conditions that may complicate or exacerbate alcohol withdrawal and to ensure that alcohol withdrawal is the most likely cause of the problems. Such physical examination and history information should relate to vital signs (tachycardia, tachypnea, fever, and hypertension), general status (tremors, diaphoresis, and trauma), the cardiovascular system [arrhythmia, congestive heart failure (CHF), and coronary artery disease (CAD)], the gastrointestinal (GI) system (GI bleeds, liver disease and related stigmata, and pancreatitis), the neurologic system (nystagmus, gait, neuropathy, focal defects, global confusion, and altered mental status), and psychiatric issues (disorientation, anxiety, depression, mania, and memory).

Although none of this is diagnostic for alcohol withdrawal or DTs, it can provide additional insight into other causes or potential complicating features since many people with alcohol dependence have comorbid conditions. Next, laboratory testing and imaging should be used similarly to investigate complicating factors and to optimize the potential for swift recovery. Serum blood alcohol is an important value to obtain, since withdrawal symptoms with alcohol still in the body would suggest that the withdrawal will worsen as the alcohol continues to decrease. Liver and renal function tests should be obtained since metabolic dysfunction can potentially complicate or exacerbate the withdrawal. Furthermore, a urine drug screen can be utilized if there is suspicion of additional drug use.

A complete blood count with differential and comprehensive metabolic panel should be obtained to evaluate potential concurrent infection, electrolytes, and blood glucose. Electrolytes and glucose should be corrected to minimize complications. Additionally, if concurrent infection is suspected, then investigation into the location should occur.

Infection can greatly increase morbidity during withdrawal and DTs. Potential studies may include chest radiograph, urinalysis, lumbar puncture, and more as deemed appropriate. Finally, computed tomography (CT) of head or cervical radiography may be utilized if head or neck trauma is evident or suspected.

## Treatment

Mortality for patients experiencing DTs can be as high as 15%, so it is important to evaluate and treat the patient appropriately in order to minimize complications and facilitate recovery. Mortality most commonly results from arrhythmias, pneumonia, or the failure to identify the underlying problem that led to the cessation of alcohol use. As previously mentioned, the workup should attempt to rule out any other causes or complicating factors and then treat those accordingly. This includes treating concurrent infections, workup for pancreatitis, hepatitis, or CNS injury correcting electrolyte abnormalities and removing any exacerbating medications.

Furthermore, many alcohol-dependent patients are also nutritionally deficient and dehydrated. This can be exhibited by inadequate levels of various vitamins, as well as hypoglycemia and ketoacidosis from depleted glycogen stores. Thiamine is a common deficiency in this population and should be replaced along with multivitamins, glucose, and IV fluids. Note that it is critical to administer the thiamine prior to giving glucose since glucose utilization can cause a decrease in thiamine and potentially precipitate Wernicke encephalopathy.

The mainstay of assessment and therapy for alcohol withdrawal is the revised CIWA-Ar.[1] This is the most well-validated tool for alcohol withdrawal when used properly in the correct circumstances. First, it is important to be sure that the patient is truly suffering from alcohol withdrawal and not some other cause for decreased arousal, altered mental status, or delirium. Additionally, it has not been validated for complex medical or surgical patients, but instead it should be used for patients in detoxification units, psychiatric units, or medical/surgical wards. CIWA-Ar is a survey or checklist that evaluates 10 items: nausea and vomiting, anxiety, tremor, sweating, auditory disturbances, visual disturbances, tactile disturbances, headache, agitation and clouding of sensorium. Each of the first nine categories is rated on a scale from 0 to 7, while the last item is rated from 0 to 4. With a total (i.e., worst) possible score of 67, any score >15 implies moderate-to-severe alcohol withdrawal and requires hospital admission and treatment. Mild withdrawal includes scores from 8 to 15, in which pharmacological therapy is still pertinent, but hospital admission may or may not be needed depending on prior history or episodes of alcohol withdrawal. Those with scores under 8 will not need hospital admission or drug therapy for the alcohol withdrawal episode.

The utilization of the CIWA-Ar criteria not only assesses the severity of the alcohol withdrawal state, it also guides the treatment. Benzodiazepines, such as chlordiazepoxide, diazepam, and lorazepam, are given at varying doses and frequencies depending on the severity of withdrawal determined by the CIWA-Ar protocol. Reassessment is continued as the withdrawal state resolves over the course of hours to days. It should be apparent that the patient will begin to require lower and less frequent medication doses as the withdrawal episode improves.

It is suggested that the patient is well enough for discharge when three sequential CIWA-Ar assessments deem it no longer necessary for benzodiazepine treatments. Throughout this process, the patient must be monitored closely as complications of alcohol withdrawal and DTs include over sedation, although the most common conditions leading to morbidity and mortality in this group are cardiac arrhythmias and respiratory failure even in the setting of appropriate medical treatment. Patients at highest risk for complications include those with severe fever, fluid and electrolyte abnormalities, concurrent illness, trauma, pneumonia, hepatitis, pancreatitis, alcoholic ketoacidosis, or Wernicke-Korsakoff syndrome. This is an opportunity to assess willingness to change, suggest alcohol rehabilitation opportunities, and introduce possible adjunctive medical therapies (e.g., disulfiram, naltrexone, acamprosate, and topiramate). The best possible outcome after such alcohol withdrawal episodes would be finding the support and resolution to overcome alcohol-dependence and avoid any similar episodes in the future.

## EXCITED DELIRIUM

The nation's ERs are seeing increasing numbers of patients who are using synthetic, designer drugs. The name "excited delirium" is a controversial name that is not widely accepted; however, the symptoms and consequences of the drug use it refers to can be very real and every emergency provider should be aware of the possibility for a patient to present symptoms of delirium, agitation, anxiety, hallucinations, speech disturbances, elevated core temperature, and resistance to pain that may be due to acute toxicity of dangerous illicit drugs. This condition is also known as Excited Delirium syndrome when it results in sudden death from cardiac or respiratory arrest.

Head trauma and alcohol withdrawal may be contributing factors to this high morbidity and mortality, but the most common precipitating factor is the use of cocaine, Phencyclidine (PCP), and bath salts. "Bath salts" refers to the informal "street name" for a family of designer drugs often containing substituted cathinones, which have effects similar to amphetamine and cocaine. Their white crystals often resemble legal bathing products like epsom salts but are chemically disparate from actual bath salts (Fig 1). Bath salts packaging often states "not for human consumption" in an attempt to avoid the prohibition of these products.

Other "street names" for this drug are Ivory Wave, Purple Wave, Vanilla Sky, and Bliss. ACEP accepts Excited Delirium as a unique syndrome. The signs and symptoms of excited delirium include severe disorientation, hyper-aggression, tachycardia, paranoia, hallucinations, forceful and incoherent speech, severe hyperthermia, and profuse sweating even in cold weather. Most of the time, the person is found naked with all or some of the symptoms described above. Majority of the fatal case reports are of males who are involved in acute drug use, especially psychostimulants such as cocaine, PCP, and methamphetamine.

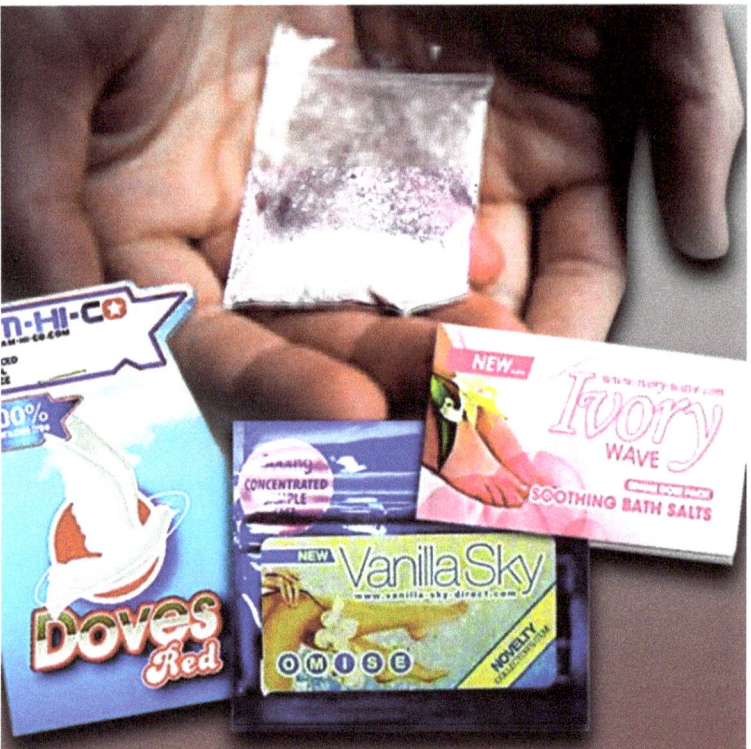

**Fig. 1:** Bath salts are similar to amphetamines.

## REFERENCE

1. Sullivan JT, Sykora K, Schneiderman J, et al. Assessment of alcohol withdrawal: the revised clinical institute withdrawal assessment for alcohol scale (CIWA-Ar). Br J Addict. 1989;84(11):1353-7.

## FURTHER READING

1. Domino FJ, Baldor RA, Golding J, Stephens MB. The 5-Minute Clinical Consult 2019. Philadelphia: Wolters Kluwer; 2018.
2. http://en.wikipedia.org/wiki/Excited_delirium.
3. http://en.wikipedia.org/wiki/Bath_salts_(drug).

## CASE STUDY 43: STROKE

*Time lost is brain lost.*

—**American Stroke Association**

Neurology

*Time is muscle; time is kidney; time is brain; time is everything in an emergency.*

—**Badar M Zaheer**

## CASE HISTORY

A 60-year-old white female is brought to the emergency department (ED) by her husband with sudden onset of right upper extremity (RUE) weakness that began while she was preparing breakfast in the morning. The husband became concerned when the patient could not talk in response to questions. Screening tools were used and patient seems to understand what is being said but cannot respond (Figs. 1 and 2). Patient has history of medication-controlled hypertension. The patient's father died of a stroke at the age of 70 after living with hypertension for several decades, her mother is in her 80s and completely healthy.

## PHYSICAL EXAMINATION

- *Neurologic examination*: Cranial nerves (CN) II–VI, VIII–XII are intact with right facial nerve palsy. She can wrinkle her forehead. Droop noted on the right side of the mouth. No lid weakness noticed.
  - *Motor*: Flaccid hemiparesis noted on the right side
  - *Sensory*: No light touch sensation in RUE

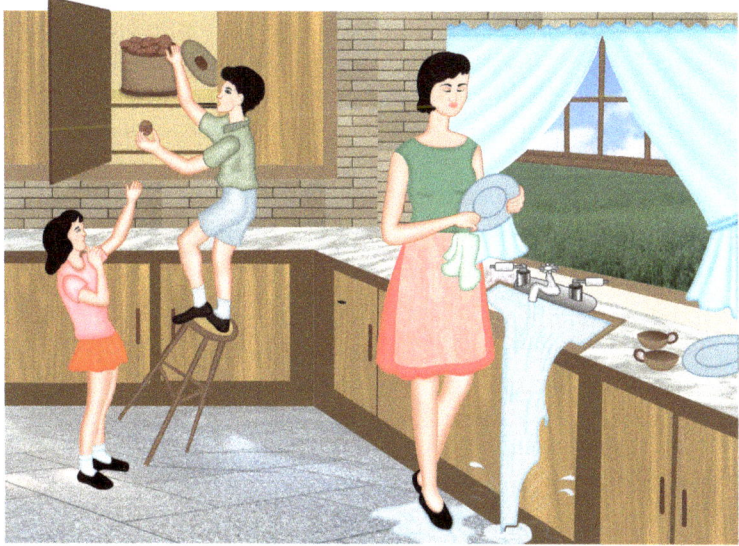

**Fig. 1:** Screening tool; patients must be able to identify the problems in the situation.
*Source:* www.ninds.nih.gov/doctors/NIH_Stroke_Scale.pdf.

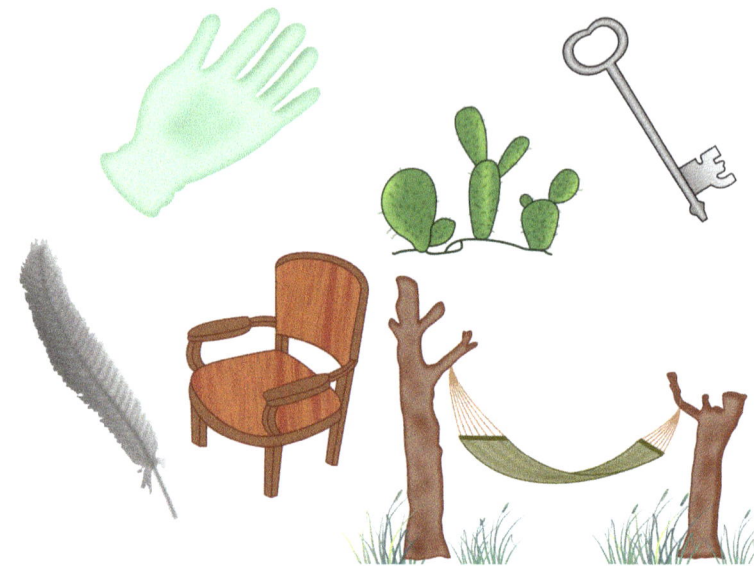

**Fig. 2:** Screening tool; patients are asked to identify the objects in the picture.
*Source:* www.ninds.nih.gov/doctors/NIH_Stroke_Scale.pdf.

- *Reflexes*: No deep tendon reflexes (DTR) of right lower extremity (RLE). Babinski reflex is present on the right big toe. Corneal and gag reflexes are normal.
- *Cerebellar*: Slight truncal ataxia to the right side and gait disturbance
- *Visual/neglect*: Lost vision and neglect on the right side of the eye
- *Language*: Dysarthria, expressive aphasia and no receptive aphasia
- *Level of consciousness*: Slightly somnolent and responds to verbal stimuli.
- Rest of the physical examination is normal.

## DIAGNOSTIC WORKUP

- The preferred initial (and most sensitive) test available to detect blood in the brain: Noncontrast head computed tomography (CT) scan. See Flowchart 1 for hemorrhagic versus ischemic stroke
  - Negative for ischemia within first 48 h after onset of symptoms
- *Accurate test for ischemia*: Available
- Diffusion-weighted magnetic resonance imaging (MRI) is done for cerebral ischemia detection.
- Search for embolic source by doing an echocardiogram, carotid duplex scan, and 24-h Holter monitoring
- Initial blood test is done to check for inherited hypercoagulability

**Flowchart 1:** Types of stroke.

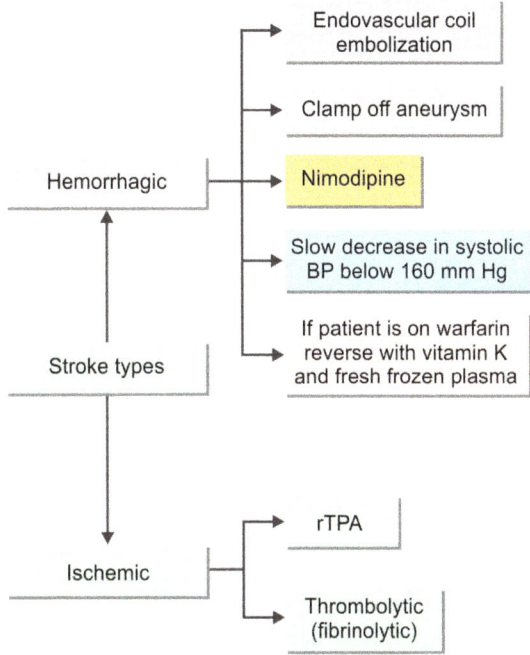

- Electrocardiogram (ECG) may help to show ischemia or inverted T-waves.
- Bubble study on echocardiogram to detect cardiac defect and function. The bubble echocardiogram shows better results than a conventional echocardiogram. Watch on Youtube http://www.youtube.com/watch?v=3dssbDeow50.

## MANAGEMENT

A diagnosis of acute ischemic stroke and acute onset of focal neurologic deficit is made. The course of treatment suggested for this patient was tissue plasminogen activator (tPA) since there were no hemorrhages found and it was within 2 h of the onset of symptoms (the typical time limit is 4.5 h from symptom onset). As a rule of thumb, patients presenting with ischemic stroke should be appropriately triaged and IV alteplase started within 1 h of patient arrival. The patient was administered tPA: 0.9 mg/kg body weight. Follow the guidelines from http://www2.massgeneral.org/stopstroke/tpaDoseCalc.aspx. A repeat neurologic examination was performed 90 min following treatment and showed increased speech and use of the right arm. The patient was eventually discharged to a rehabilitation hospital on day 7 and scheduled for a follow-up examination in 3 months.

## DIFFERENTIAL DIAGNOSIS

The differential diagnosis for presentations concerning for acute stroke include epileptic seizures and postictal subdural hematoma, tumor, hyponatremia, hypocalcemia, hepatic encephalopathy, Wernicke–Korsakoff syndrome, hypoglycemia, hyperglycemia, alcohol, illicit drugs, head injury, encephalitis, cerebral abscess, hypertensive encephalopathy, peripheral nerve lesion, multiple sclerosis, Creutzfeldt–Jakob disease, and subarachnoid hemorrhage.

## TREATMENT

### Golden Hour of Acute Ischemic Stroke (Fig. 3)

Acute ischemic stroke is an extremely serious medical emergency. In a typical large-vessel acute ischemic stroke, 1.9 million neurons may be lost each minute without medical management. Rapid intervention is crucial in the management of acute ischemic stroke. Door to treatment in ≤60 min is the standard of care recognized by professional medical associations involved in the treatment of acute ischemic stroke (Fig. 3).

- *tPA*: Administered in <3 h from onset of symptoms, better neurologic function in 3 months post-CVA
- *CI to tPA*: Stroke or serious head trauma <3 months ago
  - *Hemorrhage:* Gastrointestinal/genitourinary (GI/GU) <3 weeks ago
  - Surgery <2 weeks ago
  - History of intracranial hemorrhage

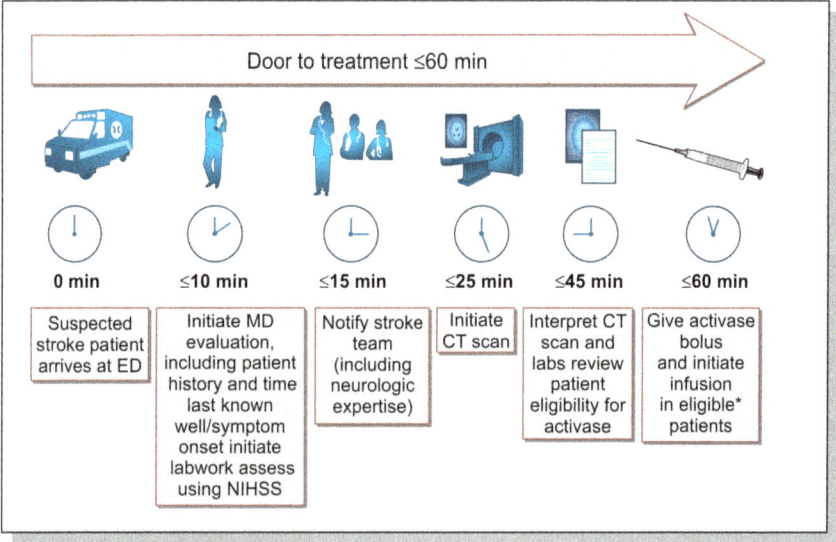

**Fig. 3:** Golden hour for thrombolytic therapy.
*Source:* Adapted from http://www.ninds.nih.gov/news_and_events/proceedings/ stroke_proceedings/recs-emerg.htm#emergency; and Jauch EC. American Heart Association guidelines for cardiopulmonary resuscitation and emergency cardiovascular care. Circulation 2010;122(18 suppl 3):S818-28.

- Arterial puncture <1 week ago
- Lumbar puncture <1 week ago
- BP >185/110 mm Hg.

## Checklist before tPA Therapy

Checklist before starting tPA therapy is shown in Box 1.

> **Box 1:** Checklist before starting tPA therapy.
>
> 1. Check the indications below that apply:
>    ☐ Patient is 18 years of age or older.
>    ☐ Time of symptoms onset can be identified accurately.
>    ☐ Thrombolytic therapy can be started within 3 h of symptom onset.
> 2. If all the boxes in Step 1 are checked, then review the absolute CIs below and check the ones that apply:
>    ☐ Head CT scan today showing intracranial bleeding
>    ☐ Head CT scan today shows no intracranial bleeding, but the clinical presentation is suspicious for subarachnoid hemorrhage.
>    ☐ Head CT scan today shows multilobar infarction (hypodense area greater than one third the area of the cerebral hemisphere).
>    ☐ Any of the following within the past 3 months; intracranial or intraspinal surgery, serious head trauma, or a witnessed seizure
>    ☐ Witnessed seizure since the onset of symptoms
>    ☐ BP higher than 185 mm Hg (systolic) or higher than 110 mm Hg (diastolic)
>    ☐ Arterial puncture at noncompressible site within past 7 days.
>    *Risk of hemorrhage*:
>    ☐ Evidence of active internal bleeding
>    ☐ Patient has an arteriovenous malformation, aneurysm, or neoplasm
>    ☐ Prior history of intracranial bleeding.
>    ☐ Laboratory evidence of a coagulopathy (e.g., platelet count < 100,000/μL)
>    ☐ Patient on Coumadin and INR ≥1.7, or patient received heparin in past 48 h and aPTT above normal range.
> 3. If none of the boxes in Step 2 are checked, review the relative CIs below and check any that are considered an unacceptable risk:
>    ☐ Major surgery or serious trauma in past 14 days
>    ☐ GI or urinary tract bleeding within past 21 days
>    ☐ Acute MI in past 3 months or post-MI pericarditis
>    ☐ Blood glucose <50 mg/dL or >400 mg/dL.
>    If all boxes in Step 1 are checked, and no boxes in Steps 2 and 3 are checked, then give thrombolytic therapy.

*Source*: Adapted from American Heart Association Guidelines for cardiopulmonary resuscitation and emergency cardiovascular care. Part 9: Adult stroke. Circulation 2005;112: IV111-20.

- *Current use of anticoagulants*: Platelets <100,000/mm$^3$ coagulopathy, prothrombin time (PT) is >15 s
  - *Heparin*: It is given but no clear benefit
  - Increased risk of bleeding
  - *Strongest indication*: Acute thrombosis
  - *Used only with higher risk of recurrent stroke*: Risk from side effects offsets benefit of treatment
- Atrial fibrillation, basilar artery thrombosis, stroke in evolution.

## Antiplatelet Therapy
### Endovascular Therapies

Since the publication of MR CLEAN study in 2014, the main treatment of stroke beyond 4.5 hours from onset of symptoms has become endovascular therapy. When administered within 24 hours of symptom onset, early endovascular therapy with stent retriever has proven benefit in mortality and morbidity. This was also demonstrated by the DAWN group, indicating that time is essential in salvaging brain tissue. Both studies have emphasized the importance of promptly administrating intravenous Alteplase, regardless of the decision to pursue endovascular therapy. Alteplase therapy should immediately follow a non-contrast head CT scan in selects patients meeting criteria. Additional imaging can be obtained afterwards.

- *Aspirin*: It is a first line drug most useful in secondary prevention of ischemic stroke
- 24 h post-tPA, dipyridamole, if continue to have recurrent CVA on aspirin alone
- *Clopidogrel*: Known allergy to aspirin.

## Surgical Interventions

- *Carotid endarterectomy*: Occlusion of <70% of arterial lumen and symptomatic lesion. Mechanical thrombectomy (Fig. 4)
- *Alternative*: Carotid stenting (Fig. 5).

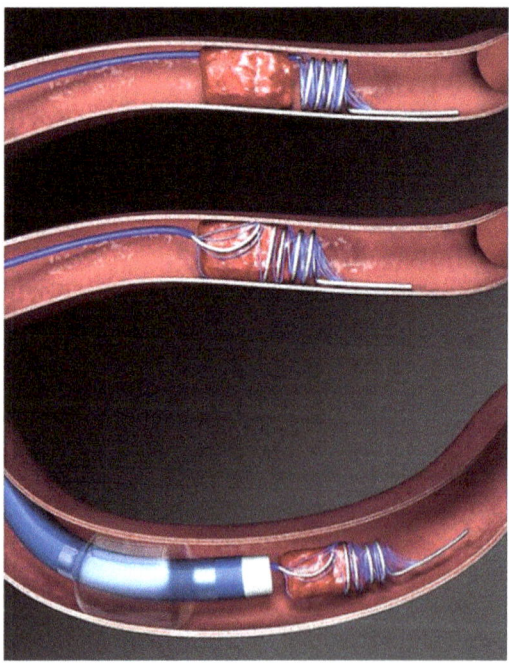

**Fig. 4:** Mechanical thrombectomy.
*Source: Courtesy of Wikipedia*: http://en.wikipedia.org/wiki/File:Merci_L5.jpg.

# Neurology

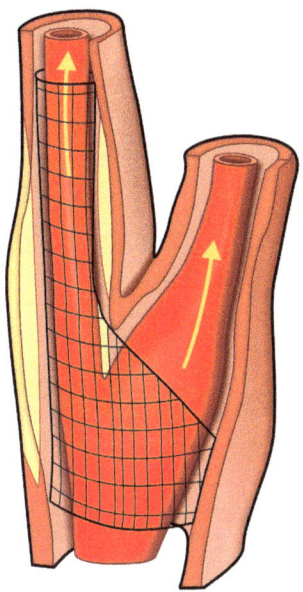

**Fig. 5:** Stents and angioplasty.
*Source: Courtesy of Wikipedia*: http://en.wikipedia.org/wiki/File:Merci_L5.jpg.

*Question:* Does adding endovascular procedures to intravenous tissue plasminogen activator (tPA) improve outcomes for patients with stroke?
*Answer:* Local delivery of tPA extracting the thrombus or stenting (endovascular therapies) showed no benefit in a randomized clinical study and in other two clinical trials which reaffirmed the ineffectiveness of this procedures (Figs. 4 and 5).[1,2] None of the above procedures are as effective as intravenous tPA which provides modest benefit, if the patients are correctly selected.

## PRACTICE PEARL

The Emergency MD needs to be able to diagnose accurately and acts upon certain CT findings without specialist (e.g., radiologist) assistance, because many disease processes are time-dependent and require immediate lifesaving action. Do not forget the mnemonic while reading the CT (Box 2).

| Box 2: Mnemonics for CT study. | | |
| --- | --- | --- |
| B | Blood | Blood |
| C | Can | Cisterns |
| B | Be | Brain |
| V | Very | Ventricles |
| B | Bad | Bone |

Head—"Blood Can Be Very Bad," where blood = blood, can = cisterns, be = brain, very = ventricles, and bad = bone.

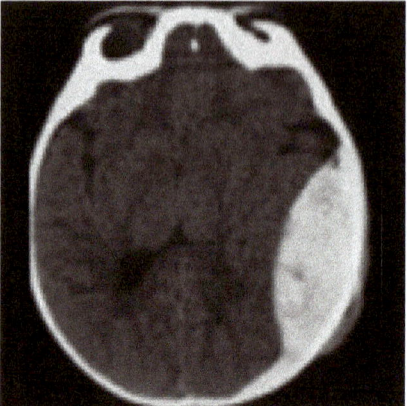
**Fig. 6:** Epidural hematoma: Elliptical/lens shaped.

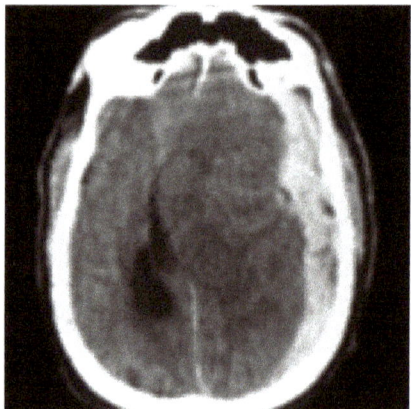
**Fig. 7:** Subdural hematoma: Crescent.

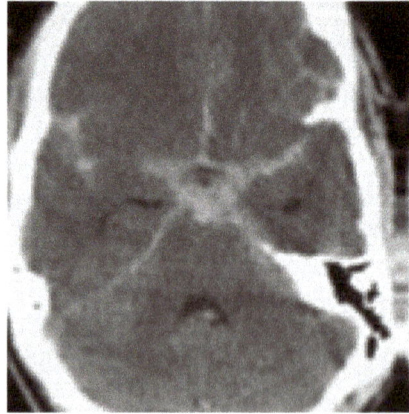
**Fig. 8:** Subarachnoid hemorrhage: Star shaped, Texas "The Lone Star Flag."

## Blood
- Presence of blood, its location, and spread (Figs. 6 to 8)
- Acute bleeding absorbs X-rays and they become white (hyperdense).

## Cisterns
Examine the cisterns which are collections of CSF protecting the brain. Look for asymmetry, presence of blood, and effacement.

## Brain Matter
- Look for asymmetry and midline shift. Trace the falx as your guidance
- Identify white hyperdense areas associated with blood IV contrast, or any calcifications
- Look for hypodense areas which are associated with fat, air, ischemia or tumor.

## Ventricles
Look at third and fourth ventricles for asymmetry and dilatation and for hemorrhage.

## Bone
On CT scans, cortical bones of the skull have the highest density. It is best viewed on separate bony windows when looking for fractures or tumors.

## Public Awareness and Public Education
The acronym FAST should be used to educate the public about stroke (Fig. 9).

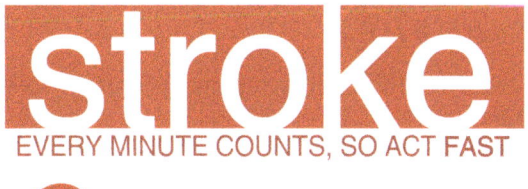
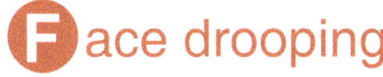
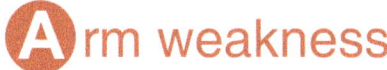
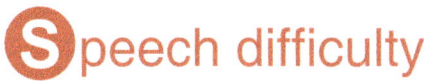
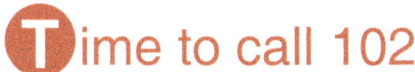

**Fig. 9:** Warning signs of stroke as per National Stroke Association.

## REFERENCES

1. Kidwell CS, Jahan R, Gornbein J, et al. A trial of imaging selection and endovascular treatment for ischemic stroke. N Engl J Med. 2013;368(10):904-14.
2. Kidwell CS, Jahan R, Gornbein J, et al. A trial of imaging selection and endovascular treatment for ischemic stroke. N Engl J Med. 2013; 368(10):914-23.

## FURTHER READING

1. 2018 AHA/ASA Stroke Early Management Guidelines. American College of Cardiology. https://www.acc.org/latest-in-cardiology/ten-points-to-remember/2018/01/29/12/45/2018-guidelines-for-the-early-management-of-stroke. Accessed July 18, 2018.
2. NIH Stroke Scale/Score (NIHSS). MDCalc. https://www.mdcalc.com/nih-stroke-scale-score-nihss. Accessed July 18, 2018.

## CASE STUDY 44: BELL'S PALSY

### CASE HISTORY

A 30-year-old male is presented to the emergency department (ED) with a sudden onset of right-sided facial weakness and right eye irritation. He woke up with these symptoms. He denies any preceding history of viral syndrome or trauma. Past medical history is negative.

### DIAGNOSIS

Facial nerve palsy (Bell's palsy) (Fig. 1).

### SIGNS AND SYMPTOMS

Common signs are excessive tearing, unilateral facial drooping, and inability to wrinkle the forehead.

### DISCUSSION

Bell's palsy is a diagnosis of exclusion. Other causes of facial nerve palsy include Lyme disease, tumors of the temporal bone, Ramsay Hunt syndrome, and acoustic neuromas. The onset of Bell's palsy is sudden, and the symptoms can range from weakness to complete paralysis for more than a week; however, sensations are intact. It is usually preceded by a viral infection but not always.

Associated symptoms may include pain behind the ear, ipsilateral loss of taste sensation, decreased or increased lacrimation, and hyperacusis. Majority of the patients recover within a few months. However, if the symptoms do not resolve in 6 months, laboratory studies, imaging studies, or

# Neurology

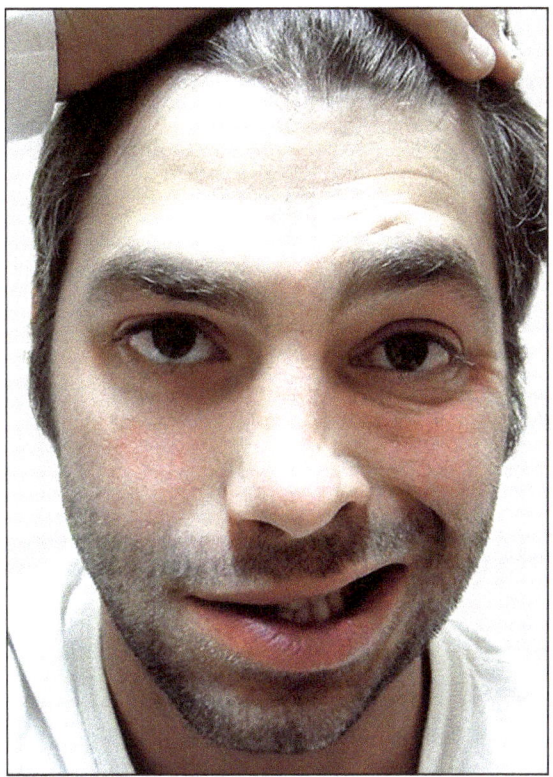

**Fig. 1:** Male patient with Bell's palsy.
*Courtesy:* Wikimedia.org.

motor-nerve conduction studies should be considered. Bell's palsy is secondary to complete destruction of the facial nerve nucleus (lower motor neuron lesion) itself or its facial nerves' branches, whereas upper motor neurons of the motor cortex or connection between cortex and facial nucleus show contralateral paralysis of lower face only.

Keep in mind that Bell's palsy is a diagnosis of exclusion. First rule out a cerebrovascular event. If any nerve is involved other than the facial nerve (CN7) then Bell's palsy is ruled out. A patient with symptoms similar to Bell's palsy but with sparing of the forehead is concerning for acute stroke. Also, since the chorda tympani exits, CN7 before the inflammation of the nerve taste is typically spared.

## TREATMENT
- Use an eye patch while sleeping to prevent corneal drying and abrasions
- Frequent application of artificial tears every hour while awake

- Massaging the weakened muscles might improve muscle tone
- Corticosteroids and antiviral agents, such as acyclovir (oral) should be started as soon as possible or at least within a week of the onset of the symptoms.
- If medical therapy is unsuccessful, surgical decompression of the facial nerve might be helpful.

## FURTHER READING

1. Bell's Palsy Fact Sheet. National Institute of Neurological Disorders and Stroke. https://www.ninds.nih.gov/Disorders/Patient-Caregiver-Education/Fact-Sheets/Bells-Palsy-Fact-Sheet. Accessed July 18, 2018.
2. Lyme Disease. Centers for Disease Control and Prevention. https://www.cdc.gov/lyme/signs_symptoms/. Published October 26, 2016. Accessed July 18, 2018.

## CASE STUDY 45: SEIZURE DISORDERS IN CHILDREN

## CASE HISTORY

A 5-year-old child is presented in the emergency room (ER) with a chief complaint of seizures which were tonic clonic, lasted <5 min, and were bilateral. On examination, vital signs are temperature of 104°F, heart rate 120 bpm, blood pressure 80/30 mm Hg, and oxygen saturation 99% on room air. This is the first episode and the parents were terrified.

### Family History

Father had similar episode when he was a child.

## DIAGNOSTIC WORKUP

- Septic workup is done.
- Blood, urine culture, and complete blood count (CBC) were negative.

## TREATMENT

Conservative treatment is followed. Ice packs and Tylenol are given to control fever and diazepam suppository is also given. The child is >18 months, so lumbar puncture is not advisable. No computed tomography (CT) is required. Anticonvulsive drugs are not indicated for simple seizure. Electroencephalogram (EEG) is advised on an outpatient basis.

## DISCUSSION
### Differential Diagnosis of Seizures in Children
- Fever/febrile seizures
- Epidural and subdural infections
- Meningitis or encephalitis
- Epidural hematoma
- Sepsis or bacteremia
- *Epilepsy type*: Rolandic (or benign focal epilepsy with centrotemporal spikes) are the most common in children. The diagnosis can be confirmed when the characteristic centrotemporal spikes are seen on electroencephalography (EEG). Typically, high-voltage spikes followed by slow waves are seen. The prognosis for rolandic seizures is invariably excellent, with probably <2% risk of developing absence seizures. Given the benign nature of the condition and the low seizure frequency, treatment is often unnecessary.

Seizures in children are commonly seen in emergency department. Definition of status epilepticus has changed. Previously, we used to define status epilepticus as continuous seizures lasting >30 min or more than two sequential seizures without full recovery of consciousness in between the seizures. Now, we agree that a shorter period of seizure activity can also result in neuronal injury and that seizure activity is unlikely to terminate by itself after 5 min. A duration of longer than 5 min is the criteria for status epilepticus especially if the seizure type is generalized convulsive disorder which does not resolve spontaneously in 3–5 min. Our major goal in the ER is to provide rapid control of the seizure activity in order to prevent neurologic injury. In prehospital, status epilepticus intramuscular (IM) midazolam is equally effective as compared to intravenous (IV) administration of benzodiazepines.

In conclusion, for subjects in status epilepticus, IM midazolam is as safe and effective as IV lorazepam for the hospital seizure physician.
*Courtesy:* National Institute of Neurological Disorders and Stroke and others and Clinical Trials.gov.

### Infantile Spasms
A more subtle form of pediatric seizure that occurs primarily in infants <1 year of age. These seizures are difficult to diagnose as they typically present as brief episodes of partial muscle twitches accompanied by an inability to make eye contact and interact with the parent rather than a full on tonic clonic seizure. Symptoms most commonly occur in clusters when the infant awakes and changes in respiratory rate and heart rate may occur. Due to the

risk of chronic developmental disability in untreated children, infants presenting with these puzzling symptoms often warrant pediatric neurology consult or admission for video EEG monitoring and follow up with an experienced pediatric neurologist.

## Intravenous Keppra Levetiracetam

Keppra can also be effective for acute status epilepticus treatment which is frequently given by neurologists in acute seizure management. A Keppra load may be given along with benzodiazepines in order to suppress status epilepticus. Benzodiazepines are still the recommended first-line therapy. Intravenous valproic acid (VPA) can be used effectively also for acute seizure control, safely in children. Intravenous VPA is safe and effective in treating acute seizures in emergency department for children. The dose of midazolam is for IM use is 0.2 mg/kg of body weight. Atomized or buccal midazolam can be given in a dose of 0.2–0.5 mg/kg of body weight. When there is a great risk of permanent neurologic injury without delay, it is better to use intraosseous line placement after giving IM, nasal or buccal medication (Versed) when IV line is not possible.

### Background

Early termination of prolonged seizures with intravenous administration of benzodiazepines improves outcomes. For faster and more reliable administration, paramedics increasingly use an intramuscular route.
**Question:** If intravenous access is not available, how good are intramuscular benzodiazepines?
**Answer:** Intramuscular midazolam was shown in this trial to be an acceptable alternative route for acute seizure control.

## FURTHER READING

1. ⟨http://www.epmonthly.com/cme/current-issue/pediatric-seizures-/1/⟩.
2. Silbergleit R, Durkalski V, Lowenstein D, et al. Intramuscular versus intravenous therapy for prehospital status epilepticus. N Engl J Med 2012;366(7):591-600.
3. ⟨http://en.wikipedia.org/wiki/Rolandic_epilepsy⟩.

# CASE STUDY 46: SEIZURE DISORDERS IN ADULTS

## CASE HISTORY

A 48-year-old male patient was brought to the emergency department (ED) after being involved in a motor vehicle accident. His vehicle rolled over multiple times and landed in a ditch; the airbag did not deploy. The paramedics noted severe damage to the front of the car. Vital Signs (VS): BP = 110/85 mm Hg, HR = 140 bpm, $R$ = 24 breaths/min, saturating 98% on 15 L via nonrebreather mask. During transport to the ED, the paramedics noted a seizure involving tonic clonic movements of all four extremities. Lorazepam 2 mg IV was given and resolved the seizure. Upon arrival, the Glasgow coma scale score was 8 and blood sugar was 75 mg/dL. Pupils were 3 mm and reactive. Normal tone was present in all four extremities and reflexes were 2 + throughout. The remainder of the examination was unremarkable. A computed tomography (CT) head was performed and revealed a large right frontal intraparenchymal hemorrhage. The Emergency MD then spoke to the neurosurgeon and the OR was prepared for the arrival of the patient.

## DISCUSSION

Traumatic brain injury results from direct or indirect forces to the brain. Direct injury is caused by the force of an object striking the head or penetrating injury. Indirect injuries result from acceleration and deceleration forces that result in the movement of the brain within the skull.

## MANAGEMENT

- Initially stabilize the patient by following Advanced Trauma Life Support (ATLS) guidelines and administer 100% oxygen.
- A patient with Glasgow Coma Scale of 8 or lower warrants orotracheal intubation for airway control.
- Slow and sustained careful blood pressure monitoring is necessary. It should be maintained around a mean arterial pressure (MAP) >90 mm Hg. If hypertensive, 25-30% reduction of MAP may be achieved carefully.
- As an intracranial bleed is identified, an immediate neurosurgery consult is obtained and the trauma team is alerted and awaiting the patient's arrival in the receiving hospital.
- For signs of increased intracranial pressure (ICP), elevate the head of the bed to 15-30°. Maintain MAP > 90 mm Hg and maintain adequate arterial oxygenation.
- For ICP, hyperventilate to maintain a $p\text{CO}_2$ 26-30 mm Hg; however, do not hyperventilate too aggressively as this increases the risk of cerebral ischemia. A mannitol 0.25-1 g/kg intravenous (IV) bolus may be started; however, the effects take up to 30 min to decrease ICP.

Other first line treatments include sedation, CSF drainage, osmotic diuretics. If initial attempts to decrease ICP fail, patient may require emergency decompression by trephination which is rarely done these days unless

neurosurgical intervention is not available and the patient cannot be safely transferred
- For seizure prophylaxis, use anticonvulsants in consult with neurosurgery. May use benzodiazepines, or fosphenytoin with a loading dose of 18–20 mg/kg
- Use prophylactic antibiotics such as ceftriaxone 1 g IV q12 h if patient has basilar skull fracture or penetrating injury.

## FURTHER READING

1. Ma OJ, Cline D. Emergency Medicine Manual. New York: McGraw-Hill, Medical Pub. Division; 2004.

# CASE STUDY 47: AUTONOMIC DYSREFLEXIA

## CASE HISTORY

An 18-year-old teen athlete who was driving with other teens was involved in a motor vehicle crash, hitting a pole. He unfortunately sustained upper spinal cord injury at the T6 level. He is currently wheelchair bound with loss of bladder and bowel control. He uses straight catheterization of the bladder every 4–6 h, for relief. The patient presents with sudden onset severe headache, blurring of vision, and vomiting along with profuse sweating and the redness (erythema) in the upper extremities. His heart rate is 55 bpm and his blood pressure (BP) is 220/115 mm Hg.

## DISCUSSION

Autonomic hyperreflexia is characterized by the sudden onset of headache and hypertension in a patient with a lesion above the T6 spinal level. There may be associated bradycardia, sweating, dilated pupils, blurred vision, nasal stuffiness, flushing, or piloerection. It usually occurs several months after the injury and has an incidence as high as 85% in quadriplegic patients. Frequently, it subsides within 3 years of injury, but it can recur at any time. Bowel and bladder distention are common causes. Hypertension is the major concern because of associated seizures and cerebral hemorrhage.

Autonomic hyperreflexia is associated with spinal cord injury patients (usually T6 or above) sometime after initial injury:
- Vasculature has adapted to loss of sympathetic tone.
- BP normalized
- Loss vasodilatory response to increased BP.
  Autonomic nervous system reflexively responds with arteriolar spasm.
- Increased BP

- Stimulates peripheral nervous system (PNS)
- Results in bradycardia
- Peripheral and visceral vessels unable to dilate.

## CLINICAL PRESENTATION

- Paroxysmal hypertension
- Headache
- Blurred vision
- Sweating and flushed skin above level of injury
- Increased nasal congestion
- Nausea
- Bradycardia
- Distended bladder or rectum.

Autonomic hyperreflexia is a reaction of the autonomic (involuntary) nervous system to overstimulation. This reaction may include high BP, change in heart rate, skin color changes (pallor, redness, blue-gray skin color), and excessive sweating.

## CAUSES

The most common cause of autonomic hyperreflexia is spinal cord injury (SCI) because the types of stimulation that are tolerated by healthy people can create an excessive response from the nervous system of a SCI patient.

Other causes include medication side effects, use of stimulants such as cocaine or amphetamines, Guillain–Barré syndrome, subarachnoid hemorrhage, severe head trauma, and other brain injuries.

A number of conditions have symptoms as autonomic hyperreflexia but have a different cause:
- Carcinoid syndrome is a disease caused by abnormalities of hormone-producing cells in the lungs and the gut
- Neuroleptic malignant syndrome is a condition which causes muscle stiffness, high fever, and drowsiness. This is caused by combinations of certain medications
- Serotonin syndrome is caused by an abnormal release of serotonin from the brain
- Thyroid storm is caused by production of too much thyroid hormone.

## EXAMINATIONS AND TESTS

### Signs

Signs often seen on examination include:
- Dilated pupils
- Flushed (red) skin above the level of SCI

- High BP
- Bradycardia or tachycardia.

### Tests

Tests may include
- Blood and urine tests
- Brain pictures including head CT scan or magnetic resonance imaging (MRI)
- Electrocardiography (ECG)
- Lumbar puncture
- Spine pictures, particularly MRI
- Tilt-table testing
- Toxicology screening to look for stimulants
- X-ray.

## TREATMENT

This condition is life-threatening, so it is important to quickly identify and treat the problem. A person with symptoms of autonomic hyperreflexia should sit up with their head raised and tight clothing should be removed. Treatment will be based on the cause. If medications or drugs are causing the symptoms, the drugs must be stopped and any underlying illness must be treated.

If a slowed heart rate is causing the symptoms, anticholinergic medications may be helpful. Very high BP must be treated quickly but carefully. A sudden severe drop in BP can occur and can cause further issues. Commonly used emergency drugs for high BP include nifedipine, nitroglycerin, phenoxybenzamine hydrochloride, mecamylamine, and diazoxide.

A pacemaker may be needed for certain unstable heart-related situations.

## PROGNOSIS

Prognosis is dependent on the underlying cause. If medications are the cause, patients usually recover with withdrawal of the medication. If other factors are the cause, prognosis depends on the successful treatment of the underlying condition.

## COMPLICATIONS

Complications may occur as a result of medications used to treat the hyperreflexia. If the pulse rate drops severely, cardiac arrest can result.

Prolonged, severe high BP may cause seizures, ocular hemorrhage, stroke, or death.

## PREVENTION

Prevention of autonomic hyperreflexia includes avoiding medications that cause this condition or make it worse. In SCI patients, there are a number of steps to avoid this complication including avoiding letting the bladder become too full, keeping pain levels low, and practicing proper bowel care to avoid stool impaction.

## HISTORICAL CASE

Richard Marvin Hansen (Fig. 1) is a famous Canadian athlete, who was the final torchbearer in the Winter Olympics of 2010 and also spoke during its opening ceremony. When he was 15, he was riding with his friend in a pickup truck and the truck swerved and hit a tree. From this accident, he received an SCI. Now he runs the Rick Hansen Foundation, a nonprofit foundation, which has generated >$200 million for SCI-related programs. The goal is to effect the changes in clinical practice necessary to achieve the best possible outcome for victims of SCI.

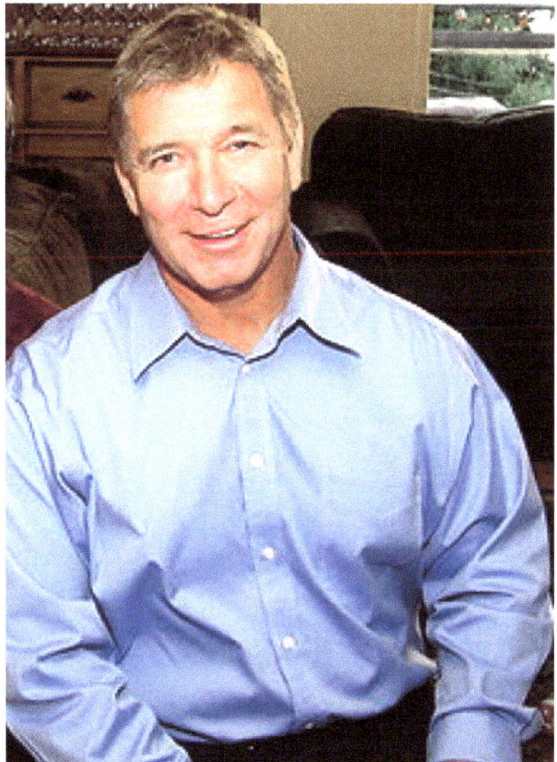

**Fig. 1:** Richard Marvin Hansen.

## FURTHER READING

1. http://www.ncbi.nlm.nih.gov/pmc/articles/PMC1743257.
2. http://en.wikipedia.org/wiki/Rick_Hansen.
3. Bycroft J. Autonomic dysreflexia: a medical emergency. Postgrad Med J. 2005;81(954):232-5.
4. Ediz L, Al B, Hiz O. An emergency medical situation in rehabilitation medicine: autonomic dysreflexia. J Acad Emerg Med. 2010;9(4):175-8.

# CHAPTER 7

# Endocrine

## CASE STUDY 48: THYROID STORM

*Remember the 4 Ps in the management of thyroid storm.*

—Badar M Zaheer

### CASE HISTORY

#### History of Present Illness

A 47-year-old Navajo native American female living on an Indian Reservation in Arizona is presented to the emergency department with her husband. She has chief complaint of fearfulness and a sudden onset of feeling as though her heart is going to explode out of her chest. **She is also febrile, tachycardic, and tachypneic.** She is also presented with difficulty in speaking due to a stiff jaw.

#### Past Medical History

She was suffering from hypertension since age of 40 years. She was being treated with hydrochlorothiazide (HCTZ) tablets 25 mg/day for the past 7 years with no renal organ involved.

#### Medications

- Daily HCTZ, per oral (PO), 25 mg
- Traditional indigenous herbal supplements.

### PHYSICAL EXAMINATION

#### General Appearance

Patient is apprehensive, delirious, obtunded, anxious, in distress, restless, and irritable to staff and family members. Patient vomits and has diarrhea several times during the encounter.

## Vital Signs

Her vital signs are temperature 104°F, blood pressure 210/110 mm Hg, heart rate 180 bpm, respiratory rate 30 breaths/min, oxygen saturation 99%, height 66 in, weight 160 lb, and body mass index 25.8 kg/m².

## Head and Neck

- No evidence of trauma, tumor, facial edema, carotid bruits, or thyroid nodules
- Diffuse goiter seen
- *Mental status*: Delirious, obtunded, anxious, and irritable. No head injury
- *Pupillary size*: 3 mm, symmetric, reactive to light, and accommodation. Sclera is icteric with dry oral mucus.
- Patient has rigidity of the jaw and has difficulty and hesitancy in articulate due to discomfort.
- Fine silky hair.

## Cardiac Examination

- Point of maximal impulse is palpated at the left fifth intercostal space at the point of intersection with the left midclavicular line.
- Heart auscultated at apex and base tachycardic, irregular rhythm, and forceful impulse.
- *Heart sounds*: S4 gallop, S1, S2, and prominent systolic flow murmur.

## Pulmonary Examination

- No wheezes, rales, or rhonchi
- *No evidence of consolidation*: No bronchial breath sounds or egophony
- *No increased work of breathing*: No retraction, no accessory muscle use
- Abdominal breathing and tachypnea.

## Abdominal Examination

Negative.

## Neurologic Examination

- Obtunded, apprehensive, irritable, and anxious
- Intact cranial nerves II–XII; difficulty in opening jaw to test masseter muscle is noted
- Sensation, reflex, cerebellar function found intact.

## Laboratory Tests

- *Thyroid*: Free T4 levels are elevated and thyroid stimulating hormone (TSH) levels are reduced.

- CBC and BMP are within normal limits
- EKG shows sinus tachycardia.

## DISCUSSION

- A thyroid storm is a rare but life-threatening clinical scenario that is caused by severe thyrotoxicosis. Most cases are caused by an acute event such as surgery, infection, trauma, parturition, or excessive iodine intake.
- Thyroid storm can also manifest in patients with long-standing untreated hyperthyroidism, it can be the initial presentation of a thyroid disorder such as toxic multinodular goiter, solitary toxic adenoma, or Graves disease.
- Most patients with thyrotoxicosis will have hyperpyrexia; therefore, a normal temperature in the context of thyroid storm may indicate a comorbid infection.
- If you suspect thyroid storm with congestive heart failure, always obtain an echocardiogram prior to administering beta-blockers. If the echo shows the CHF is secondary to high-output failure, you can still use beta-blockers with caution.

## IMPRESSION

*Thyroid storm*: Patient seemed to have had hyperthyroidism that did not receive medical attention and the recent upper respiratory infection has precipitated the condition.

## DIFFERENTIAL DIAGNOSIS

- Hypertensive crisis
- Hypertensive emergency
- Acute pulmonary edema
- Heat stroke
- Malignant hyperthermia
- Sepsis/septic shock
- Sympathomimetic toxicity
- Tachyarrhythmia
- Pheochromocytoma.

## TREATMENT

### Supportive Therapy

- Intravenous (IV) normal saline, 200 cm$^3$/h
- IV dextrose 5% in 0.45% saline, 200 cm$^3$/h
- IV Glucocorticoids (steroids) are given

- Oxygen is provided, cooling blankets are used
- Management can be summarized by remembering the 3 Ps and 2 Ss:

    P—Propranolol to reduce β-adrenergic symptoms and quell peripheral conversion of T4 to T3.

    P—Propylthiouracil (PTU) to reduce thyroid hormone synthesis and also assist propranolol in decreasing peripheral conversion of T4 to T3. It is advised to wait 1 h before giving **Lugol's solution in order for the PTU to prevent further thyroid hormone synthesis.**

    P—Potassium iodide to reduce hormone release S.

    P—Prednisone (steroids) to decrease peripheral T4 to T3 conversion.
- Supportive care should always be provided as necessary.

## Medication

- PTU × 100 mg/2 h (antithyroid drug) or 20 mg of methimazole every 4–6 h, orally, or via nasogastric tube (the high doses if antithyroid medication are justified due to the high risk of mortality associated with thyroid storm as well as the reduced intestinal absorption that is likely in this patient population).
- Iodine (inhibit thyroid hormone release)
- Propranolol is given to control tachycardia, a 40 mg IV push or 60–80-mg orally is recommended with close monitoring of heart rate
- Dexamethasone IV 4 mg × 3 (inhibit prostaglandin H release; impair peripheral T4 to T3 conversion; provide adrenal support) alternatively 100 mg/8 h of IV hydrocortisone can be given to patients with life-threatening thyrotoxicosis.

For the rare patients with contraindications to taking thionamides (previous effects of agranulocytosis or hepatotoxicity when taking thionamides, or because of drug allergy), surgery is the treatment of choice after being stabilized and treated with beta-blockers, glucocorticoids, bile acid sequestrants, and iodine.

## FOLLOW-UP

The patient was transferred to another hospital after being stabilized, and a follow-up call confirmed that the patient survived and was transferred to a medical floor after being 24 h in the intensive care unit.

Further follow-up indicates antithyroid agent was stopped 10 days prior to treatment and following radioactive iodine treatment. She was then stabilized and put on daily levothyroxine after radioactive ablation therapy. She is scheduled for a full physical examination in 2 weeks.

## CASE STUDY 49: DIABETIC KETOACIDOSIS

## CASE HISTORY

### Basic Information
Patient is a 15-year-old Caucasian male.

### History of Present Illness
A 15-year-old confused white male is brought to the emergency room (ER) on Friday night by his parents who state that the patient suffers from anorexia, profound nausea, repeated vomiting, epigastric pain, and shortness of breath for almost 24 h. Parents report starting early this week because patient had an incredible increase in appetite and complained of extreme thirst and increased volume of urination during the night.

The patient looks direly ill as he enters the ER; his skin and mucous membranes look extremely dry. His respirations are labored. He has decreased skin turgor, decreased reflexes, and characteristic acetone like breath odor.

*Laboratory results:*
- Glucose: 850
- Sodium: 125
- Potassium: 4.5
- Bicarbonate: 5
- BUN: 30
- pH: 7.1
- $PCO_2$ (mm Hg) 17.

## DISCUSSION

This clinical presentation is typical of diabetic ketoacidosis. It is a metabolic emergency. Delay in treatment may result increase morbidity and mortality. Diabetic ketoacidosis (DKA) may present as an initial presentation of type 1 diabetes in 25% of cases. Majority of the cases are of type 1 diabetes, but some patients with type 2 diabetes may also present with DKA under severe physiologic distress. Most of the patients will present with the classical symptoms of polyuria, polydipsia, polyphagia, and fatigue. Other may present with respiratory difficulty because of metabolic acidosis. Some others may present with idiopathic symptoms such as severe abdominal pain. The precipitating factors are usually infection, stress, travel, dehydration. Some patients may present with altered sensorium and history is unobtainable. The hallmark of DKA is a combination of hyperglycemia, elevated anion gap, and serum bicarbonate level below 20 mEq/L. Usually, there is no correlation between the severity of hyperglycemia and the severity of ketoacidosis. Ketones in the serum and the blood and urine will be positive.

## MANAGEMENT

As the name itself indicates, DKA is diabetes (hyperglycemia) + ketosis + acidosis (metabolic). Except in the rare cases of anuric patient, the absence of ketones in the urine reliably excludes the diagnosis of DKA. Patients in DKA can have significant fluid deficits, sometimes up to 5–10 L. Shock is fairly common and must be managed right away with crystalloid infusion to prevent organ damage. Adults with clinical shock should receive an initial 2 L bolus of normal saline with frequent reassessments. In children, shock is treated with 20 mL/kg of normal saline. Although there is a possibility of overhydrating that can present substantial complications later in the course of treatment, rectifying shock is a more concern. If shock is not treated right away, it will contribute to severe acidosis.

### Insulin

- 0.1 U/kg intravenous (IV) push, then 1 L/kg/h by continuous infusion. Decrease dose rate 50% when serum $HCO_3$ rises above 16 mEq/L
- Do not try intramuscular injections which are painful and less reliably absorbed when the patient is in shock. The combination of treatment of rehydration and insulin will usually lower serum glucose much faster than ketones are cleared. In any event, insulin infusion should continue until the anion gap returns to normal. When the serum glucose falls between 200 and 300 mg/dL (11.1–16.7 mmol/L), dextrose infusion should be added to prevent hypoglycemia. Insulin binds to IV tubing, so a thorough flush with a drip solution is necessary.

### Fluids

Start with 0.9% NS, 1 L/h for the first 2 h. Follow with 0.45% saline at 250–500 mL/h. Total fluid deficit is usually 50–100 mL/kg. Simply reversing shock with normal saline and then infusion of half normal saline at 2–3× the maintenance dose is usually sufficient.

### Potassium

Usually, the potassium deficit is quite large. But the serum potassium may still show low, normal, or even high. If potassium is initially elevated, look and treat for hyperkalemia based on the EKG findings. You can continue giving fluids without potassium until the serum potassium returns normal.

If the initial potassium is normal or low, potassium can be given immediately. Magnesium supplementation may be necessary sometimes to help the patient to retain potassium.

## Phosphate

Usually, phosphate supplementation is not required and has little impact. But, if the phosphate depletion is severe enough where it falls below 1 mg/dL, then it may be necessary for replacement therapy. Recommended dose is 7.7 mg/kg over 4 h.

## Sodium Bicarbonate

Causes more harm than good. Supplementation is not recommended regardless of the severity.

## Pathophysiology

- Severe insulin insufficiency resulting in decreased glucose uptake leading to hyperglycemia and osmotic diuresis which results in electrolyte depletion, dehydration, and acidosis
- *Increased proteolysis*: Increased nitrogen loss and increase in amino acids leading to gluconeogenesis and glycogenolysis resulting in hyperglycemia
- Lipolysis leading to increase in glycerol and free fatty acid levels.
  - Glycerol contributing to gluconeogenesis and glycogenolysis
  - Increased free fatty acids cause ketogenesis which leads to ketonemia, then ketonuria and finally, acidosis.

## Findings in DKA (Table 1)

- Leukocytosis without toxic granulations, secondary to release of stress hormones
- Hemoconcentration secondary to dehydration, if hematocrit (HCT) <35% of suspected blood loss
- Serum amylase elevation in 40%–80% cases; no relation to severity, morbidity, or mortality
- *Renal amylase/creatinine clearance ratio*: Raised without clinical symptoms of acute pancreatitis
- Serum lipase: Normal
- Abnormal values for SGOT, SGPT, lactate dehydrogenase (LDH), and other liver enzymes in 33% cases
- No correlation between serum hepatic enzymes levels and severity of abdominal symptoms
- Reversible hepatocellular damage, sufficient to allow release of cytosolic enzymes
- Fatty infiltration of liver and reduced hepatic perfusion may contribute.

**Table 1:** Features of diabetic ketoacidosis and hyperosmolar hyperglycemic nonketotic state.

| Characteristics | Diabetic ketoacidosis | Hyperosmolar hyperglycemic nonketotic state |
|---|---|---|
| Type | DM 1 | DM 2 |
| Age at onset | 15–30 | 50–70 |
| Precipitating factor | Acute illness, initial presentation for new onset DM 1 | Chronic/major illness, inadequate insulin dosage, CVA, MI, sepsis |
| Blood glucose levels (mg/dL) | 200–300 | 600–1,000 (can be higher) |
| Ketosis | Present | Absent |
| Insulin levels | Low | Normal to high |
| Signs and symptoms | Kussmaul respirations, acetone (fruity) breath, emesis, abdominal pain, dyspnea, polydipsia, polyuria | Confusion, lethargy, polyuria, polydipsia, dyspnea, altered mental status |
| Water loss (liter) | 3–5 | 5–10 |
| Osmolality | <350 mOsm/kg | >350 mOsm/kg |
| Mortality | 5–10% | 40–60% |

## CASE STUDY 50: SYNDROME OF INAPPROPRIATE SECRETION OF ANTIDIURETIC HORMONE

Suspect syndrome of inappropriate antidiuretic hormone (ADH) (SIADH) in any patient with **hyponatremia**, hyposmolality, and a high urine osmolality (above 100 mOsm/kg).

### CASE HISTORY

A 70-year-old male is presented to the emergency department (ED) with significant lethargy. Patient is unable to answer questions but family informs that recently he has lost a lot of weight and has not been eating. He has been coughing more than usual and the sputum occasionally contains blood. They have been trying to get him to see a doctor, but he has been refusing. This morning when his son went to visit him at his home where he normally lives by himself, his son found him in this confused state and immediately called emergency medical services (EMS). Patient is minimally responsive and oriented only to person. Pupils are equal and reactive. Patient withdraws to pain in all four extremities. Patient is afebrile, and his blood pressure is 100/75 mm Hg, pulse rate 101 bpm, respiratory rate 22 breaths/min, and oxygen saturation level remained 93% on room air with administration of 2 L oxygen via nasal cannula.

## Laboratory Test
- Na$^+$ ↓ 120
- K$^+$ 4.7 mEq/L
- Bicarbonate (HCO$_3$) 35 mEq/L
- Serum osmolality 265 mOsm/kg (normal range 275–290)
- Urine osmolality 390 mOsm/kg (normal range >800 mOsm/kg).

## DISCUSSION

The SIADH secretion is a syndrome of hyponatremia due to inappropriate or increased secretion of ADH wherein water is retained causing hyponatremia, concentrated urine >100 mOsm/L in the face of hypotonic plasma <260 mOsm/L. The key to understanding the pathophysiology, signs, symptoms, and treatment of SIADH is the awareness that the hyponatremia is a result of an excess of water rather than a deficiency of sodium.

Common etiologies of SIADH include insults to the central nervous system such as stroke, hemorrhage, infection, and trauma. With an aging population and with polypharmacy becoming the norm it is important to rule out less common causes of hyponatremia and SIADH. Particular attention should be paid to patients with a history of lung, head and neck cancer, epilepsy, or psychiatric disorders who may be on cyclophosphamide, selective serotonin reuptake inhibitor (SSRIs), carbamazepine, or oxcarbazepine. Both have been shown to increase sensitivity of hypothalamic osmoreceptors, renal ADH receptors and upregulate the expression of aquaporin channels in the medullary collecting ducts—all of which result in increased water retention and total body water.

Recently, it has also been shown that a genetically based increased sensitivity of the vasopressin-2 (V2) receptor to ADH can result in a picture of SIADH with normal level of ADH but otherwise asymptomatic hyponatremia, and elevated osmolality of urine. These patients are often discovered incidentally with routine blood tests.

Lastly, be aware that postsurgical patients and those with severe acute infections—pulmonary disease including tuberculosis, pneumonia, and meningitis may present with a picture of SIADH.

## SIGNS AND SYMPTOMS

Anorexia, nausea, headache, vomiting, altered mental status, and seizure activity may present in acute cases depending on the severity of hyponatremia like confusion, disorientation, delirium, generalized muscle weakness, myoclonus, tremor, asterixis, hyporeflexia, ataxia, dysarthria, Cheyne-Stokes respiration, generalized seizures, and coma. Chronic hyponatremia rarely causes any acute symptoms. Symptoms may not correlate with the severity of the condition.

## DIAGNOSIS

In the absence of a single laboratory test to confirm the diagnosis, SIADH is best defined by the classic Bartter–Schwartz criteria, which can be summarized as follows:
- Hyponatremia with corresponding hypo-osmolality
- Continued renal exertion of sodium
- Urine less than maximally dilute
- Absence of clinical evidence of volume depletion
- Absence of other causes of hyponatremia
- Correction of hyponatremia by fluid restriction.

The patient's volume should be assessed clinically to help rule out the presence of hypovolemia. Imaging studies that may be considered include the following:
- Chest radiography (for detection of an underlying pulmonary cause of SIADH, like small cell carcinoma of lung).
- Computed tomography or magnetic resonance imaging of the head (for detection of cerebral edema occurring as a complication of SIADH, for identification of a CNS disorder responsible for SIADH, or for helping to rule out other potential causes of a change in neurologic status).

## MANAGEMENT

The ideal method of threating SIADH is to treat the underlying disease or cause, if possible. However, in the ED setting it is often most appropriate to focus on initial therapy to raise the serum sodium, especially in symptomatic patients. Patients with persistent SIADH require prolonged therapy and follow up.

Examples of underlying disease and other causes of SIADH include hormone replacement in adrenal insufficiency which can cause an overly rapid correction of hyponatremia, or hypothyroidism. Infections such as meningitis, pneumonia, or tuberculosis can be the cause of hyponatremia. Certain drugs, such as SSRIs, and chlorpropamide, may cause SIADH as a side effect.

Initial therapy for SIADH in the ED and the rapidity of correction of hyponatremia depend on the following:
- Degree of hyponatremia

Mild—Only water restriction <500 mL/day is enough and V2 receptor antagonist if needed.

If the sodium level is below 115 mEq/L or associated with seizures, give 3% normal saline 1 mL/kg/h to raise the sodium concentration by not >2 mEq/L/h and not >8–10 mEq/L/h in the first 24 h, to avoid central pontine myelinolysis (CPM).

If the duration of hyponatremia is unknown and the patient is asymptomatic, it is reasonable to presume chronic SIADH. In an emergency setting, aggressive treatment of hyponatremia should always be weighed against the risk of including CPM. Such treatment is warranted as follows: Second-line drugs furosemide 40 mg intravenous (IV) and demeclocycline 300–600 mg.

Avoid fluid restriction in patients with sub arachnoid hemorrhage as the resulting hypotension encourages cerebral vasospasm, alternatively, hyponatremic patients with SAH should be treated with hypertonic saline to preserve cerebral perfusion and prevent cerebral edema. It is also appropriate to initiate treatment at 20 mL/h and adjust based on serum sodium measurements every 6 h.

## FURTHER READING

1. Paul Tran T. Emergency complications of malignancy. In: Emergency medicine manual, 6th ed. McGraw-Hill Professional, 2003.
2. Steven SA, Elizabeth DA. Step-up to medicine. 2nd edn. Philadelphia, PA: Lippincott Williams and Wilkins; 2005. p. 169-70.
3. Yoo M, Bediako EO, Akca O. Syndrome of inappropriate antidiuretic hormone (SIADH) secretion caused by squamous cell carcinoma of the nasopharynx: case report. Clin Exp Otorhinolaryngol 2008;1(2):110-2.

# CASE STUDY 51: ADRENAL CRISIS/ADDISONIAN CRISIS

## CASE HISTORY

A 45-year-old man is brought to the emergency department (ED) by his wife with chief complaints of confusion and delirium. He is also been having nausea, vomiting, weight loss, and looks extremely dehydrated. He had symptoms of upper respiratory tract infection preceding this ED visit as described by his wife. Physical examination findings include a temperature of 98°F, blood pressure (BP) 68/40 mm Hg, heart rate 140 bpm, serum glucose of 34 mg/dL, and hyperpigmented skin.

## ASSESSMENT

The patient is experiencing acute adrenal insufficiency. Low serum glucose and BP are a result of low levels of glucocorticoids. The presence of hyperpigmentation of the skin is indicative of high serum levels of adrenocorticotropic hormone (ACTH) and thus primary adrenal insufficiency.

## DIAGNOSTIC TESTS

Primary laboratories should include basal ACTH, cortisol, and renin levels in addition to electrolytes. These basic laboratories often suffice to determine the physiological level of insufficiency.

It is vital to establish whether insufficiency is primary or secondary as that will dictate further workup and the likelihood of a given pathology. For example, primary insufficiency is most likely due to autoimmune adrenalitis or tuberculosis infiltration and destruction of the adrenal glands. Secondary insufficiency, however, should raise the suspicion of a pituitary etiology or acute withdrawal of exogenous corticosteroid intake.

## EMERGENCY ROOM CARE AND DISPOSITION

If suspicion for acute adrenal crisis is high, then laboratories should be drawn, but one should not wait on results to begin treatment. Treatment will consist of gaining access with a large bore intravenous (IV) and rapid infusion of 2–3 L of isotonic saline or 5% dextrose in saline followed by 4 mg of dexamethasone over 5 min. Frequent hemodynamic monitoring should be performed with attention to potential fluid overload. 4 mg dexamethasone should be readministered every 12 h. Dexamethasone is preferable because it does not interfere with cortisol and ACTH levels; however, if unavailable, 100 mg of hydrocortisone may be used and should be administered every 6 h.

### Supportive Measures should be Provided as Necessary

Once patient is stabilized, the etiology and appropriate workup for the adrenal crisis must be initiated. Isotonic saline may continue to be infused over 1–2 days. 0.1 mg fludrocortisone PO should be started once IV is stopped if there was an associated electrolyte imbalance and patient has a primary adrenal insufficiency. Oral glucocorticoid treatment should also begin once patient is stabilized.

This particular patient underwent fluid resuscitation with rapid administration of 2 L of normal saline. 50 mL of 50% dextrose was administered via IV push and hydrocortisone 300 mg IV. Patient subsequently became more awake, alert and stable. On examination, BP was 105/50 mm Hg, serum glucose 72 mg/dL, serum sodium ($Na^+$) 124 mEq/L, and serum potassium ($K^+$) 5.5 mEq/L.

The goal of the treatment is to replace crystallite fluids, glucocorticoids, and mineralocorticoids. To correct volume, glucose and sodium deficits is our object.

Hydrocortisone 100–300 mg IV every 6–8 h is sufficient to provide glucocorticoids and mineralocorticoids.

## DISCUSSION

Adrenal crisis is a life-threatening emergency of adrenal insufficiency. They usually present in a state of shock or change in mental status.

The adrenal cortex of the adrenal glands produces a number of steroid hormones: aldosterone, glucocorticoids, and androgen hormones. Aldosterone is responsible for maintaining BP and to excrete excess serum $K^+$. Its secretion is stimulated by the renin–angiotensin pathway and high serum $K^+$. Glucocorticoids are responsible for maintaining serum glucose, potentiating vasoconstriction, inhibiting inflammatory responses, and are associated with memory formation and arousal. Glucocorticoid production is controlled by the hypothalamus–anterior-pituitary–ACTH pathway. Androgens are responsible for production of sex hormones (including testosterone and estrogen) and are responsible for sexual development and other complex functions.

Aldosterone and glucocorticoids are crucial to metabolism, BP control, and electrolyte balance and their absence is incompatible with life. For this reason, adrenal insufficiency will present with symptoms related to hormonal functions and must be quickly recognized.

Adrenal insufficiency is characterized by underproduction of glucocorticoids. Glucocorticoids maintain serum glucose by stimulating gluconeogenesis, fatty acid metabolism, and amino acids breakdown. They also inhibit insulin sensitivity and thus the uptake of glucose, hence further increases serum glucose. Glucocorticoids also maintain BP in conjunction with the sympathetic system by potentiating the vasoconstrictive effects of epinephrine and norepinephrine on blood vessels. When there are insufficient glucocorticoids, low serum glucose, hypotension, and reflex tachycardia are expected.

Glucocorticoids production is stimulated by ACTH, which is secreted by the anterior pituitary under the influence of hypothalamus. Serum ACTH therefore provides us with clues to the etiology of glucocorticoid insufficiency. In primary adrenal insufficiency, the adrenal glands themselves are the origin of the problem. Because hypothalamic–pituitary–adrenal axis is intact, the lack of negative-feedback by glucocorticoids stimulates ACTH production, which translates into high circulating ACTH. Moreover, because ACTH shares homology with melanocyte stimulating hormone (MSH), the patients often present with hyperpigmentation of the skin. Primary adrenal insufficiency can arise from gradual destruction of the glands. For example, Addison disease is characterized by autoimmune destruction of the adrenal glands. Tuberculosis (TB) can disseminate to the glands. While rare in the United States, TB is the leading cause of adrenal insufficiency in the third-world countries. Because these diseases tend to be chronic, prolonged excessive ACTH may lead to hyperpigmentation. Primary adrenal insufficiency can also occur acutely. For example, Waterhouse–Friderichsen syndrome is the hemorrhage of the adrenal glands following a meningococcal septicemia, or disseminated intravascular coagulation (DIC). In this case, hyperpigmentation is not observed as ACTH elevation is not prolonged.

In contrast, secondary adrenal insufficiency is caused by deficiency in ACTH. This may arise from lesions in either hypothalamus [lack of corticotropin-releasing hormone (CRH)] or pituitary. Motor vehicle accidents, Sheehan syndrome and tumor are just some potential causes of secondary adrenal insufficiency.

However, the most common cause of acute secondary adrenal insufficiency in the Western world is chronic exogenous steroids. Chronic use of synthetic steroids depresses ACTH secretion, thus decreasing the stimulus needed for glucocorticoid production. If the patient suddenly withdraws from steroid medications, the adrenal glands are unable to ramp up the production to compensate for the sudden drop of glucocorticoids. This sudden adrenal insufficiency or adrenal crisis can present with symptoms as described by the case history. To avoid adrenal insufficiency secondary to chronic steroid use, clinicians need to gradually taper down the dosage of patients' steroid medications before completely stopping steroid therapy.

Because adrenal cortex also produces aldosterone, aldosterone deficiency and associated hyperkalemia can occur in some forms of adrenal insufficiency. In Addison disease and Waterhouse–Friderichsen syndrome, the entire adrenal cortex is damaged. Therefore, one can expect symptoms of both glucocorticoid and aldosterone deficiency. On the other hand, secondary adrenal insufficiency is due to lack of ACTH, which mainly controls the production of glucocorticoids. As a result, only isolated glucocorticoid deficiency is manifested (Fig. 1).

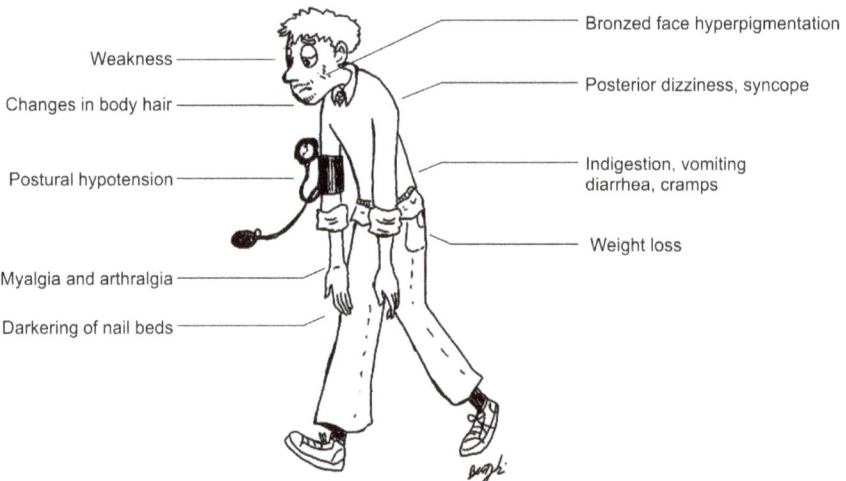

**Fig. 1:** Signs and symptoms in adrenal crisis.
*Courtesy:* Picture drawn by medical student, Bing Li, Chicago, USA (UIC-COM) specifically for 101 Clinical Cases in Emergency Room by Badar Zaheer, MD, Chicago, USA.

# CHAPTER 8

# Psychiatric Emergencies

## CASE STUDY 52: PANIC ATTACK

### CASE HISTORY

A 46-year-old male with no history of hypertension or high cholesterol is presented to the emergency room (ER). The patient's chief complaint is chest heaviness and left-arm pain that started early in the morning. He also complained of having shortness of breath at home. These symptoms lasted approximately 2 h. When they did not subside, he became very panicky. He started to breathe heavily, became lightheaded, and also had tingling around his mouth and fingertips. At this point, the patient felt like he was going to die and felt he should go to the ER. He presented to the emergency department (ED) with mild chest heaviness and pain that started again though his arm, neck, jaw, and back pain had gone away. The patient did not complain of nausea or emesis. He has been a half-pack per day smoker for the last 10 years. The patient's father had a heart attack when he was 55 years old. The patient eats spicy food and has a history of reflux. The patient does not have any headache, focal numbness, tingling, and weakness at time of presentation. He reports taking one baby aspirin at home earlier today. Serial electrocardiography (ECG) is done three times and shows normal sinus rhythm. Normal cardiac enzymes, creatine kinase (CK), creatine kinase-muscle and brain (CK-MB), and troponin are all within normal limits. The values of brain natriuretic peptide and D-dimer are also normal.

### DISCUSSION

Panic attack is a diagnosis of exclusion because the symptoms and signs mimic those of several potentially life-threatening emergency conditions like MI (myocardial infarction) and PE (pulmonary embolism). They are characterized by a surge of intense fear or discomfort. The fear reaches its climax very quickly (usually within minutes). While the patient is experiencing this fear, four or more of the following symptoms must also be observed within 10 min [according to the *Diagnostic and Statistical Manual of Mental Disorders* (DSM)-5]:[1]

- Palpitations, pounding heart, or accelerated heart rate
- Sweating
- Trembling or shaking
- Sensations of shortness of breath or smothering
- Feeling of choking
- Chest pain or discomfort
- Nausea or abdominal distress
- Feeling dizzy, unsteady, lightheaded, or faint
- Derealization (feelings of unreality) or depersonalization (being detached from oneself)
- Fear of losing control or going crazy
- Fear of dying
- Paresthesias (numbness or tingling sensations)
- Chills or hot flashes.

A panic attack that comes into the ER and is not stabilized or resolved often results in panic disorder. Panic disorder falls under the heading of anxiety disorders, which by definition are mental illnesses characterized by abnormal, pathological fear and anxiety. The DSM-5 definition for diagnosing panic disorder is as follows:[2]

(A) Both (1) and (2):
  1. Recurrent unexpected panic attacks
  2. At least one of the attacks has been followed by 1 month (or more) of one (or more) of the following:
     (a) Persistent concern about having additional attacks
     (b) Worry about the implications of the attack or its consequences (e.g., losing control, having a heart attack, "going crazy")
     (c) A significant change in behavior related to the attacks.
(B) The presence (or absence) of agoraphobia.
(C) The panic attacks are not due to the direct physiological effects of a substance (e.g. a drug abuse, a medication) or a general medical condition (e.g. hyperthyroidism).
(D) The panic attacks are not accounted for by other mental disorders, such as social phobia (e.g. occurring on exposure to feared social situations), specific phobia (e.g. on exposure to a specific phobic situation), obsessive–compulsive disorder (e.g. on exposure to dirt in someone with an obsession about contamination), posttraumatic stress disorder (e.g. in response to stimuli associated with a severe stressor), or separation anxiety disorder (e.g. in response to being away from home or close relatives).

When an ED doctor sees people like in the case above, the immediate response may be that the patient is having a heart attack. We can never assume that it is panic attack unless everything is ruled out. The initial treatment given to this patient is three baby aspirin and 1 in of nitroglycerine paste. The patient is admitted to rule out coronary syndrome, and only after the doctor had a chance to look at the chart did the symptoms appear to be more consistent with panic attack.

## TREATMENT

- First exclude life-threatening conditions
- Benzodiazepines as discussed below.

If the patient is in an acute episode, antianxiety medications (Xanax, Klonopin, Ativan) may help to alleviate symptoms and sedate the patient. Quick-acting benzodiazepines (lorazepam, alprazolam, clonazepam) may be used in addition to active support and assurance of safety.[2] The typical dose and route is 0.5-mg lorazepam given intravenously every 20 min until symptoms have subsided. The physician should remember to talk in a slow calm voice and sit down with the patient to help calm them down. A psychiatric referral is often given after the patient's acute symptoms have been relieved.

## REFERENCES

1. American Psychiatric Association. Symptoms of panic attacks. [online]. Available from http://www.psych.org/; 2012 [accessed August, 2012].
2. Domino F. The 5-minute Clinical Consult. 20th ed. Philadelphia, PA: Lippincott Williams and Wilkins; 2012. p. 952-3.

## CASE STUDY 53: PSYCHOSIS

*"One in every eight ER visits in 2007 involved either a diagnosis of a mental health or substance abuse condition."*

**—Agency for Healthcare Research and Quality**

## CASE HISTORY

A 60-year-old man who is a known, successful restaurant owner is brought to the emergency department (ED) by his family members for being isolated and suspicious of his wife having extramarital relations with another man. The man is suspecting his son to be a murderer, and the man thinks his son will murder him. He does not trust any of his family members and thinks they are stealing his property. The man often exclaims to his wife that "God has sent me here, and he told me you are stealing from me."

## DISCUSSION

Psychosis is typically seen as drastic changes in personality and a loss of contact with reality. This condition which commonly appears as the defining symptom of many mental disorders (schizophrenia, schizoaffective, delusional) is characterized by delusions and hallucinations. Auditory hallucinations are most commonly associated with psychiatric causes of psychosis, whereas visual hallucinations have organic cause. Impaired functioning and distorted view of reality may also be seen with classical cases of psychosis. Psychosis may be caused by psychological, social, and biological factors; the trick is figuring out which one is the culprit. Episodes may be caused by a variety of things not limited to alcohol, illegal drugs, brain tumor, some steroids, epilepsy, schizophrenia, and genetic abnormalities. Another possible factor that influences psychosis is migration. It has been found that people immigrating to other countries often have higher incidence of psychosis than natives.

When diagnosing psychosis, the physician should first rule out delirium, noting that psychosis should never have fluctuating consciousness or reduced clarity of awareness.[1] If biological and social factors are ruled out, diagnosis should be followed by a referral for psychological consultation to determine if another mental disorder is responsible.

Our ED physicians have limited resources on the evaluation and treatment of patients with mental health issues. American Association for Emergency Psychiatry (AAEP) is providing an online help for ER physicians. It may not be useful as a real-time quick reference guide, but nevertheless, it provides guidelines for psychiatric emergencies. Modified SAD PERSONS scale, a clinical decision-making tool, can evaluate the risk of suicide of a patient. For assessing the suicidal risk at the time of discharging a patient, this 10 question tool can be easily used by the ER physician. As the patient population in the ER for mental health condition increases, there is a greater need for developing a more standardized and a robust emergency residency program to treat and provide a proper treatment for patients with mental health issues.

## TREATMENT

*Note*: Before patients can receive antipsychotic medications, imagine and blood work must be drawn. The following tests should be obtained:
- Finger-stick glucose test is a must for altered mental status (AMS).
- CT scan non-contrast of the head for new-onset psychosis
- Urine drug screen
    - Obtain immediate EKG and troponin levels for cocaine abuse
- Complete metabolic panel
- Complete blood count to assess for sepsis
- Thyroid-stimulating hormone level
- Vitamin B12 level
- Urinalysis
- Liver function tests
- HIV and syphilis testing for high-risk populations.[1]

Atypical antipsychotic medications are the classic treatment for psychotic patients because they decrease the risk of extrapyramidal symptoms while still effectively treating the patient. Specifically, when using olanzapine and clozapine, there is less risk of hyperlipidemia, new-onset diabetes, or weight gain.[2] Typical dosing for olanzapine is 5–10-mg intramuscular (IM) with up to 3 × 10 mg injections over a 24-h period. Also, the physician may order benzodiazepines such as ziprasidone 5–20 mg IM every 4–6 h with a maximum of 40 mg in a 24-h period. Lastly, the physician must remember that a person who is diagnosed with psychosis or having an acute psychotic episode may be legally hospitalized against their will. In particular, if this patient is violent or threatening harm to themselves or others, especially if they plan to commit suicide. Also, the physician may hospitalize a patient who is malnourished or ill because they fail to feed themselves. Finally, the physician must look at things like dress being appropriate for the climate when doing intake on a patient to see if they are able to care for themselves or not.

It has now become standard of care to treat patients with acute psychosis with violent behavior with 5-2-1-cocktail, consisting of 5 mg of haloperidol, 2 mg of lorazepam, and 1 mg of benztropine mesylate.[3]

## REFERENCES

1. Marder S, Davis M. Clinical manifestations, differential diagnosis, and initial management of psychosis in adults. UpToDate. www-uptodate-com.proxy.cc.uic.edu/contents/clinical-manifestations-differential-diagnosis-and-initial-management-of-psychosis-in-adults?source; 2017.
2. Domino F. The 5-minute Clinical Consult. 20th ed. Philadelphia, PA: Lippincott Williams and Wilkins; 2012. p. 952-3.
3. Spollen III JJ. Schizophrenia. Medscape.com; 2002. www.medscape.org/viewarticle/438507.

## FURTHER READING

1. AHRQ.gov

# CHAPTER 9

# Environmental Injuries, Toxicology, and Animal Bites

## CASE STUDY 54: PEANUT ANAPHYLAXIS

*"7th Grader Dies at School Event from Food Allergy."*
—CBS News 2011

### CASE HISTORY

**Chief Complaint: Allergic Reaction**

A 13-year-old girl was rushed to the emergency department (ED) from a school event. While sitting with a group of friends and eating Chinese food, she became a vibrant red and was having difficulty breathing. She collapsed moments after and was unable to be resuscitated. At the ED, she had a feeble pulse and no breath sounds. The blood pressure (BP) was not palpable. Intravenous (IV) lines were placed, and patient was immediately intubated. Fluids, epinephrine, and benadryl were all given.

Soon afterward, the patient lost her pulse and her BP never recovered. Resuscitation attempts were unsuccessful. The patient passed away a few hours after the initial presentation.

Her family denied any previous medical history. Her mother had an uneventful course in pregnancy. She was born at full term, appropriate for gestational age (AGA) with no malformations. Her parents report that she had a peanut allergy. The school officials report that they were aware of the allergy and made sure that the Chinese food they ordered had no peanuts.

### Allergies

None known at time of presentation.

### Physical Examination

- *Skin*: Urticaria, skin flushing
- *Vitals*: BP was not measurable

- *Cardiovascular system*: Weak, decreased heart sounds
- *Respiratory system*: No breath sounds on initial presentation.

## Diagnosis

Patient has anaphylactic reaction due to peanut allergy. While the school ensures that the Chinese food ordered did not have any peanuts, many Chinese restaurants use peanut oil without considering it as a peanut product.

## Differential Diagnosis

- *Esophageal*: Globus hystericus, hereditary angioedema, foreign body aspiration (young children, especially), and angioedema
- *Endocrine*: Pheochromocytoma and malignant carcinoid syndrome
- *Hematology/oncology*: Mastocytosis, thyroid, and medullary carcinoma
- *Cardiac*: Shock, capillary leak syndrome, and myocardial dysfunction
- *Respiratory*: Pulmonary embolism
- *Neurological*: Vasodepressor (vasovagal) reaction (probably the most common masquerader) and autonomic epilepsy
- *Psychiatric*: Panic attacks and vocal cord dysfunction syndrome
- *Toxic*: Scombroid fish poisoning, monosodium glutamate poisoning, red man's syndrome, and ethanol toxicity.

# ANAPHYLAXIS

## Pathophysiology

Anaphylaxis is considered as a type 1/immunoglobulin E (IgE)-mediated allergic reaction. Sudden activation of mast cells occurs when IgE antibodies exposed to an allergen. The mast cells then release inflammatory mediators. The physiologic responses to the release of anaphylactic mediators include smooth muscle spasm in the respiratory and gastrointestinal (GI) tracts, vasodilation, increased vascular permeability, and stimulation of sensory nerve endings. Increased mucous secretion and increased bronchial smooth muscle tone, as well as airway edema, contribute to the respiratory symptoms observed in anaphylaxis. Anaphylactoid reactions have an identical clinical manifestation that results from mast cell degranulation without IgE mediation.

The frequency of anaphylaxis is increasing, and this has been attributed to the either an increased number of allergens that people are exposed to or a sterile lifestyle during childhood development. Evidence of the former is provided by the increased correlation between the rising rate of anaphylaxis and increased pollution. The lifetime prevalence of anaphylaxis is 1–2% of the population. The frequency of anaphylaxis is increasing, and this has been attributed to the increased number of potential allergens to which people are exposed.

Up to 500–1,000 fatal cases of anaphylaxis per year are estimated to occur in the United States. Estimated mortality rates range from 0.65% to 2% of patients with anaphylaxis.

## Immunologic IgE-mediated Reactions

Certain foods are more likely than others to elicit an IgE antibody response and lead to anaphylaxis. Foods likely to elicit an IgE antibody response in all age groups include: peanuts, tree nuts, fish, and shellfish. Those likely to elicit an IgE antibody response in children also include eggs, soy, and milk.

An analysis of 32 fatalities thought to be due to food-induced anaphylaxis revealed that peanuts likely were the responsible food in 62% of the cases. In placebo-controlled food challenges, peanut-sensitive patients can react to as little as 100 μg of peanut protein.[1] The Rochester epidemiology project, in agreement with earlier studies, found that food ingestion was the leading cause of anaphylaxis, accounting for as many as one-third of all cases.

Scombroid fish poisoning can occasionally mimic food-induced anaphylaxis. Bacteria in spoiled fish produce enzymes capable of decarboxylating histidine to produce biogenic amines, including histamine and *cis*-urocanic acid, which is also capable of mast cell degranulation.

## Immunologic IgE-independent Reactions

Anaphylaxis may result from administration of blood products including IV immunoglobulin, or animal antiserum, at least partly as a consequence of activation of the complement cascade. Certain byproducts of the cascade are capable of causing mast cell/basophil degranulation.

Exercise-induced anaphylaxis is a rare syndrome that can take one of two forms. The first form is ingestant dependent, requiring exercise and ingestion of particular types of food (e.g. wheat, celery) or medications [e.g. nonsteroidal anti-inflammatory drugs (NSAIDs)] to cause an episode of anaphylaxis. In these patients, exercise alone does not produce an episode, and ingesting the culprit food or medication alone does not cause an episode.

The second form is characterized by intermittent episodes of anaphylaxis during exercise, independent of any food ingestion. Anaphylaxis does not necessarily occur during every episode of physical exertion.

Anaphylaxis can be a manifestation of systemic mastocytosis, a disease characterized by excessive mast cell numbers in multiple organs. Such patients appear to be at increased risk for food and venom reactions. Alcohol, vancomycin, opioids, radiocontrast media, and other biologic agents that can degranulate mast cells directly are discouraged.

## Nonimmunologic Reactions

Certain agents, including opioids, dextrans, protamine, and vancomycin, are thought to cause direct, nonimmunologic release of mediators from mast cells. Evidence also exists that dextrans and protamine can activate several inflammatory pathways, including complement, coagulation, and vasoactive (kallikrein–kinin) systems.

Intravenously administered radiocontrast media causes an anaphylactoid reaction that is clinically similar to true anaphylaxis and is treated in the same way. The reaction is not related to prior exposure. Approximately 1–3% of patients who receive hyperosmolar IV contrast experience a reaction. Reactions to radiocontrast media usually are mild (most commonly, urticarial), with only rare fatalities reported. Risk of a fatal reaction has been estimated at 0.9 cases per 100,000 exposures.

Pretreatment with antihistamines or corticosteroids and use of low-molecular weight (LMW) contrast agents lead to lower rates of anaphylactoid reactions to IV radiocontrast media (approximately 0.5%). Consider these measures for patients who have prior history of reaction, since rate of recurrence is estimated at 17–60%. Some institutions use only LMW agents. Personnel, medications, and equipment needed for treatment of allergic reactions always should be available when these agents are administered. Obtain consent before administration.

Patients who are atopic and/or asthmatic are also at increased risk for reaction. In addition, allergic reaction is more difficult to treat in those taking beta-blockers.

Shellfish or iodine allergy is not a contraindication to the use of IV contrast and does not mandate a pretreatment regimen. As with any allergic patient, give consideration to the use of LMW contrast agents. In fact, the term "iodine allergy" is a misnomer. Iodine is an essential trace element present throughout the body. No one is allergic to iodine. Patients who report iodine allergy usually have had either a prior contrast reaction, a shellfish allergy, or a contact reaction to povidone-iodine (betadine).

Mucosal exposure [e.g. GI, genitourinary (GU)] to radiocontrast agents has not been reported to cause anaphylaxis; therefore, a history of prior reaction is not a contraindication to GI or GU use of these agents.

## WORKUP

### Presentation

Patients often describe a sense of impending doom, accompanied by pruritus and flushing. This can evolve rapidly into the following symptoms, broken down by organ system:
- *Cutaneous/Ocular*: Flushing, urticaria, angioedema, cutaneous and/or conjunctival pruritus, warmth, and swelling
- *Respiratory*: Nasal congestion, rhinorrhea, throat tightness, wheezing, shortness of breath, cough, and hoarseness
- *Cardiovascular*: Dizziness, weakness, syncope, chest pain, and palpitations

- *GI*: Dysphagia, nausea, vomiting, diarrhea, bloating, and cramps
- *Neurologic*: Headache, dizziness, blurred vision, and seizure (very rare and often associated with hypotension)
- *Others*: Metallic taste and feeling of impending doom.

## PHYSICAL EXAMINATION

The first priority in the physical examination should be to assess the patient's airway, breathing, circulation, and adequacy of mentation (e.g. alertness, orientation, and coherence of thought).

General appearance and vital signs vary according to the severity of the anaphylactic episode and the organ system(s) affected. Vital signs may be normal or significantly altered with tachypnea, tachycardia, and/or hypotension.

Patients commonly are restless due to severe pruritus from urticaria. Anxiety, tremor, and a sensation of cold may result from compensatory endogenous catecholamine release. Anxiety is common, unless hypotension or hypoxia causes obtundation. Frank cardiovascular collapse or respiratory arrest may occur in severe cases.

### Respiratory Findings

Severe angioedema of the tongue and lips [as may occur with the use of angiotensin-converting enzyme (ACE) inhibitors] may obstruct airflow. Laryngeal edema may manifest as stridor or severe air hunger. Loss of voice, hoarseness, and/or dysphonia may occur. Bronchospasm, airway edema, and mucus hypersecretion may manifest as wheezing. In the surgical setting, increased pressure of ventilation can be the only manifestation of bronchospasm. Complete airway obstruction is the most common cause of death in anaphylaxis.

### Cardiovascular Findings

Tachycardia is present in one fourth of patients, usually as a compensatory response to reduced intravascular volume or to stress from compensatory catecholamine release.

Bradycardia, in contrast, is more suggestive of a vasodepressor (vasovagal) reaction. Although tachycardia is the rule, bradycardia has also been observed in anaphylaxis (see the "Pathophysiology" Section). Thus, bradycardia may not be as useful for distinguishing anaphylaxis from a vasodepressor reaction as was previously thought. Relative bradycardia (initial tachycardia followed by diminished heart rate despite worsening hypotension) has been reported previously in experimental settings of insect sting anaphylaxis, as well as in trauma patients.[2]

Hypotension (and resultant loss of consciousness) may be observed secondary to capillary leak, vasodilation, and hypoxic myocardial depression. Cardiovascular collapse and shock can occur immediately, without any other findings. This is an especially important consideration in the surgical setting. Because shock may develop without prominent skin manifestations or history of exposure, anaphylaxis is part of the differential diagnosis for patients who present with shock and no obvious cause.

## Cognitive Findings

If hypoperfusion or hypoxia occurs, it can cause altered mental status. The patient may exhibit a depressed level of consciousness or may be agitated and/or combative.

## Cutaneous Findings

The classic skin manifestation is urticaria (i.e. hives). Urticaria can occur anywhere on the body, often localizing to the superficial dermal layers of the palms, soles, and inner thighs. Lesions are red and raised and sometimes have central blanching. Intense pruritus occurs with the lesions. Lesion borders are usually irregular and sizes vary markedly. Only a few small or large lesions may become confluent, forming giant urticaria. At times, the entire dermis is involved with diffuse erythema and edema.

In a local reaction, lesions occur near the site of a cutaneous exposure (e.g. insect bite). The involved area is erythematous, edematous, and pruritic. If only a local skin reaction (as opposed to generalized urticaria) is present, systemic manifestations (e.g. respiratory distress) are less likely. Local reactions, even if severe, are not predictive of systemic anaphylaxis on re-exposure.

Angioedema (soft-tissue swelling) is also commonly observed. These lesions involve the deeper dermal layers of skin. It is usually nonpruritic and nonpitting. Common areas of involvement are the larynx, lips, eyelids, hands, feet, and genitalia.

Generalized (whole-body) erythema (or flushing) without urticaria or angioedema is also occasionally observed.

Cutaneous findings may be delayed or absent in rapidly progressive anaphylaxis.

## Gastrointestinal Findings

Vomiting, diarrhea, and abdominal distension are frequently observed.

## DIAGNOSTIC STUDIES

Anaphylaxis is a clinical diagnosis in most cases.

## LABORATORY STUDIES

### Histamine and Tryptase Assessment

Plasma histamine levels rise within 10 min of onset but fall again within 30 min. Urinary histamine levels are generally not dependable, as this test can be affected by diet and by bacteria in the urine. Urinary histamine metabolites measurement is a better test but is not generally available.

Serum mature tryptase (previously called β-tryptase) levels peak 60–90 min after the start of an episode and may persist for as long as 5 h.

Basal levels of total and mature tryptase between episodes of anaphylaxis can be helpful to rule out systemic mastocytosis. Patients with mastocytosis constitutively produce large quantities of α-tryptase, while individuals with anaphylaxis from other causes have normal levels of α-tryptase at baseline between episodes of anaphylaxis. During anaphylaxis, a ratio of total tryptase (α and mature) to mature tryptase of 20 or greater is consistent with mastocytosis, whereas a ratio of ≤10 suggests anaphylaxis of another etiology.

Detecting the rise of histamine or tryptase levels can be difficult, and some patients might have a rise in one but not the other.

### 5-Hydroxyindoleacetic Acid Levels

If carcinoid syndrome is considered, urinary 5-hydroxyindoleacetic acid levels should be measured.

### Serological and Skin Tests

Skin testing, in vitro IgE tests, or both may be used to determine the stimulus causing the anaphylactic reaction (e.g. food allergy, medication allergy, or insect bite or sting).

These tests cannot be used for non-IgE-mediated reactions.

## INITIAL EMERGENCY DEPARTMENT INTERVENTIONS

The 2010 Joint Task Force Anaphylaxis Parameter Update, the 2011 World Allergy Organization anaphylaxis guidelines and the 2010 National Institute of Allergy and Infectious Diseases (NIAID)-sponsored expert panel report have similar recommendations for immediate treatment in the ED. It should begin with monitoring and treatment, including oxygen, cardiac monitoring, breathing, mental status, skin, and a large-bore IV with isotonic crystalloid solution. At the same time, where appropriate, the ED team should call for specialized help, particularly a resuscitation team. Further, intervention depends on severity of reaction and affected organ system(s), but the guidelines recommend the injection of epinephrine and placing the patient in a supine position (or position of comfort if dyspneic or vomiting) with the legs elevated.

## Airway Management

For the initial assessment, check the airway closely. If needed, establish and maintain an airway and/or provide ventilatory assistance. Assess the level of consciousness and obtain BP, pulse, and oximetry values. Place the patient in the supine position with legs elevated and begin supplemental oxygen.

One of the quickest and most effective ways to support ventilation involves a one-way valve facemask with oxygen inlet port [e.g. Pocket-Mask (Laerdal Medical Corporation, Gatesville, Texas) or similar device]. Artificial ventilation via the mouth-to-mask technique with oxygen attached to the inlet port has provided oxygen saturations comparable to endotracheal intubation. Patients with adequate spontaneous respirations may breathe through the mask.

Severe laryngeal edema may occur too rapidly during anaphylaxis, and endotracheal intubation may be impossible. Epinephrine may rapidly reverse airway compromise. If the edema does not reverse with epinephrine, an endotracheal tube should be inserted.

In extreme circumstances, cricothyrotomy or catheter jet ventilation may be lifesaving when orotracheal intubation or bag/valve/mask ventilation is not effective. Cricothyrotomy is much easier that tracheostomy and is recommended if no surgical staff is immediately available. Wheezing or stridor indicates bronchospasm or mucosal edema.

Treatment with epinephrine and inhaled β-agonists is effective for these indications. Inhaled β-agonists are used to counteract bronchospasm and should be administered to patients who are wheezing.

Corticosteroids can be used, but they do not have effect until several hours after the administration. Aminophylline can be more effective than corticosteroids in refractory bronchospasm.

For bradykinin-mediated angioedema (including angioedema due to ACE inhibitors), antihistamines and corticosteroids are probably not effective. Epinephrine may be tried in severe cases, but airway intervention may be needed.

## Cardiac Monitoring

Cardiac monitoring is indicated due to the epinephrine and steroid use.

### Intravenous Access

The IV line should be of large caliber due to the potential requirement for large-volume IV fluid resuscitation. Isotonic crystalloid solutions (i.e. normal saline, Ringer's lactate) are preferred. A keep-vein-open (KVO) rate is appropriate for patients with stable vital signs and only cutaneous manifestations. If hypotension or tachycardia is present, administer a fluid bolus of 20 mg/kg for children and 1 L for adults. Further fluid therapy depends on patient's response.

*Epinephrine Administration*

Epinephrine should be rapidly administered as a subcutaneous (SC) or intramuscular (IM) injection at a dose of 0.01 mL/kg of aqueous epinephrine 1:1,000 (maximum adult dose, 0.3–0.5 mL). The dose may be repeated q 5–10 min if there is persistence or recurrence of symptoms. Endotracheal epinephrine should be considered if IV access is not possible during life-threatening reactions.

## Histamine Administration

Administration of H1 and H2 receptor antagonists is also recommended in the initial treatment of anaphylaxis.
- Administer diphenhydramine 25–50 mg IV or IM
- Cimetidine 300 mg IV over 3–5 min, or ranitidine 50 mg IV, should be given initially; subsequent doses of H1 and H2 blockers can be given orally q 6 h for 48 h.

*Corticosteroids*

Corticosteroids are not useful in the acute episode because of their slow onset of action; however, they should be administered in most cases to prevent prolonged or recurrent anaphylaxis. Commonly used agents are hydrocortisone sodium succinate 250–500 mg IV q 4–6 h in adults (4–8 mg/kg for children) or methylprednisolone 40–250 mg IV in adults (1–2 mg/kg in children).

## β-Agonists

Aerosolized β-agonists [e.g. albuterol, 2.5 mg, as-needed [pro re nata (PRN)] every 20 min] are useful to control bronchospasm.

*Atropine and Dobutamine*

*Additional useful agents in specific circumstances:* Atropine for refractory bradycardia, dopamine for refractory hypotension (despite volume expansion), and glucagon in patients on β-blocking drugs.

## DISCUSSION

It is important to remember that anaphylaxis can be caused by often unpredictable causes. There have been instances where even ketchup has resulted in life-threatening anaphylactic shock. The author has personally seen medical staff crash within moments of eating French fries and ketchup.

## Food Allergy Scenarios

- A medical assistant went to a fast-food restaurant and had an anaphylactic reaction to a component in her ketchup. As her condition worsened, she stopped breathing and was transported to the hospital via helicopter.

- A young girl orders Chinese food at a sleepover, unaware that it contains peanuts. She experiences a fatal anaphylactic reaction.
- A nurse, with a history of asthma, was intubated several times in an intensive care unit following exposure to a perfume.

## Public Education

The general public should know the importance of carrying EpiPen's or epinephrine autoinjector. People with known allergies should always EpiPen's or epinephrine autoinjector to preventable fatality (Fig. 1).

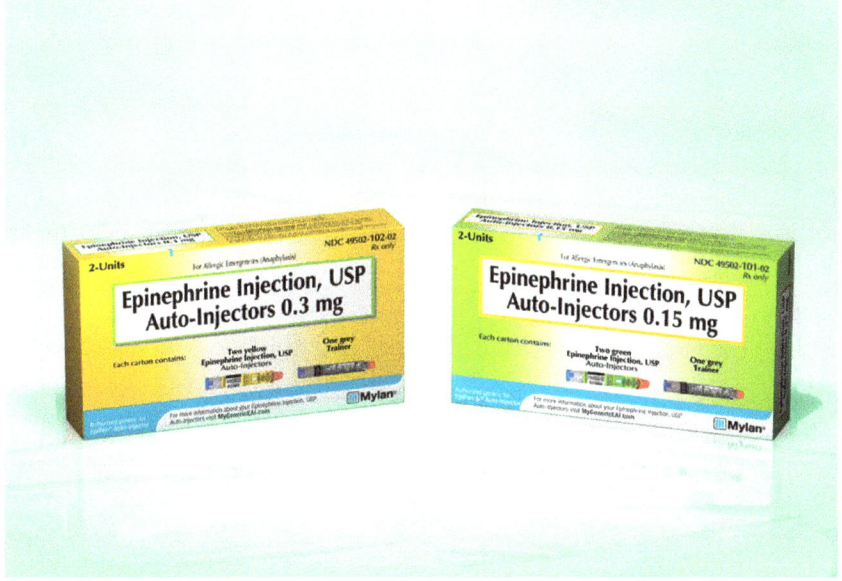

Fig. 1: Epinephrine autoinjector.

## REFERENCES

1. Asthma and Allergy Foundation of America. http://aafa.org/display.cfm?id=4&sub=83; 2013.
2. J Allergy Clin Immunol 2013. http://www.jacionline.org/.

## CASE STUDY 55: ELECTRICAL INJURY

## CASE HISTORY

A 70-year-old male and his 25-year-old son were working on an irrigation system for their farm. When the son tried to attach the system to electricity, he was shocked, his system was assaulted by 220 V and immediately went into cardiac arrest (Fig. 1). The father brought his son, the sole breadwinner for the family, into the emergency department in full cardiac arrest, and he was pronounced dead.

## DISCUSSION

*Electric current exists in two forms*: Alternating current (AC) and direct current (DC). AC involves electrons flowing back and forth whereas in DC, the electrons flow in one direction only. AC is more dangerous than DC, because AC causes tetanic muscle contractions and the "locking on" phenomenon. The depth of electrical injury is related to the intensity and magnitude of the electric current. Ohm's law states that current = voltage/resistance (Fig. 2).

## PATHOPHYSIOLOGY

Direct necrosis of the myocardium from the electrical injury causes vasoconstriction, and ischemia which in turn will release excessive catecholamine leading to cardiac dysrhythmias. Even a small current can produce cardiac dysrhythmia like asystole and ventricular tachycardia. Burns are

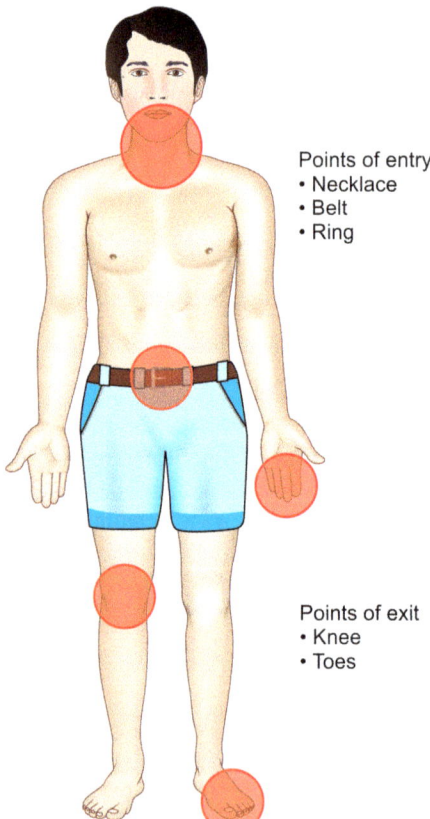

**Fig. 1:** A 25-year-old man assaulted by 220 V.

## Ohm's Law

$$\text{Current (amps)} = \frac{\text{Voltage}}{\text{Resistance}}$$

Since muscles, mucous membranes, blood vessels, and nerves have low resistance. They are the preferred pathway of electrical current.

**Fig. 2:** Ohm's law.

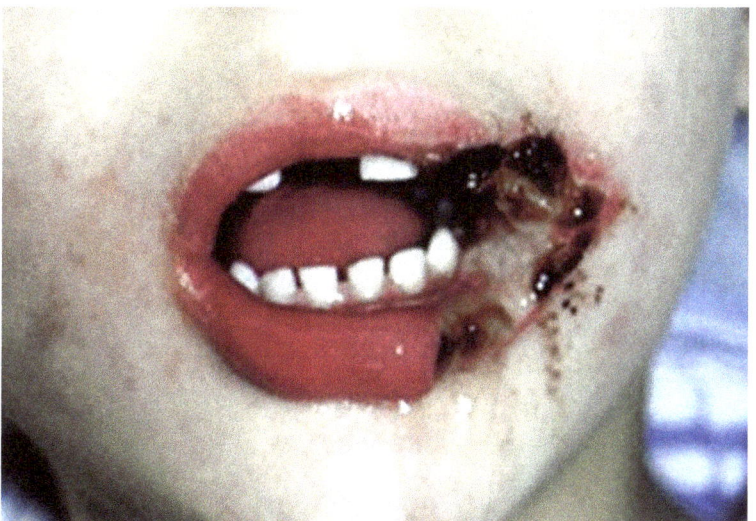

**Fig. 3:** Electrical injury caused by chewing or biting electrical cords.

very common after high voltage electrical injury. Flesh burns from electrical injuries are flame burns because they are caused by ignition of clothing from electrical heat. In children, the most common form of electrical injury is caused by chewing or biting electrical cords (Figs. 3 and 4). These cases present as perioral edema and eschar formation; the bleeding from perioral burns can be significant. Thorough physical examination is necessary to look for any entry and exit wounds.

## TREATMENT

Immediate intravenous fluids are needed to establish fluid balance in all burn patients. Fluid resuscitation should be titrated to adequate urine output according to the Parkland formula shown in Figure 5A. Some patients may need admission to specialized burn units. Burns on both hands indicate electrical injury path going through the heart; this has a very poor prognosis (Fig. 5B).

Arrhythmias occur in approximately 15% of the patients with electrical injuries. However, sudden cardiac death can occur in these patients prior to

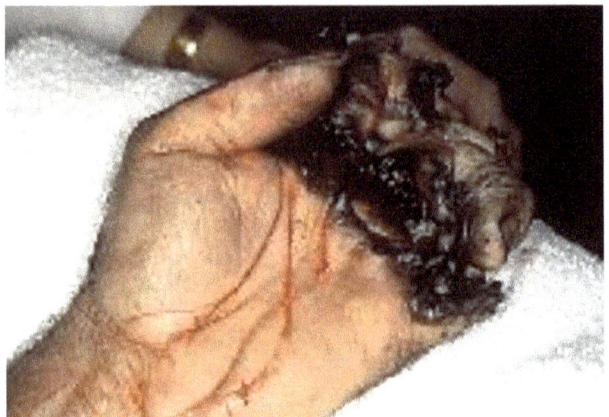

**Fig. 4:** Flesh burns from electrical injury.

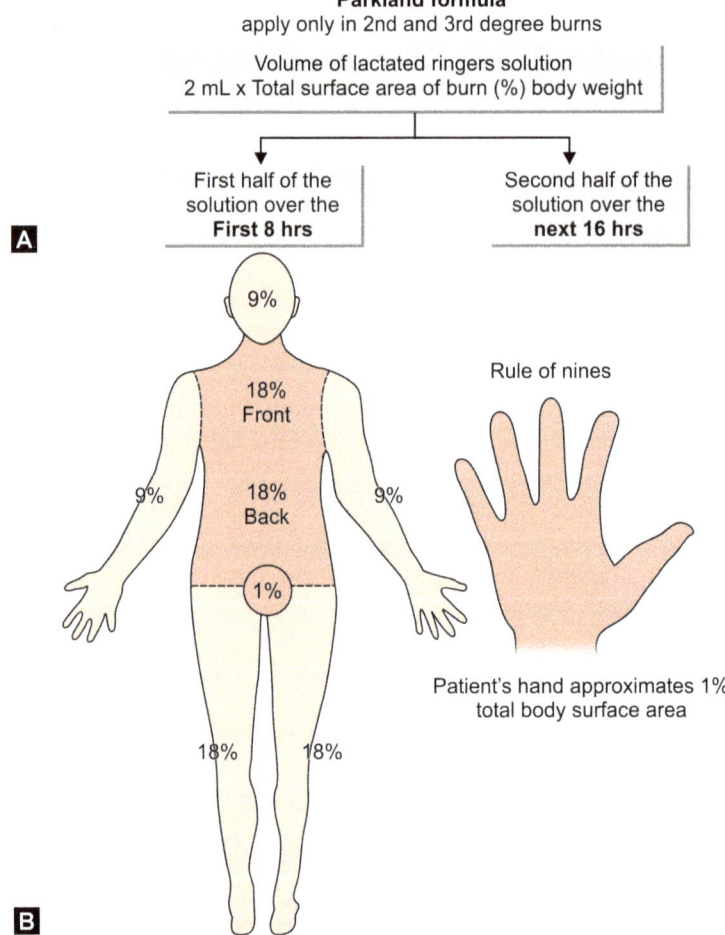

**Figs. 5A and B:** (A) Parkland formula; (B) Rule of nine.

hospitalization due to ventricular fibrillation or asystole. The following three complications must be always monitored:
- Acute kidney injury due to hypovolemia
- Rhabdomyolysis from massive tissue necrosis
- Acute compartment syndrome due to deep electrothermal injury and edema

Hence, the following tests should be ordered immediately:
- Complete blood count (CBC)
- Comprehensive metabolic panel (CMP)
- Cardiac enzymes, including troponin-I and CK-MB
- EKG
- CK levels
- Urine monitoring for myoglobinuria

## CASE STUDY 56: EDEMA OF LIP AND TONGUE

### CASE HISTORY

A 56-year-old woman is presented to the emergency department with severe edema of the lips, tongue, and difficulty in breathing. Symptoms started suddenly after dinner. Patient's temperature is 100°F, and she has elevated blood pressure (BP). She is tachycardic, tachypneic, and her $O_2$ saturation level is 90% on room air. The patient is treated with oxygen, epinephrine 0.5 mg subcutaneously, and Solu-Medrol 125 mg intravenously. Patient started feeling better in a few minutes.

Patient has no history of allergy to food, medication, or environment. There is no previous history of atopic eczema or asthma. Past medical history has significant hypertension for which the patient is taking lisinopril 25 mg daily. Patient is treated in the emergency room and discharged with oral steroids, Zyrtec, and beta-blocker and told to discontinue her medication. The next day the patient presented with the same symptoms: recurrent facial edema, and swelling of lips and tongue. The treatment is repeated with epinephrine, Solu-Medrol 125 mg BID, oxygen, and Benadryl 25 mg BID, and she is transferred to telemetry unit for stabilization and observation. She is discharged 3 days after treatment and diagnosed with angioneurotic edema secondary to angiotensin-converting enzyme (ACE) inhibitor use. Patients with fulfillment allergic response, angioedema, and airway compromise should be admitted and observed for >48 h and closely monitored following discharge.

### DISCUSSION

ACE inhibitors are used for controlling BP, treating congestive heart failure, prevention of strokes, and prevention and progression of chronic kidney disease in diabetes or hypertension. ACE inhibitors are absolutely contraindicated in pregnant patients because they may cause birth defects. Patients with bilateral renal artery stenosis are also a contraindication for the use of ACE inhibitors. Cough and increase in potassium levels, dizziness, and drowsiness are the main side effects for ACE inhibitors. The most serious and fatal side effects are kidney failure and serious allergic reaction (Figs. 1 and 2).

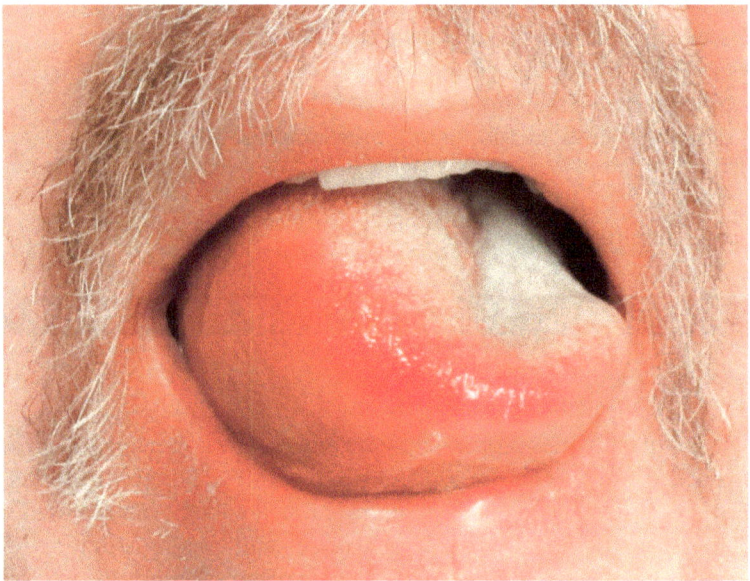

**Fig. 1:** ACE inhibitor-induced angioedema affecting half the tongue. (ACE: angiotensin-converting enzyme.)

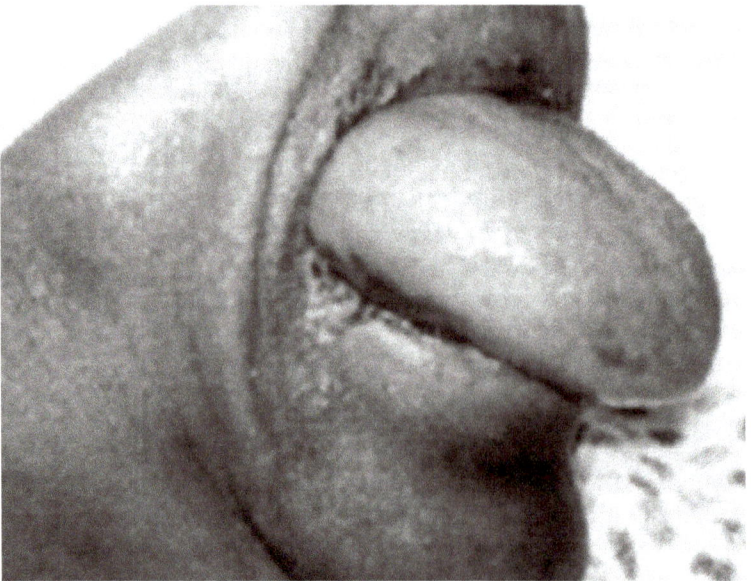

**Fig. 2:** Angioedema affecting the tongue.

It can be anticipated, and early treatment intervention and withdrawal of the medication will prevent the morbidity and mortality secondary to ACE inhibitor use.

## CASE STUDY 57: LIGHTNING INJURY

## CASE HISTORY

A 35-year-old male who was working on top of floor of the high-rise building during a thunderstorm came out to watch the thunderstorm. All of a sudden, a lightning strike (Fig. 1) happened throwing the person to the ground. He was brought by the paramedics by ambulance to the emergency department. He is in cardiac arrest secondary to direct lightning strike. He was cardioverted. Immediate cardiopulmonary resuscitation (CPR) started and continued in spite of the fact that his pupils were fixed and dilated. Patient regained consciousness and started breathing spontaneously. There is no evidence of head and spinal cord injuries. He was bleeding from the left ear most likely secondary to rupture of the tympanic membrane (50% incidence). Electrocardiogram (ECG) and computed tomography (CT) head show negative results. Examination of the back in the thoracic area shows a fern-like skin pattern of the injury (Fig. 2). There is no evidence of compartment syndrome, and neurological examination is normal. Intravenous (IV) fluids, normal saline are established for fluid resuscitation to have optimal urine output.

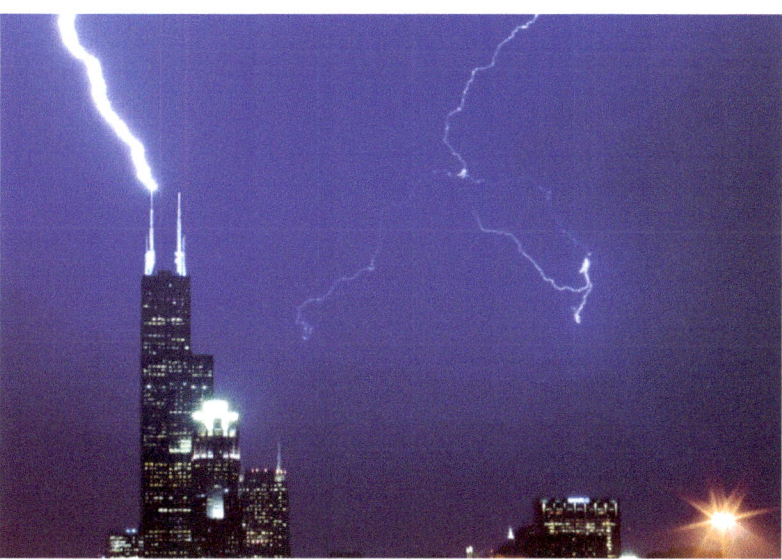

**Fig. 1:** Willis Tower in Chicago hit by lightning.

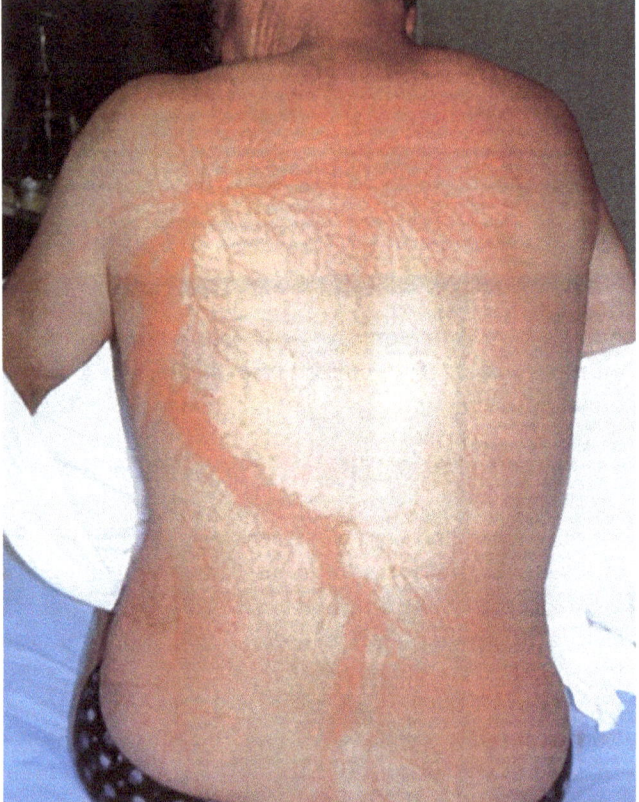

**Fig. 2:** Lichtenberg figure (pathognomonic of lightning).

## DISCUSSION

Differences between lightning and electrical injury have been described in Table 1.

## MANAGEMENT/TREATMENT

Usually there will be multiple casualties at the time of lightning injury. Injuries typically take place on stormy days in outdoor locations or near high-rise buildings. Burns—linear, punctate, or fern-like pattern—are telltale clues. Rupture of the tympanic membrane with bleeding in the ear canal is also a very significant finding in the diagnosis of lightning strike. Immediate resuscitation as carried out on trauma patients is necessary. Acute compartment syndrome can be managed by the ED physician along with a surgical consult.

**Table 1:** Differences between lightning and electrical injury.

| | Electrical injury | Lightning |
|---|---|---|
| Type of current | Alternating current | Direct current |
| Occurrence | Common | Very rare |
| Fatality | Variable | 25% |
| Direction of flow | Electrons flow back and forth the circle | Electrons flow in only one direction |
| Effects | More dangerous because it can cause tetanic contractions | Extremely high voltage and single intense muscle contraction that throws the victims causing fracture and spinal injury |
| Duration | Prolonged | Brief |
| Types of injury | "Locking on" phenomenon: Preventing the victims from the electrical source and prolonged exposure of the current | • Direct strike (most common and dangerous)<br>• Side flash (other victims affected from the transmission of current from the first victim)<br>• Ground current or strike potential<br>• Flash over phenomenon |
| Complications | | |
| • Renal | Renal failure secondary to rhabdomyolysis/myoglobinuria | Rare |
| • Cardiac | Dysrhythmia more common immediately after exposure | *Cardiac arrest*: Asystole |
| • Respiratory | Respiratory arrest rare | Respiratory arrest common secondary to injury to respiratory center in the medulla |
| Cataracts | Rare | Common |
| Tympanic membrane rupture | Rare | Common |
| Skeletal injury | Fractures common | Fractures rare |

## SPECIAL CONSIDERATIONS

In situations with mass casualties, medical care is first administered to patients who have the greatest chance of survival. However, in electrical injuries, one must first treat the patient who appears lifeless or dead. Since these patients are often young, CPR must be started immediately and continued for a prolonged period, regardless of initial rhythm. Patients with asystole have been known to have better prognosis. This technique is known as reverse triage.

Airway, breathing, circulation, disability, and exposure (ABCDE) should be followed by ECG, CT scan and tetanus, diphtheria, and pertussis (Tdap) vaccine are given if necessary. Visual acuity needs to be documented because cataracts are a common complication from this type of injury.

A multidisciplinary approach must be undertaken with nephrology for rhabdomyolysis and acute kidney injury, ENT for tympanic membrane perforation, and ophthalmology for cataracts development (Fig. 3).

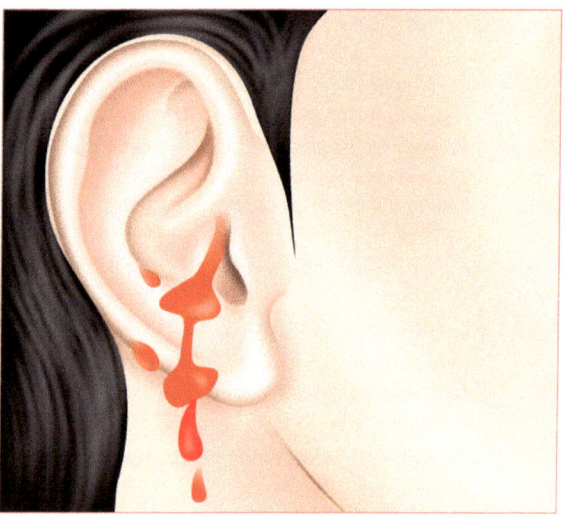

**Fig. 3:** Bleeding from ear is a significant finding from electrical burns.

## CASE STUDY 58: BEE STING

### CASE HISTORY

### Chief Complaint
Patient cannot speak and comes in gasping for air.

### History of Present illness
A 50-year-old Latino male rushes into the emergency department with swollen neck and mouth. His throat is closing up, disabling him from breathing. Patient was eating lunch outside with sweetened lemonade. Shortly after lunch, patient realized a bee sting on his right hand dorsum.

## Past Medical History

*General health:* Good
*Adult illness*: Asthma controlled with inhaler, bB
*Immunization history*: Up-to-date
*Screening history*: Annual primary care physician (PCP) visits
*Exercise*: Sports
*Tobacco:* None
*Alcohol*: Glass of wine on weekends
*Drugs*: None
*Medications*: Pro re nata (PRN) bB inhaler for asthma attack
*Allergies*: Penicillin.

## REVIEW OF SYSTEMS

*General*: Fatigue, weak, fever. No weight change, chills, or night sweats.
*Skin*: Itching, swelling, and rashes on right hand dorsum. No skin, hair, and nail changes. No sores, lumps, or moles.
*Eyes*: Redness, tearing, itching of conjunctiva. Reading glasses. No contact lenses. No blurriness or acute visual loss.
*Nose or Sinuses*: Stuffiness. No rhinorrhea, sneezing, itching, allergy or epistaxis.
*Mouth/Throat/Neck*: No bleeding gums, hoarseness or sore throat. Laryngeal edema.
*Cardiac*: Dropping blood pressure. Peripheral edema. No murmurs, angina, palpitations, dyspnea on exertion, orthopnea, or paroxysmal nocturnal dyspnea.
*Respiratory*: Shortness of breath, wheezing, dyspnea, asthma, and cough. No sputum, hemoptysis, pneumonia, bronchitis, emphysema, or tuberculosis.
*Vascular*: Peripheral edema. No claudication, varicose veins, thrombosis, or emboli.

## PHYSICAL EXAMINATION

*General*: A 50-year-old Latino male in distress. Dressed in suit with clean hygiene.
*Vitals*: BP 90/70 mm Hg, pulse rate 120 bpm, respiratory rate difficulty in breathing, temperature 37.6°C.
*Skin*: Rash, swelling, and redness.
*Eyes*: Pupils equal and reactive to light and accommodation, tearing, conjunctival injection. Anicteric sclera. No fundal papilledema.

No hemorrhage. Lids normal. Extraocular movement normal. Visual fields and acuity normal.
*Nose*: Symmetrical. Nontender. Discharge present. Mucosa swollen. No inflammation of turbinate. Frontal and maxillary sinus nontender.
*Mouth/throat*: Good hygiene. No dentures. No erythema, exudate, or tonsillar enlargement. Laryngeal edema.
*Lungs*: Bronchoconstriction, cough, dyspnea, wheezing, asthma exacerbation. Chest symmetry with respirations. No crackles, vocal fremitus, whispered pectoriloquy, and diaphragmatic excursion.
*Vascular*: Edema. Weak 1+ bilateral peripheral pulses. No bruit, jugular venous distention, and varicose veins.
*Lymphatic*: No lymphadenopathy.
*Neurologic*: Within normal limits.

## ASSESSMENT PLAN

### Impression

*Type I hypersensitivity reaction*: Anaphylaxis induced by a bee sting. Wheals and hives. Laryngeal edema. Hypotension. Tachycardia. Dyspnea. Gastrointestinal change.

## TREATMENT

The first and foremost important treatment for a severe allergic reaction is an intramuscular (IM) injection of 0.3–0.5 mg of epinephrine. This needs to be repeated as required. Corticosteroids are also very important and routinely used to decrease inflammation. Methylprednisolone (Solu-Medrol) 125 mg can be the starting dose in adults. Antihistamines such as diphenhydramine are used for treating systemic reactions. Cetirizine should be used in patients not requiring IV medications, as it has a similar onset of action and longer duration.

Local reaction treatment:
- Apply a cold, damp washcloth to the area
- For itching symptoms, take cetirizine (Zyrtec)
- Ibuprofen/acetaminophen can be used to reduce pain.

## DIFFERENTIAL DIAGNOSIS

- Asthma
- Syncope
- Panic attack.

## CONCLUSION

Type I hypersensitivity reaction mediated by IgE and mast cell activation resulting in wheals and hives.

*Acute urticaria*: Localized, cutaneous anaphylaxis. Hemodynamically stable without hypotension.

## COMMON CAUSES

*Allergic reaction*: To medication, insect bites, foods, and emotions.
*Medication*: Aspirin, nonsteroidal anti-inflammatory drugs (NSAIDs), morphine, codeine, penicillins, phenytoin, quinolones, and angiotensin-converting enzyme inhibitor (ACE-I).
*Food*: Peanuts, shellfish, tomatoes, and strawberries.
*Contact*: Latex

## Alert

Most deaths due to anaphylaxis occur within 30 min to 1 h of insect bite or sting (Fig. 1). Carrying an epinephrine autoinjector is a lifesaving practice, and all paramedics and healthcare providers should carry epinephrine (Fig. 2). Airway management is a main priority in the cases of anaphylaxis with angioedema (Fig. 3). Treating hypertension with recumbent position with legs elevated will help the victim.

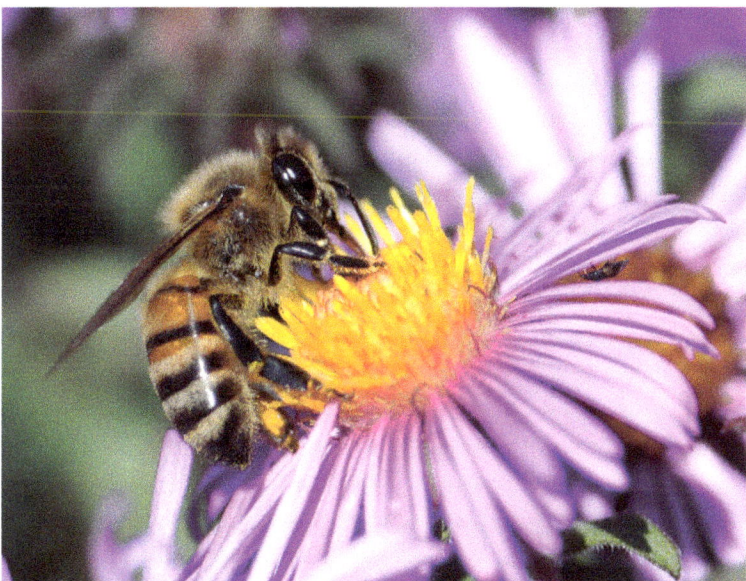

**Fig. 1:** European honey bee.
*Source:* Accessed from wikipedia.org.

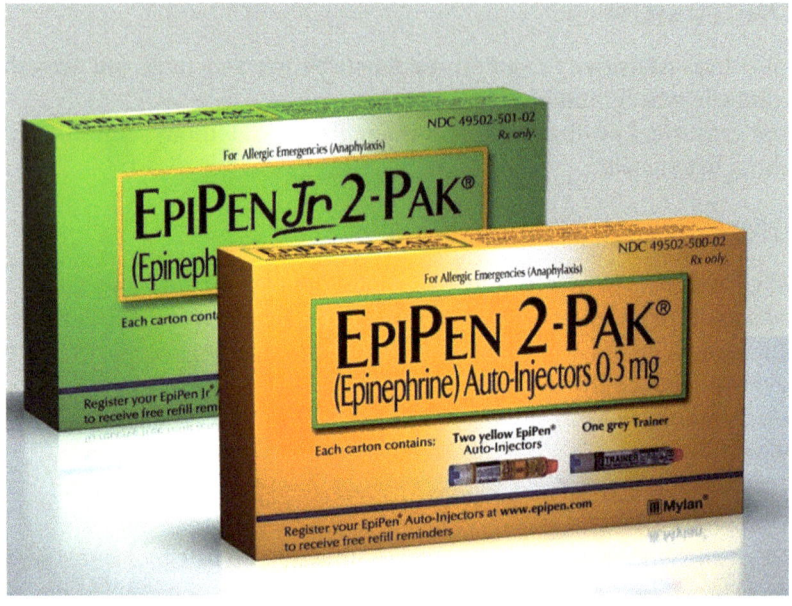

**Fig. 2:** Epinephrine autoinjector.
*Source:* www.epipen.com.

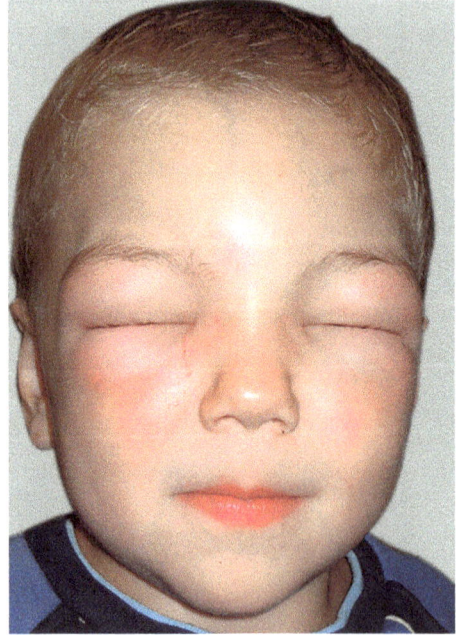

**Fig. 3:** Periorbital swelling.
*Source:* Accessed from wikipedia.org.

## PREVENTION

- Protective clothing
- Avoid common insect habitats and be aware of them, if possible
- Insect repellents which are not effective for bees and spiders
- *N,N-diethyl-m-toluamide (DEET)*: Most effective for mosquitoes, ticks, biting flies, fleas, and chiggers
- Permethrin is an insect toxin if impregnated in clothing, will help prevent mosquito bites, tick bites, flies, and chiggers
- Identify still present in skin, remove by flicking or scraping away from skin.

## CASE STUDY 59: LYME DISEASE

## CASE HISTORY

A 22-year-old male who had been camping in Wisconsin Dells, Wisconsin is presented to the emergency room with a history of tick bites, complaints of feeling weak and tired, fever with chills, characteristic rash, generalized body ache, and headache for the past 3 days. He had a tick bite which he removed himself. He does not remember how long the tick was attached to his body. It seems to have been attached for >24 h.

## DISCUSSION

The Centers for Disease Control and Prevention (CDC) defines erythema migrans as an expanding red macule or papule that must reach ≥5 cm in size with or without central clearing (Figs. 1A to C). As for the Infectious Diseases Society of America (IDSA) guidelines, this rash is sufficient to make the diagnosis of Lyme disease in the absence of laboratory confirmation.

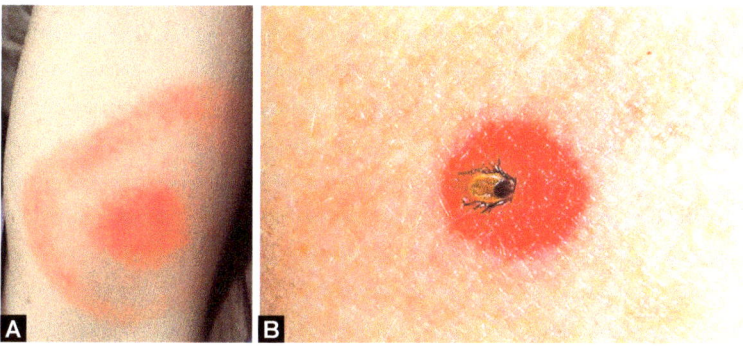

**Figs. 1A and B:** Erythema migrans.

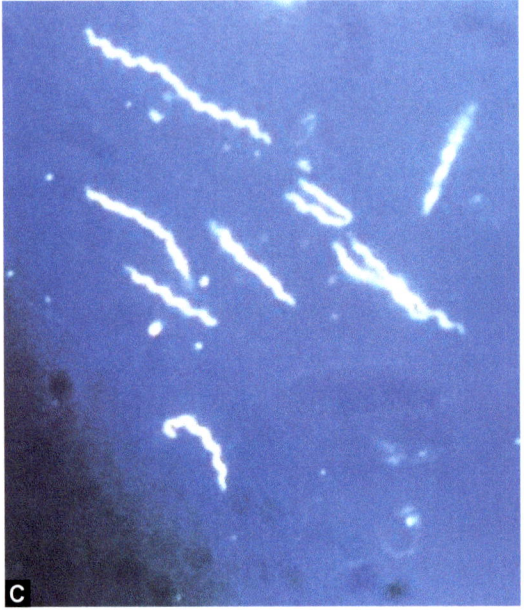

**Fig. 1C:** Lyme Disease Microscopy showing *Borrelia burgdorferi*.

## DIAGNOSTIC WORKUP

See Flowchart 1.

**Flowchart 1:** Diagnostic workup.

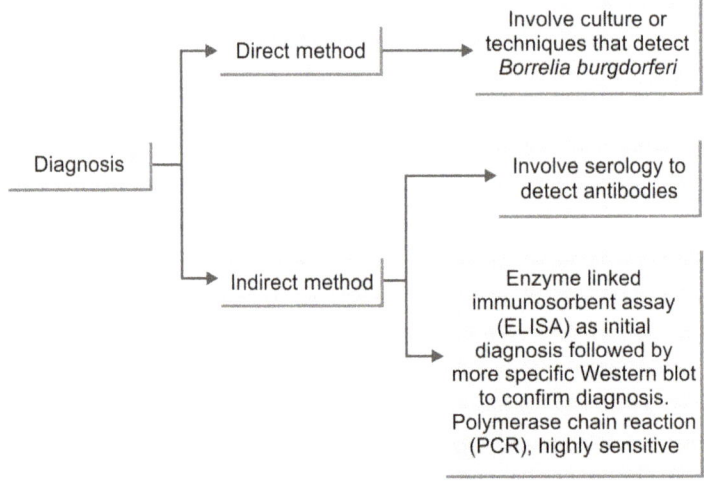

## PREVENTION

Tick bites can be prevented to reduce the risk of Lyme disease. The most common risk factor for acquiring Lyme disease is working outdoors near old stone walls and areas of low-lying shrubs or grasses in endemic regions. Personal protection strategies after outdoor activities include
- Wearing protective clothing such as long-legged and long-sleeved clothing
- Using a tick repellant on skin or clothes
- Regular checks on clothing for ticks
- Taking a bath and placing clothes in a dryer after outdoor trips
- Avoid tick abundant areas: New England, mid-Atlantic states, and upper Midwest.

In addition, a randomized controlled trial indicates that prophylaxis, with a single 200 mg dose of Doxycycline for a recognized bite even when suspicion is low, is highly effective in preventing the development of Lyme disease.

## TREATMENT

The treatment plan for Lyme disease is discussed in Flowchart 2.

**Flowchart 2:** Treatment plan.

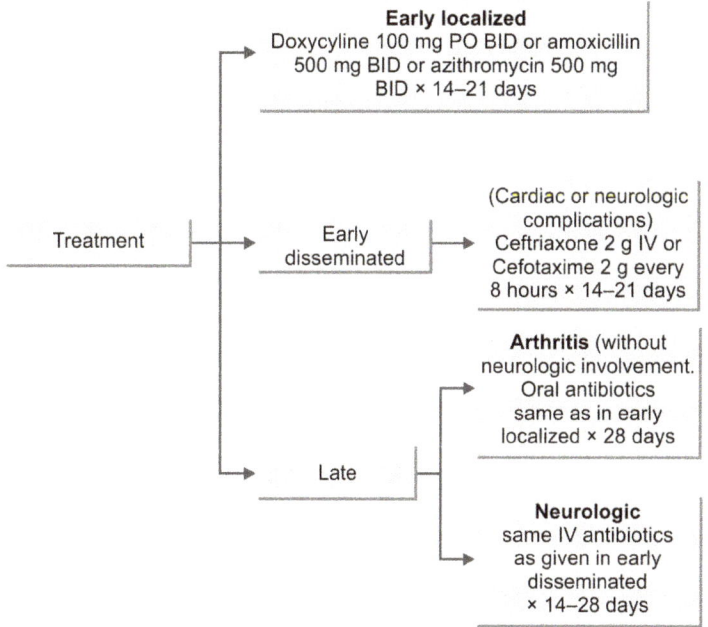

## FURTHER READING

1. Nadelman RB. N Engl J Med 2001;345:79-84. July 12, 2001. DOI: 10.1056/NEJM200107123450201.

## CASE STUDY 60: ORGANOPHOSPHATE POISONING

### CASE HISTORY

Patient is a 34-year-old farmer who was working in his cornfield in Indiana spraying insecticide. While spraying his cornfield, he started to notice a tingling numbness, profuse sweating, salivation, lacrimation, coughing, palpitations, increased heart rate, increased urinary frequency, and abdominal pain. He was in a confused state and having muscle cramps. He is brought into the emergency room after 30 min of this exposure. On arrival to the emergency room, he is decontaminated by giving a full body shower in the designated decontamination room to avoid further contact with the chemical. Stat (immediately) 2 mg of atropine intravenous (IV) is given under cardiac monitoring and repeated once more. Also, pralidoxime (2-PAM or 2-pyridine aldoxime methyl chloride) 1 g is given every 6 h.

### ORGANOPHOSPHATE POISONING
#### Mechanism

Organophosphates irreversibly bind to cholinesterase molecules. On the other hand, carbamates form a reversible bond with cholinesterase. Inhibition of cholinesterase enzymes leads to signs and symptoms of cholinergic crisis or excess. Exposure occurs most commonly through the dermal or oral routes. Frequently, hydrocarbons are present in the vehicle, and if ingested, this must be considered as part of the toxic picture.

#### Clinical Effects

The clinical manifestations are mediated through two primary systems: muscarinic and nicotinic.

*Muscarinic Effects*

These include salivation, lacrimation, urination, gastrointestinal distress, bronchorrhea, bradycardia, bronchospasm, abdominal cramping, and miosis.

*Nicotinic Effects*

These include altered mental status (AMS), hypertension, tachycardia, and muscle cramps.

#### Laboratory Tests

Treatment should be guided by the signs and symptoms of toxicity. However, plasma and red blood cell (RBC) cholinesterase levels are rarely available at hospitals. If available, RBC cholinesterase levels give a better reflection of what is happening at the nerve terminal. These values are generally only of value in retrospect. Fifty percent cholinesterase activity has mild toxicity. In a range of 10–20%, it shows moderate toxicity and if <10% shows severe toxicity.

## Treatment

### Initial Resuscitation

Patients with severe AMS need 100% $O_2$, and ET tube placement. This should be followed by
- IV Atropine
- IV PAM
- Volume resuscitation.

In organophosphate poisoning, IV Atropine is given in 2 mg increment boluses until heart rate is >80 bpm, SBP >80 mm Hg, and a clear chest. Salivation, lacrimation, and urination will start slowing down, but this should not be the criteria to guide therapy. The most important endpoint is the improvement of respiratory function and decreased secretions.

The dose should be "enough" or until atropinization occurs. Pralidoxime (2-PAM) 1 g is given every 6 h in cases where atropine is required for treatment (Fig. 1). It works in organophosphate poisoning by dephosphorylating the cholinesterase enzyme permitting it to function. Currently, WHO

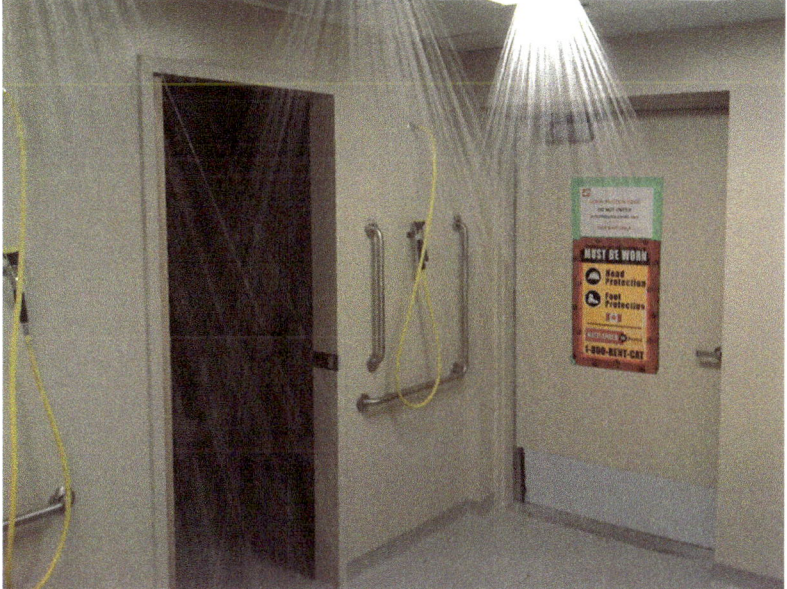

**Fig. 1:** Emergency department decontamination shower.

recommends using IV bolus therapy of pralidoxime with ≥30 mg/kg in adults and 25–50 mg/kg for children based on severity of symptoms. Avoid using PAM without atropine.

Volume resuscitation with isotonic crystalloid should be concurrently given.

## Center for Disease Control and Prevention Recommendations

### Critical Care Area

Every emergency department should have a decontamination room equipped with high pressure showers as shown in Figure 1. Decontamination is a critical part of managing dermal exposures.

If appropriate decontamination efforts have been completed before entry to the critical care area, there should be no need for special equipment or precautions, such as covering floors and walls with plastic or shutting off the ventilation system. However, if the patient has ingested a chemical, then prepare to isolate toxic vomitus quickly (see "Ingestion Exposure" as shown in Figure 2).

Chemical burns have characteristics that are different from thermal burns. The extent and depth of injury in a chemical burn often is not apparent

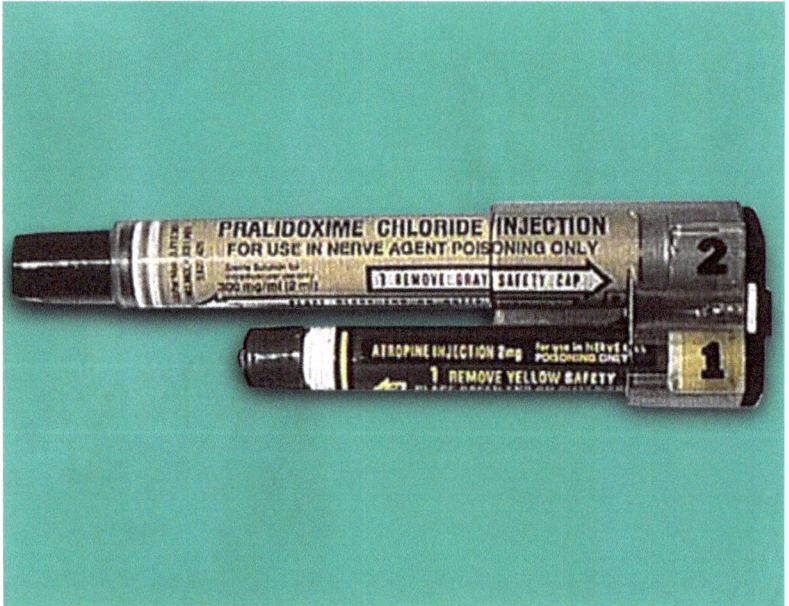

**Fig. 2:** Atropine and pralidoxime chloride injections.

immediately; severity is frequently underestimated. Circulating fluid loss can occur as with thermal burns. In addition, absorption of a corrosive chemical may cause acute or delayed systemic toxicity.

Patients with exposure to a highly corrosive, penetrating, oily, or persistent chemical exposure may require additional decontamination to prevent further injury and systemic absorption. Common sites of residual contamination include the armpits, groin, buttocks, hair, ears, nostrils, and under the fingernails and toenails. Usually, these patients do not pose a risk of secondary contamination if they have undergone the basic decontamination, but if the material is highly contaminating (e.g. organophosphate pesticides, radioactive dust), caregivers should wear gowns and gloves to protect themselves. Use plain liquid soap or shampoo for cleansing the skin.

## Skin and Eye Contact

Skin and eye contact can occur with solids, liquids, or gases. Corrosive agents can cause direct damage to tissues by various mechanisms including low or high pH, chemical reaction with surface tissue, or removal of normal skin fats (defatting) or moisture (desiccant effect). Chemicals can also be absorbed systemically through the skin. This is more likely to occur when the normal skin barrier is disrupted (e.g. with a chemical burn or a traumatic injury) or if the chemical is highly fat-soluble (e.g. organophosphate and organochlorine pesticides).

## Central Nervous System

The brain is affected by many drugs and chemicals. Depressants (e.g. chloroform, hydrocarbon solvents) cause a generalized decrease in brain activity that may result in headache, dizziness, confusion, lethargy, stupor, or coma. Some early effects of depressants may appear to be stimulatory, producing euphoria, and giddiness (similar to beverage alcohol). Severe depression of the brainstem can cause respiratory arrest and cardiovascular collapse.

Central nervous system stimulants [e.g. Dichlorodiphenyltrichloroethane (DDT), other chlorinated hydrocarbon insecticides, organophosphates] can cause agitation, anxiety, delirium, and seizures. Excessive muscular activity associated with seizures can result in hyperthermia.

## Dermal

The skin provides a relatively impermeable protective barrier against excessive fluid losses from the body or inward movement of microorganisms, allergens, and chemicals. Many chemicals disrupt the integrity of the skin by killing cells or removing fats from the skin. The barrier effect also may be lost by thermal burns or traumatic injuries. Disruption of the normal protective barrier can allow easier entry of chemicals into the systemic circulation.

In addition, systemic illness can occur even without skin damage because many fat-soluble chemicals (e.g. some organophosphate insecticides) can penetrate intact skin.

*Support Zone*

As the support zone is set up away from the dangers of physical hazards or chemical exposure, contamination is not a serious problem in this area. Generally, personnel in the support zone does not require special protective clothing as long as victims have been decontaminated properly.

One important exception is exposure to a potent organophosphate pesticide or similar chemical; the support zone team should wear disposable aprons or gowns and latex gloves.

## FURTHER READING

1. SP Kalantri, Sumedh Jajoo. WHO. http://medind.nic.in/jaw/t11/i1/jawt11i1p1.pdf.
2. U.S. Department of Human Services, Public Health Service, Agency for Toxic Substance and Disease Registry. Medical management guidelines for acute chemical exposures. [Online]. Available from wonder.cdc.gov/wonder/prevguid/p0000016/p0000016.asp; 1992 [accessed August, 2012].

## CASE STUDY 61: IRON POISONING IN CHILDREN

## BACKGROUND

Iron is a common accidental and intentional poisoning. It can carry a high morbidity and is one of the greatest causes of fatality in the pediatric age group from poisoning.

## MECHANISM

Excessive iron is corrosive to the gastrointestinal (GI) system and can lead to hemorrhage. It can cause direct vasodilation leading to hypotension. It can affect most organs. It is a direct mitochondrial poison—where it gets concentrated, disrupts oxidative phosphorylation and causes free radical formation leading to cell death. In the liver, it causes "cloudy swelling" of the hepatocytes.

## TOXIC DOSE

It is important to determine the elemental content of iron in each tablet (Tables 1 and 2).

**Table 1:** Elemental iron content of various iron formulations.

| Formulation | Elemental iron content (%) |
| --- | --- |
| Ferrous fumarate | 33 |
| Ferrous sulfate | 20 |
| Ferrous gluconate | 12 |

**Table 2:** Approach of treatment according to the dose of elemental iron uptake.

| Elemental iron dose | Suggested management |
| --- | --- |
| <20 mg/kg | Treat at home |
| >40 mg/kg (or lower if symptomatic) | Refer to hospital |

## STAGES OF IRON TOXICITY

- *0-6 h*: Nausea, vomiting, abdominal pain, diarrhea, and hematemesis (in severe cases) can occur.
- *Up to 12 h*: A quiescent or danger phase occurs. One may develop a false sense of security in this phase.
- *Starting at 6-12 h*: This is the most serious phase including shock, GI hemorrhage, and hepatic toxicity.
- *Weeks later*: This is the recovery phase where liver will be regenerated, if recovery has occurred. Gastric and intestinal stricture may be found at this time.

## LABORATORY TESTS

Iron levels should be obtained at 4 h postingestion. Peak levels >500 µg/dL are considered toxic. Total iron binding capacity (TIBC) will be falsely elevated and is not necessary to be drawn. If the iron level exceeds the TIBC, this confirms toxicity but if not present does not exclude the toxicity.

Electrolytes may reveal an increased anion gap and metabolic acidosis. White blood count and glucose levels >15,000/mm$^3$ and 150 mg/dL, respectively, have previously been correlated with a toxic iron level. A recent study has shown these parameters to be unreliable; therefore, if these values are present, they may suggest toxicity but if absent does not rule it out. An X-ray of kidneys, ureters, and bladder (KUB) should be ordered to look for retained tablets. A positive KUB has been suggested as an indication for whole bowel irrigation with a polyethylene glycol electrolyte lavage solution (Golytely).

## TREATMENT

- Supportive care: Fluid resuscitation and cardiac monitoring
- Bowel irrigation/gastric lavage in limited cases

- IV or IM deferoxamine: Iron chelating agent of choice, with a standard dose of 15 mg/kg/h administered over 6 h. Indications include shock, altered mental status, persistent GI symptoms, overdose >60 mg/kg, metabolic acidosis.

Contact American Association of Poison Control Centers at 1-800-222-1222 for acute poisoning advice. Document the reference number given by poison control and follow their recommendations. Each country has its own poison control center for free 24-h advice. Parents and physicians can reach them anytime.

Deferoxamine therapy is optimally done as an intravenous infusion at 10–15 mg/kg/h. A "vin-rose" color is a marker that iron is being removed from the body and excreted in the urine. However, the only important markers to follow are the persistence of an anion gap or low PH. Once this has resolved, deferoxamine can be discontinued. The deferoxamine should be used until the patient is free of systemic toxicity. It generally should not be used beyond 24 h because of the risk of developing delayed acute respiratory distress syndrome (ARDS) from deferoxamine toxicity.

## PREVENTION

An iron overdose is the leading cause of fatalities in children <6 years of age. Unintentional overdose of prenatal vitamins and pure iron preparations of ferrous sulfate tablets are the most common cause as the tablets are brightly colored and have the appearance of candy (Fig. 1). Safety locks on medicine

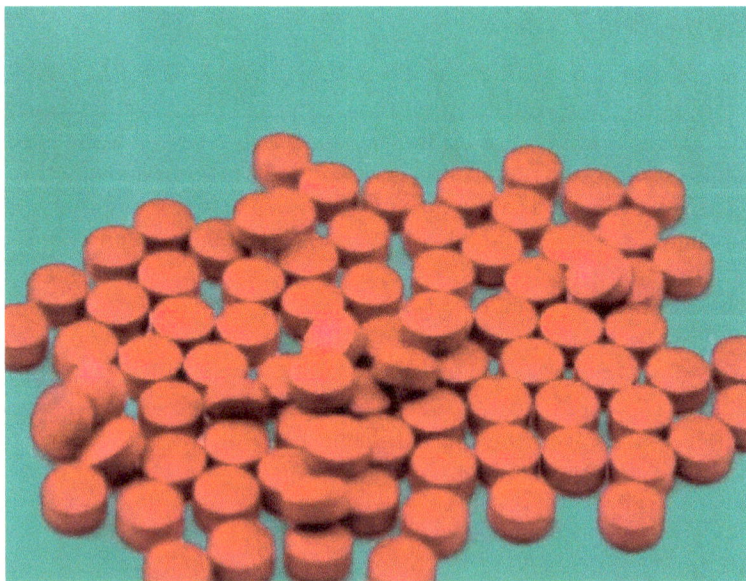

**Fig. 1:** Iron tablets

cabinets and properly sealed medicine containers are advised to prevent iron overdose. Fatal toxicity has been associated with >60 mg/kg of elemental iron ingestion.

Children perceive iron tablets as candy. One tablet is considered serious or fatal.

WHO. http://www.who.int/nutrition/topics/TOR_consultant_indicator_trained_ifasupplementation/en/.

## CASE STUDY 62: CARBON MONOXIDE POISONING

### CASE HISTORY

A 40-year-old male who was working in the garage for 2–3 h on his car, without opening the garage because of cold weather, is brought to emergency department for severe headache, nausea, and vomiting.

Carbon monoxide (CO) is an odorless, colorless gas that accounts for approximately 400 deaths annually. It is known as "the great imitator" and can typically cause vague symptoms mimicking other illnesses such as viral syndromes. CO is formed by incomplete combustion of carbonaceous fuels.

### MECHANISM

There are four major mechanisms of toxicity:
- Binding directly to hemoglobin causing a shift in the oxygen dissociation curve to the left
- Direct cardiovascular depression
- Inhibition of cytochrome
- Lipid peroxidation (free radical generation).

### CLINICAL EFFECTS

Symptoms impact all organ systems. Headache is the most common presenting symptom seen in patients with carbon monoxide poisoning. Patients also often nausea, vomiting, dizziness, and fatigue. This may be misdiagnosed as viral syndrome. They may present with altered mental status as well. Levels do not necessarily correlate with signs and symptoms; the guidelines are given in Table 1.

### LABORATORY TESTS

Generally, a level >10% of carboxyhemoglobin (COHb) confirms poisoning in smokers and a level higher than 5% confirms poisoning in a nonsmoker.

**Table 1:** Signs and symptoms associated with carbon monoxide poisoning and correlated carboxyhemoglobin levels.

| COHb% | Signs and symptoms |
|---|---|
| 0 | None |
| 10 | Frontal headache |
| 20 | Throbbing headache |
| 30 | Impaired judgment, nausea, dizziness visual disturbance, fatigue |
| 40 | Confusion, syncope |
| 50 | Coma, seizures |
| 60 | Hypotension, respiratory failure |
| 70 | Death |

Levels are as discussed above. Other important evaluations include creatine phosphokinase for the risk of rhabdomyolysis, electrocardiography and cardiac enzymes for ischemia, neuropsychiatric testing and pulse oximetry or arterial blood gases (ABG). Findings of ABG include a normal $PaO_2$, a falsely elevated calculated oxygen saturation and a decreased measured oxygen saturation. Standard pulse oximetry cannot be used to rule out carbon monoxide poisoning.

## TREATMENT

Remove the patient from the source of exposure and administer high-flow 100% oxygen and immediate attention should focus on the airway, breathing, and circulation. Cardiac monitoring and IV line should be established.

Hyperbaric oxygen is indicated for more severe poisoning. Hyperbaric therapy is aimed at lowering the potential for delayed neuropsychiatric sequelae.

### Indications for Hyperbaric Therapy

- History of coma or loss of consciousness*
- COHb >25
- COHb >40, if transfer to chamber is required
- Symptoms persisting >4 h in spite of oxygen therapy
- Abnormal neuropsychiatric testing
- Neonates
- Pregnancy with a level >10*
- Low pH <7.2.

---

* Noncontroversial indications.

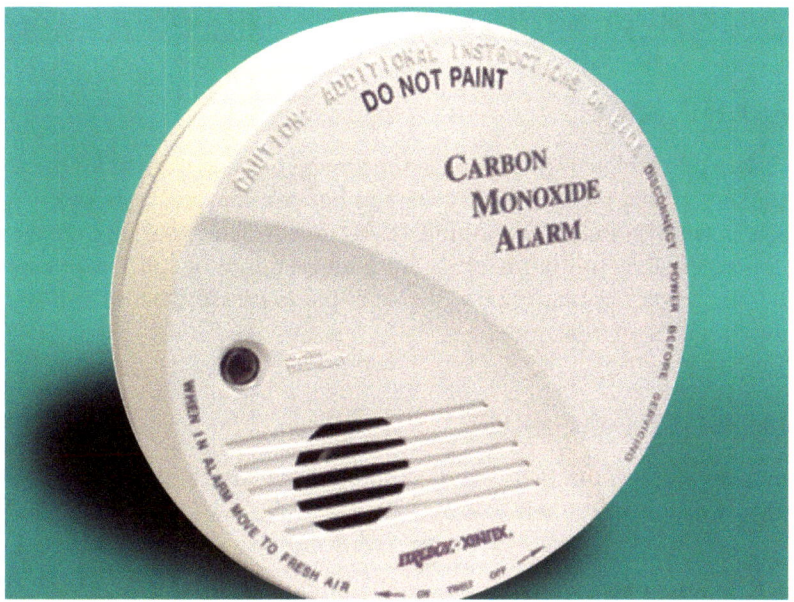

**Fig. 1:** Carbon monoxide alarm.

## PREVENTION

You can prevent carbon monoxide exposure:
- Have your heating system, water heater, and any other gas, oil, or coal burning appliances serviced by a qualified technician every year
- Install a battery-operated or battery back-up CO detector in your home (Fig. 1) and check or replace the battery when you change the time on your clocks each spring and fall. If the detector sounds, leave your home immediately and call 911 (United States) or 100 (India)
- Seek prompt medical attention if you suspect CO poisoning and are feeling dizzy, light-headed or nauseous
- Do not use a generator, charcoal grill, camp stove, or other gasoline or charcoal-burning device inside your home, basement, or garage or near a window
- Do not run a car or truck inside a garage attached to your house, even if you leave the door open
- Do not burn anything in a stove or fireplace that is not vented
- Do not heat your house with a gas oven.

## FURTHER READING

1. http://www.cdc.gov/co/guidelines.htm.

## CASE STUDY 63: HEAT EMERGENCY

## CASE HISTORY

A 19-year-old athlete is presented to the emergency department for the chief complaint of very high fever, very dry and hot red skin, and tachycardic with feeble pulse with shallow breathing. He is confused and delirious. On arrival to the emergency room, his vitals are a temperature of 106.2°F, pulse rate 150 bpm, respiratory rate 22 breaths/min, blood pressure 90/40 mm Hg, $O_2$ saturation 98% on room air.

## DIAGNOSTIC WORKUP

Complete blood count (CBC) and comprehensive metabolic panel (CMP) is drawn and also urine analysis is performed.

## Differential Diagnosis

See Table 1.

**Table 1:** Heat-related injuries.

| Sunburn | Heat cramps | Heat exhaustion |
|---|---|---|
| Red skin, pain, possible swelling, blisters, fever, headaches | Pain normally in leg and abdominal muscles, profuse sweating | Victim must lie down in a cool area. Remove clothing. Apply cool, wet clothes. Use a fan or air conditioner. If victim is conscious, give water. Allow victim to consume water slowly every 15 min. Do not give water if victim is nauseated. If there is vomiting, seek medical attention |
| Remove oils that may be blocking pores by taking a shower. Be sure to not allow the body to cool naturally. For any blisters that occur, apply a dry, sterile dressing and seek medical attention | Take victim to cooler environment, ease muscle spasms by lightly stretching and massaging gently, every 15 min give half a glass of cool water (liquid should not contain caffeine or alcohol) If victim is nauseated, do not give any more liquids | |

# DIAGNOSIS (FLOWCHART 1)

Flowchart 1: Types of heat stroke.

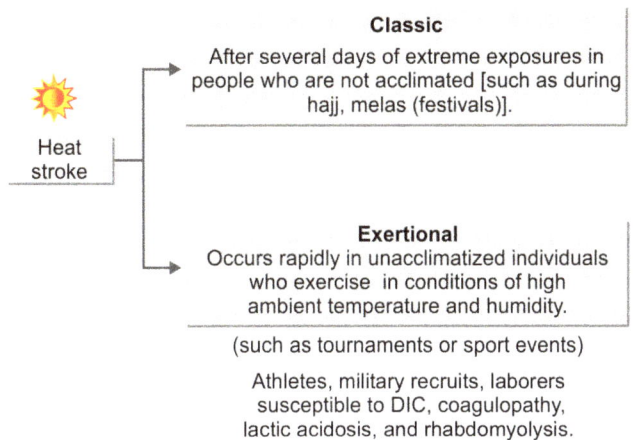

# TREATMENT (FLOWCHART 2)

Move victim to cooler room, remove clothing, intravenous (IV) fluid resuscitation, attempt body immersion in ice water, and cooling the skin via evaporation by spraying water over the patient and via convection by using fans. Immersing the hands and forearms in ice cold water is necessary, watch for breathing problems, apply ice packs, and deal with extreme caution. Aspirin, salicylates, ibuprofen, acetaminophen, and dantrolene are all not effective and can cause more harm.

Central venous pressure (CVP) monitoring is necessary in extreme heat exhaustion and heat stroke. Immunomodulators like corticosteroids can be

Flowchart 2: Treatment plan.

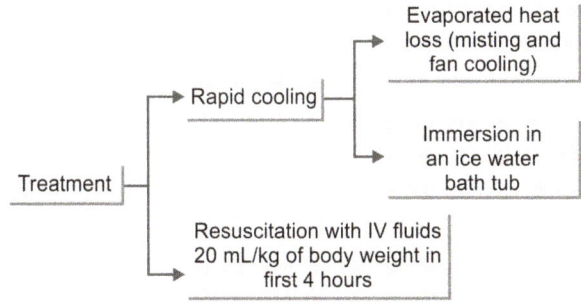

Note: Stop cooling when temperature is 102°F (38.9°C)

used if necessary. Iced gastric, bladder, or peritoneal lavage may also prove helpful in severe situations.

Altered mental status, agitation, and shivering can be suppressed by administering 1–2 mg IV benzodiazepines, such as Lorazepam. This will also aid in core body temperature cooling.

In order to minimize risk of iatrogenic hypothermia, continuous monitoring of rectal temperature is mandatory. Cooling efforts must be stopped once the rectal temperature reaches 38–39°C.

Recently, alternative cooling methods have been used, including water ice therapy (WIT) in which the patient lies supine on stretcher placed on top of an ice water tub. This was shown to be 70% as effective as cold-water immersion.

## FURTHER READING

1. https://www.uptodate.com/contents/severe-nonexertional-hyperthermia-classic-heat-stroke-in-adults?source=search_result&search=heat%20stroke&selectedTitle=1~58.
2. https://www.ncbi.nlm.nih.gov/pubmed?term=19653575.

## CASE STUDY 64: AMPHETAMINES OVERDOSE

## CASE HISTORY

An 18-year-old student of 12th grade is brought to the emergency department by his parents early one morning for "behaving oddly." He reportedly stayed awake all night studying for one of his final examinations. His mother found him early in the morning making spaghetti for himself in the kitchen. Her son was extremely anxious and could not sit still or calm himself. At presentation, the boy is very talkative but emotionally labile. His temperature is 38.3°C, heart rate 120 bpm, respiratory rate 20 breaths/min, and blood pressure 140/90 mm Hg. His skin is flushed, and his pupils are dilated. Mild hyperreflexia is noted on physical examination.

## DIFFERENTIAL DIAGNOSIS

- Substance abuse or amphetamines abuse
- Sepsis
- Encephalitis
- Meningitis or brain abscess
- Neuroleptic malignant syndrome (NMS)
- Malignant hyperthermia.

Environmental Injuries, Toxicology, and Animal Bites

## DISCUSSION

- Hyperthermia has a broad differential, and drugs of abuse should be kept in mind.
- Watch for rhabdomyolysis, disseminated intravascular coagulation (DIC), and multiorgan failure after hyperpyrexia.
- Amphetamines result in dopamine, norepinephrine and serotonin release, and catecholamine surge.

## SYMPTOMS

- Patient may present with altered mental status, agitation, seizures, palpitations, chest pain, nausea, vomiting, and diarrhea (Fig. 1).
- Severe hyperpyrexia
- Hyponatremia.

## TREATMENTS

Amphetamine overdose patients should be treated based on the severity of symptoms. The main goal is to reduce core body temperature, rehydration, and sedation. Cardiac monitoring may be needed to monitor for arrhythmias.

If amphetamine was ingesting within 1 h, oral activated charcoal can be given. Supportive care with intravenous (IV) fluids and cooling is recommended.

Severely intoxicated patients can become extremely agitated or violent and should be sedated with IV benzodiazepines (Midazolam 2.5-5 mg or Lorazepam 2-4 mg IV). IM injection may be used if IV access is not possible.

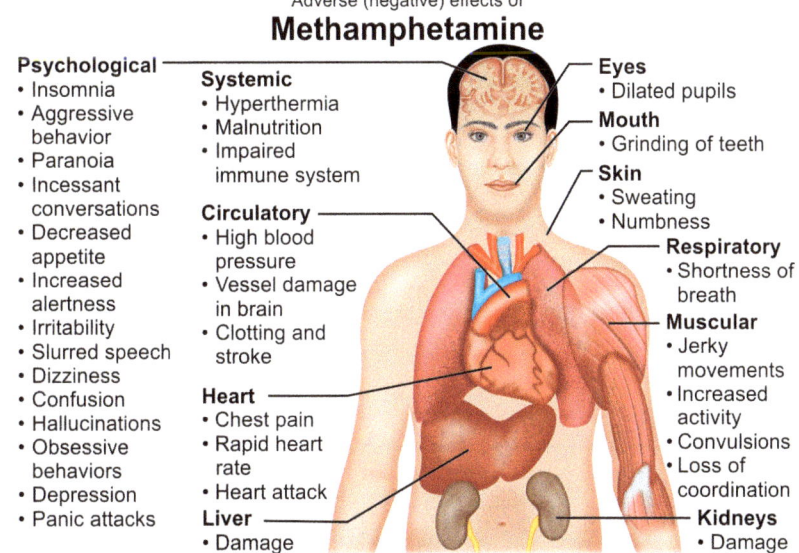

**Fig. 1:** Adverse effects of amphetamine overdose.

Benzodiazapine (BDZ) dosing can be repeated every 8–10 min depending on patient response. A second benzodiazepine or adjunctive second-generation antipsychotic agents such as ziprasidone 10 mg IV or haloperidol 5–10 mg IV may be used if the first drug has minimal effect after more than two doses.

Patients with severe hyperthermia (core body temperature >104°F) should be immediately cooled down with cooling blankets and cooled IV fluids. Aggressive sedation, neuromuscular paralysis, and fluid resuscitation may also be utilized. Antipyretics have no role treatment of amphetamine induced hyperthermia.

Hypovolemic patients should be resuscitated with isotonic saline and should be monitored for fluid overload. In the cases of metabolic acidosis or rhabdomyolysis, patients should be treated with aggressive IV fluids with a urine output of ≥1-2 mL/kg/h.

Benzodiazepines help decrease blood pressure; however, if hypertension persists, labetalol, nitroprusside, nitroglycerine, and phentolamine may be used. Cardiac monitoring should be done on all patients with symptoms of chest pain or presence of underlying ischemic heart disease.

## COMPLICATIONS

- Rhabdomyolysis
- DIC
- Renal failure
- Hepatic necrosis
- Gastrointestinal bleeding
- Diarrhea
- Risk of vasculitis
- Neuropsychiatric abnormalitis
- Damage to dopaminergic and serotonergic neurons
- Cardiomyopathy.

## FURTHER READING

1. https://online.epocrates.com/diseases/34141/Amphetamine-overdose/Treatment-Approach.
2. https://www.uptodate.com/contents/methamphetamine-acute-intoxication?source=search_result&search=amphetamine%20overdose&selectedTitle=1~150#H9.

## CASE STUDY 65: MARIJUANA (CANNABIS) ABUSE

## CASE HISTORY

A 16-year-old girl is caught smoking marijuana with friends by her parents. She is now in the emergency department for assessment. She admits to smoking marijuana with these same friends on two other occasions over the past

6 months. She has also been to two parties where alcohol was available, and she states that she drank fewer than two beers at each event. She denies tobacco use and use of any other illicit drugs. She states that she is sorry that she "broke her parent's trust" and says she is motivated to remain abstinent.

## DISCUSSION

Marijuana is a prevalent substance of abuse among teenagers and adults.[1] Two out of every five Americans admit to having tried marijuana in their lifetime, and one in ten have used in the past year. Marijuana is made with mixture of dried parts of the Cannabis sativa plant and is usually smoked. Street names include pot, weed, bud, herb, ganja, hashish, grass, and bhang (Fig. 1). Marijuana smoked as cigarettes are referred to as joints, whereas pipes used to smoke it are called bongs. When cigars are used, they are referred to as blunts.[2]

Marijuana is the most commonly used illegal drug with a higher admission rate to treatment programs than all other drugs combined. Although marijuana is typically thought to be a milder drug, it can have systemic, multiorgan effects, and it can have a profound impact on all areas of one's life including their personal life and employment. The active ingredient in marijuana is Δ-9-tetrahydrocannabinol (THC). Marijuana today has three times as much THC as that sold 20 years ago, making it much more potent. Puff for puff, smoking marijuana is more dangerous than smoking cigarettes, and its use has been linked to head and neck cancer.

Users often feel relaxed, have feelings of euphoria, increased heart rate, poor balance and coordination, slow reaction time, disorientation, and panic. After the effects begin to fade, users begin to feel sleepiness, depression, and distrust or paranoia. Long-term marijuana use can impair learning

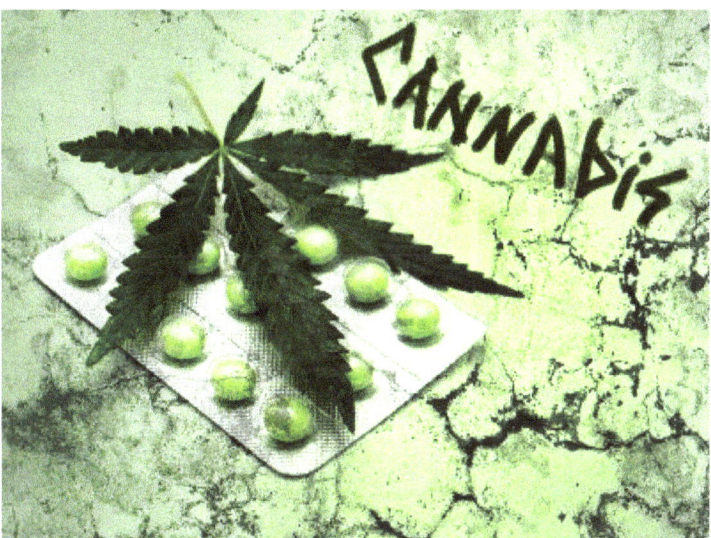

**Fig. 1:** Marijuana preparation in tablet form.

and memory, and lower grades and poor work performance can result when people use marijuana.[3]

Legally, marijuana has been used to treat several medical conditions including glaucoma, nausea that occurs with AIDS and cancer treatments, and the pain caused by multiple sclerosis. Marinol is the prescription form which contains marijuana's active ingredient of THC. Marinol is mainly used to treat nausea and vomiting.

## TREATMENT

Mild intoxication can be managed by placing patient in a dark quite room and reassurance. Benzodiazepines, such as Lorazepam is helpful.

Severe intoxication with violent behavior can be managed with combination therapy using second-generation antipsychotics like risperidone and haloperidol.

Recent studies have shown that Canabanoid Hyperemesis Syndrome (CHS) can be effectively and efficiently managed with capsaicin cream, which is a derivative of chili peppers belonging to Genus Capsicum.[4]

## PREVENTION

The best method for marijuana abuse is prevention. Abstinence greatly increases the chance for a successful recovery. Patients may benefit from seeing a psychiatrist or psychologist for cognitive behavioral therapy to control their addiction.

## REFERENCES

1. Fine KS. Substance use and abuse. In: Pediatric board recertification review. Philadelphia, PA: Lippincott Williams & Wilkins; 2008. p. 159-70.
2. National Institute on Drug Abuse. DrugFacts: marijuana. [Online]. Available from www.drugabuse.gov/publications/infofacts/marijuana; 2010 [accessed September, 2012].
3. National Institute on Drug Abuse. MedlinePlus: marijuana. [Online]. Available from www.nlm.nih.gov/medlineplus/marijuana.html; 2012 [accessed September, 2012].
4. EPmonthly.com. October 18, Vol. 25. No. 10

## FURTHER READING

1. https://www.uptodate.com/contents/cannabis-marijuana-acute-intoxication?source=search_result&search=marijuana&selectedTitle=1~150#H455 434711.

## CASE STUDY 66: HEROIN ABUSE

## CASE HISTORY

An 18-year-old female is presented to the emergency department (ED) unresponsive via emergency medical services (EMS). According to EMS, her parents called 911 after finding her unresponsive in her bedroom. They say, she had recently been exhibiting strange behavior at home, but they did not know she had been using drugs until they found her unresponsive with needles lying next to her on the floor. They could barely tell if she was breathing but were able to find a faint pulse. En route, EMS started her on nasal cannula, placed two large bore intravenous (IV) lines, and administered Narcan subcutaneously. They noted that her breathing improved somewhat, but that she was still unresponsive. Vitals are temperature of 37°C, blood pressure 100/70 mm Hg, pulse rate 60 bpm, respiratory rate 8 breaths/min, and $O_2$ saturation level 85% on nasal cannula. Physical examination reveals an unconscious female with unreactive pinpoint pupils and several track marks on her forearms bilaterally. The airway cart is prepared while the patient is administered 2 mg of naloxone intravenously. Patient's respiratory rate improves, and she starts to regain consciousness. Two minutes later, another dose of 2-mg naloxone is administered. Now, the patient is awake and alert, sitting up in bed and vomiting. Laboratory tests, urine analysis, and urine drug screening are ordered, and the patient is admitted for further monitoring of withdrawal effects.

## DISCUSSION

Heroin is an illegal, highly addictive street drug.[1] It is commonly taken intravenously but may be administered in other forms also (Figs. 1 and 2).

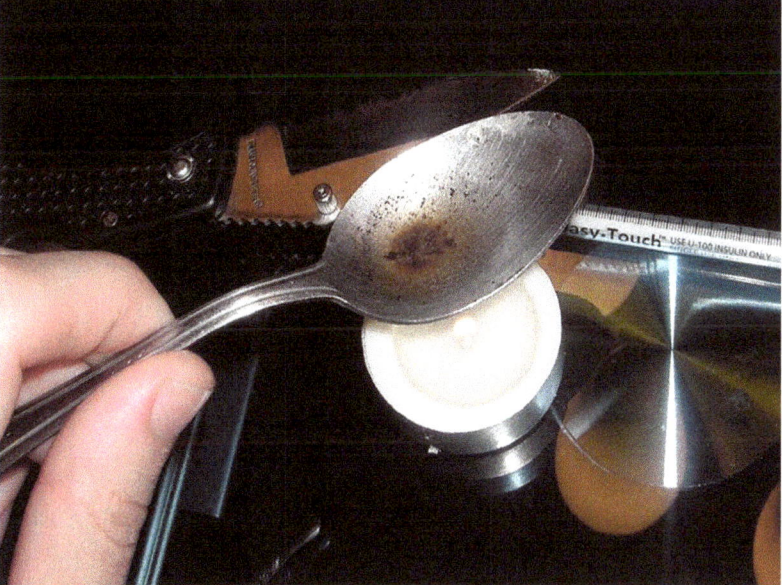

**Fig. 1:** Preparing heroin for injection.
*Source:* www.wikipedia.com.

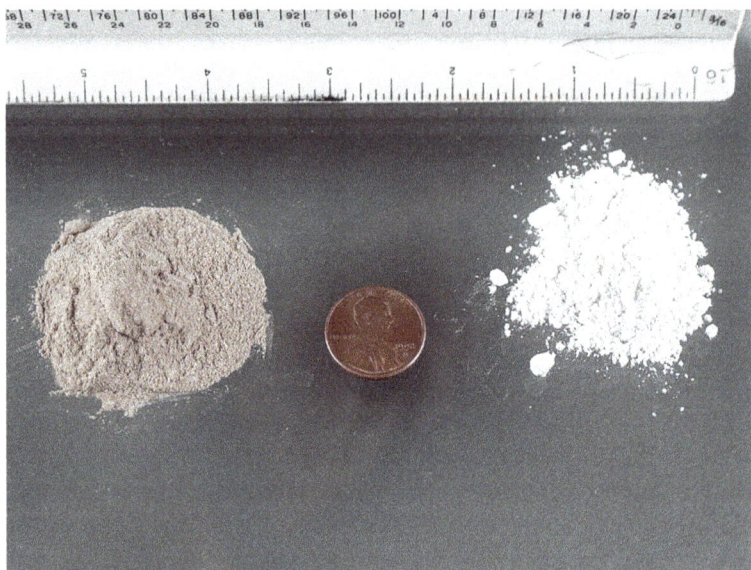

**Fig. 2:** Heroin comes in brown or white powder.
*Source:* Drug Enforcement Agency, United States of America.

Street names include junk, smack, and skag. It is made from morphine which occurs naturally in the seed pods of poppy plants. Patients experience a sense of euphoria when using this drug. Over time, patients develop a tolerance and require more and more of the substance to achieve the same effect.

Symptoms of overdose include lack of breathing, shallow breathing, or slow and difficult breathing.[2] Patients may also have dry mouth, pinpoint pupils, tongue discoloration, low blood pressure, weak pulses, bluish colored nails and lips, constipation, intestinal spasms, coma, delirium, disorientation, drowsiness, and muscle spasticity. Skin examination may reveal track marks, or marks from "popping" heroin on the skin.

Overdoses may be made more severe when the heroin is mixed with other drugs.[3] This may make treatment and recovery much more difficult.

## TREATMENT

Treatment should include airway support, fluids, laxatives, and naloxone. Naloxone is an opioid antagonist which can reverse the effects of the opioid. This can be very useful in cases where breathing or mental status is altered. However, naloxone may also precipitate severe withdrawal effects. Effects should be seen from naloxone within 5 min. Naloxone may be given 0.4–2 mg IV every 2–3 min pro re nata (PRN) or when necessary. It may also be given intramuscularly, subcutaneously, or via endotracheal tube or started on continuous infusion. If symptoms occur, naloxone may be administered every

1–2 h. However, if there is no response initially after 10 mg, an alternative diagnosis should be considered.

Although naloxone nasal spray has shown no clear benefit in clinical trials with cardiac arrest patients, rapid naloxone nasal spray can be lifesaving for patients that have a pulse and severe hypoventilation with respiratory depression.

Treatment for withdrawal involves supportive care. Clonidine may be used to reduce symptoms of anxiety, agitation, myalgias, sweating, rhinitis, and abdominal cramping. Buprenorphine is also a promising medication for treating withdrawal symptoms and in fact has been shown to shorten the length of detoxification. Suboxone is the commercial name for buprenorphine combined with naloxone. It is used to treat opioid dependence. This is a high alert medication because it can cause significant harm to patients if used incorrectly.

Due to the severe withdrawal effects, methadone is often used to control these symptoms. The dose of methadone is then slowly decreased over time. Methadone is an opioid agonist that does not cause the same high of heroin but limits withdrawal because it acts at the same receptors. Methadone has a very long half-life and may be taken only once a day in order to help patients live a more normal, symptom-free life.

## REFERENCES

1. MedlinePlus. Heroin. [Online]. Available from www.nlm.nih.gov/medlineplus/heroin.html; 2012 [accessed September, 2012].
2. MedlinePlus. Heroin overdose. [Online]. Available from www.nlm.nih.gov/medlineplus/ency/article/002861.htm; 2012 [accessed September, 2012].
3. Medscape. Heroin toxicity clinical presentation. [Online]. Available from emedicine.medscape.com/article/166464-clinical#a0217; 2011 [accessed September, 2012].

## FURTHER READING

1. MedlinePlus. Heroin withdrawal. [Online]. Available from www.nlm.nih.gov/medlineplus/ency/article/000949.htm; 2012 [Accessed September, 2012].
2. http://www.justice.gov/dea/pr/multimedia-library/image-gallery/images_heroin.shtml.

## CASE STUDY 67: ALKALINE BURNS

## INTRODUCTION

The following is a case report showing comparison of acid and alkaline burns sustained by patients involved in industrial accidents.

Alkaline burns are often more damaging than acid burns due to the subsequent liquefaction necrosis that occurs at the site of injury. This involves denaturation of proteins and saponification of fats, which allows extensive tissue penetration. The patient in this case is presented to the emergency department (ED) with sodium hydroxide burns to approximately 18% of his body, encompassing mainly the right leg. The patient was treated with irrigation of the wound, intravenous (IV) fluids, and pain relief before transfer to a burn unit.

The damage from hydrofluoric acid burns results from the corrosiveness of the free hydrogen ions and the tissue penetration and coagulation necrosis caused by the acid. It additionally causes systemic toxicities due to depletion of total body calcium and magnesium, which results in enzymatic and cellular dysfunction. Most deaths are due to cardiac arrhythmias caused by hypocalcemia, which subsequently causes hyperkalemia.

## CASE REPORT 1

A 26-year-old male is presented to the ED after a chemical burn injury to the right lower extremity. He had been standing on top of a chemical tank at work when he slipped and his leg fell into the tank, which was filled with sodium hydroxide.

He has no past medical history and social history is significant only for chewing tobacco.

On initial presentation, he has a blood pressure (BP) of 132/76 mm Hg, pulse rate of 89 bpm, respiratory rate of 20 breaths/min, and temperature of 97.9°F. He is found to have second degree burns to approximately 18% of his body encompassing the right leg and right lower quadrant of the abdomen (Fig. 1). He has blistering throughout the right leg and an area of black eschar on the right calf.

The wound is immediately irrigated with sterile saline, and he is started on IV normal saline at 200 mL/h. Additionally, he is given 30 mg of toradol IV for pain relief. Vital signs remain stable, and he is transferred to a burn unit.

## CASE REPORT 2

A 29-year-old male is presented to the ED after a chemical burn injury to the right upper extremity. He had been working in a chemical plant when he dropped a container of hydrofluoric acid and sustained a splash injury.

He has no past medical history, and social history is significant only for occasional alcohol use.

On initial presentation, he has a BP of 137/72 mm Hg, pulse rate of 91 bpm, respiratory rate of 20 breaths/min, and temperature of 98.8°F. He is found to have second degree burns to approximately 9% of his body encompassing the right arm. He has blistering throughout the right arm.

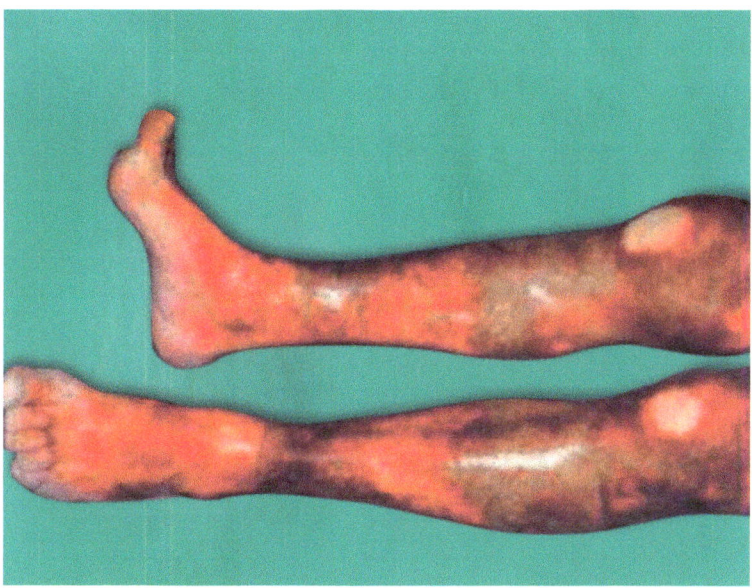

**Fig. 1:** Cement burns are one type of alkaline burn.
*Source:* Reprinted with permission from tunneltalk.com.

The wound is immediately irrigated with sterile saline and 2.5% calcium gluconate gel is applied. He is started on IV normal saline at 200 mL/h and is given 30 mg of Toradol IV for pain relief. Vital signs remain stable, and he is transferred to a burn unit.

## DISCUSSION

The pathophysiology of chemical burns involves three zones of local response. The zone of coagulation is the point of maximum contact and is the site of irreversible damage due to coagulation of proteins. Surrounding this area is the zone of stasis, which is an area of decreased tissue perfusion. This area is potentially salvageable, if proper resuscitation is started quickly. Finally, there is zone of hyperemia in which there is increased perfusion. This zone will recover as long as prolonged hypoperfusion and sepsis do not develop.[1]

Sodium hydroxide is an extremely corrosive substance. Although it does not cause systemic toxicity, it causes severe burns to any area of body with which it comes in contact. It is especially damaging to the eyes due its ability to hydrolyze protein.

## TREATMENT

The standard of care is to notify poison control and get chemical information from safety data sheets (SDS) located on the chemical container or

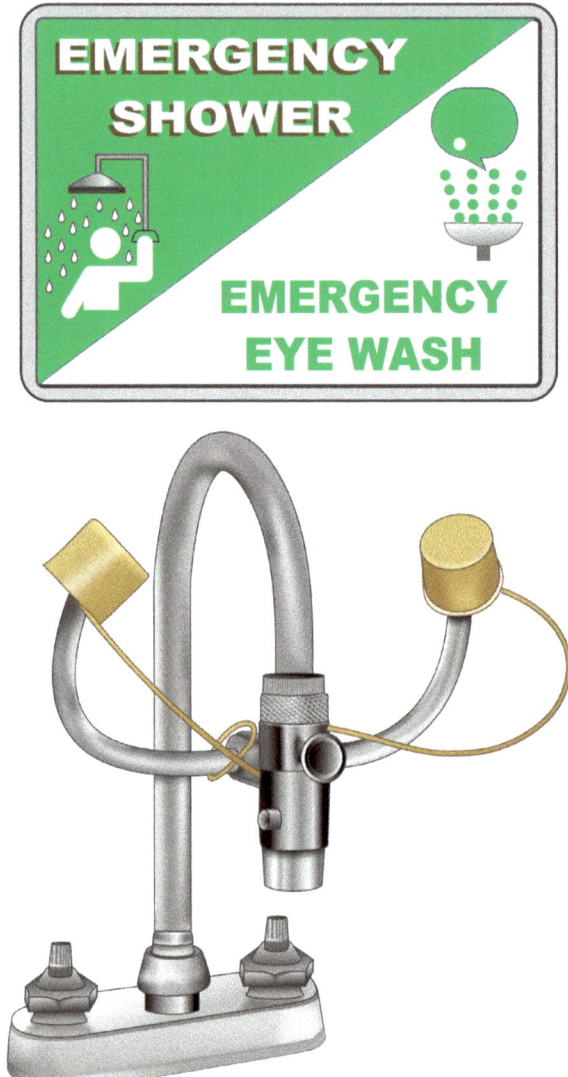

**Fig. 2:** Emergency eye wash tool.
*Source:* https://www.gemplers.com/product/109424/ANSI-compliant-Faucet-mounted-Eyewash-Station.

factory material SDSs (MSDS) required by law. OSHA (Occupational Safety and Health Administration) can be reached at 1-800-321-6742 (OSHA) to report emergencies, unsafe working condition, and any health violations (Fig. 2).

Any chemical burn treatment focuses on irrigation of the wound to decrease the length of exposure to the substance and fluid resuscitation to account for losses from the burned areas. There has been some research regarding whether neutralization with a weak acid would improve outcomes in alkaline burns. For hydrofluoric acid burns, it is additionally important to apply calcium gluconate cream to the wound in order to neutralize the hydrofluoric acid.[3] It is also essential to monitor electrolytes and telemetry as arrhythmia due to hyperkalemia is a common cause of death.

In unfortunate cases of ocular alkali burns, prompt and aggressive treatment with an emergency eye wash/irrigation, a broad spectrum topical antibiotic (e.g. fluoroquinolone) should be applied to the eye as soon as irrigation is completed. A stat emergent ophthalmology consult is warranted.

As far as long-term treatments for all types of burns are concerned, there have been monumental advances in use of artificial skin for replacement after extensive burn injuries. The grafts are able to restore many of the physiological functions and anatomical structure of the skin, thus improving long-term outcome.

## REFERENCES

1. Hettiaratchy S, Dziewulski P. Pathophysiology and types of burns. BMJ 2004; 328:1427-9.
2. Matsuno K. The treatment of hydrofluoric acid burns. Occup Med (Lond) 1996;46:313-7.
3. Tompkins RG, Burke JF. Progress in burn treatment and the use of artificial skin. World J Surg 1990;14:819-24.

## FURTHER READING

1. PPE last choice for safety. http://www.tunneltalk.com/Safety-Sep10-PPE-last-resort.php. [Accessed 3/28/2013].
2. Andrews K, Mowlavi A, Milner SM. The treatment of alkaline burns of the skin by neutralization. Plast Reconstr Surg 2003;111:1918-21.
3. https://www.uptodate.com/contents/topical-chemical-burns?source= search_result&search=alkali%20burn&selectedTitle=1~65#H6.
4. https://www.osha.gov/html/Feed_Back.html.

CHAPTER **10**

# Sexually Transmitted Infections

## CASE STUDY 68: PELVIC INFLAMMATORY DISEASE

### CASE HISTORY

A 23-year-old female is presented to the emergency department (ED) with left lower quadrant (LLQ) abdominal pain for 1 day. She reports a history of multiple sexual partners and was treated for chlamydia 1 year ago. Her only medication is oral contraceptive pills. On examination, her vital signs are temperature 101°F, pulse rate 87 bpm, respiratory rate 16 breaths/min, and blood pressure 118/78 mm Hg. On physical examination, she has moderate LLQ tenderness on palpation but no rigidity or guarding. She has cervical motion tenderness on bimanual examination.

### CASE DISCUSSION

Pelvic inflammatory disease (PID) is an infection of the reproductive tract (Fig. 1) and begins in the lower genital tract and ascends into the endometrium, adnexa, or peritoneal cavity. This can lead to salpingitis, endometritis, tubo-ovarian abscess (TOA), perihepatitis, or focal pelvic peritonitis. It is almost always caused by *Neisseria gonorrhoeae* or *Chlamydia trachomatis* but 30–40% are polymicrobial. Risk factors for PID include multiple sexual partners, sexual abuse, adolescence, presence of other sexually transmitted diseases, douching, and intrauterine devices. It is uncommon in pregnancy but can lead to fetal loss, if it occurs in the first trimester. Long-term complications include ectopic pregnancy, infertility, and chronic pain.

### CLINICAL PRESENTATION

The most common feature is lower abdominal pain. Other symptoms include vaginal discharge, vaginal bleeding, dyspareunia, urinary discomfort, fever, nausea, and vomiting. Peritoneal signs may also be present. Patients presenting

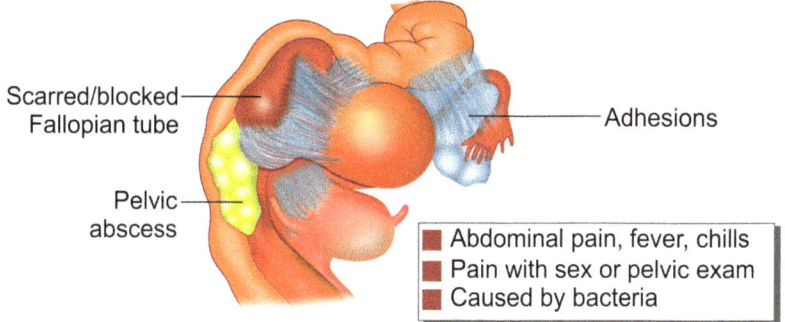

**Fig. 1:** Anatomy of female reproductive system.

with right upper quadrant pain with jaundice should be suspected of having Fitz–Hugh–Curtis syndrome or perihepatitis.

## DIAGNOSIS

Diagnosis begins with a pregnancy test, wet prep, and endocervical swabs for gonorrhea and chlamydia. Elevation of white blood cell count, erythrocyte sedimentation rate, and C-reactive protein also suggest the diagnosis. A pelvic ultrasound can be used to detect TOA. It is important to remember that PID may mimic surgical conditions such as appendicitis, cholecystitis, and ovarian torsion. Differential diagnosis also include diverticulitis, ectopic pregnancy, spontaneous or septic abortion, ovarian cyst, pyelonephritis, and renal colic.

Box 1 lists the Center for Disease Control and Prevention recommended diagnostic criteria for PID.

---

**Box 1:** CDC diagnostic criteria for PID.

*PID should be suspected and treatment is initiated if:*
- Patient is at risk of PID

  and

- Patient has uterine, adnexal or cervical motion tenderness with no other apparent cause
- Findings that support the diagnosis
- Cervical or vaginal mucopurulent (green or yellow) discharge
- Elevated erythrocyte sedimentation rate or C-reactive protein
- Laboratory confirmation of gonorrheal or chlamydial infection
- Oral temperature of 101°F (38.3°C) or greater
- White blood cells on vaginal secretion saline wet mount
- Most specific criteria for the diagnosis
- Endometritis on endometrial biopsy
- Laparoscopic abnormalities consistent with PID
- Thickened, fluid-filled tubes apparent on transvaginal ultrasound or magnetic resonance imaging.

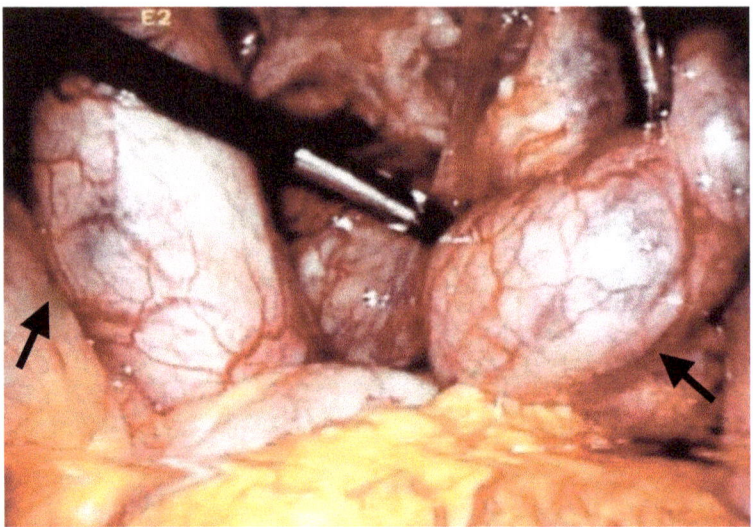

**Fig. 2:** Pyrosalpinx in PID. (PID: pelvic inflammatory disease).
*Source:* Reproduced with permission from RSNA.org, Oak Brook, Illinois, USA.

## TREATMENT

Treatment should begin with adequate analgesia and hydration. The need for inpatient management should be based on toxic appearance, inability to tolerate oral medication, inability to exclude alternative surgical diagnoses (Fig. 2), pregnancy, adolescence, immunosuppression, or suspected anaerobic infection due to intrauterine devices, suspected abscess, or recent instrumentation. If TOA is diagnosed, 60–80% of patients will respond to antibiotics alone while the remainder will require drainage. Patients managed on an outpatient basis should follow up within 72 h, and the patient and sexual partner should complete the full course of treatment in order to prevent reinfection. Preventive counseling and human immunodeficiency virus (HIV) testing should also be provided.

The following are options for outpatient antibiotic therapy:
- Ofloxacin 400 mg PO twice a day (BID) for 14 days or levofloxacin 500 mg PO four times a day (QID) for 14 days with/without metronidazole 500 mg PO BID for 14 days
- Ceftriaxone 250 mg intramuscularly (IM) once or cefoxitin 2 g IM once and probenecid 1 g PO × 1 + doxycycline 100 mg PO BID for 14 days with/without metronidazole 500 mg PO BID for 14 days.

If managed as an inpatient, the following treatment options are recommended.
- Cefotetan 2 g intravenously (IV) q12 h or cefoxitin 2 g IV q6 h with doxycycline 100 mg IV or PO q12 h
- Clindamycin 900 mg IV q8 h with gentamicin 2 mg/kg IV loading dose followed by 1.5 mg/kg q8 h

- Ofloxacin 400 mg IV q12 h or levofloxacin 500 mg IV q24 h, and doxycycline 100 mg PO or IV q12 h with/without metronidazole 500 mg IV q8 h or ampicillin-sulbactam 3 g IV q6 h.

## OTHER COMMON SEXUALLY TRANSMITTED INFECTIONS

### Syphilis

Syphilis is caused by *Treponema pallidum* and is acquired through sexual contact. Early local infection presents as a painless pustule which later ulcerates to form a chancre. This is known as primary syphilis and can spontaneously heal within 3–6 weeks even without treatment. Secondary syphilis manifests weeks to months after the chancre develops and presents with constitutional symptoms (fever, headache, malaise, adenopathy), maculopapular rash, condylomata lata (moist, painless, white wart-like lesions) (Fig. 3), gastrointestinal abnormalities, and hepatitis.

*Treatment*

The treatment of choice is a single dose of 2.4 million units of IM penicillin G.

### Human Immunodeficiency Virus (HIV)

HIV is a blood-borne disease transmitted through sexual contact, IV drug use, and maternal infection. CD4+ counts are used measure disease progression. The acute symptomatic stage is known as the acute retroviral syndrome. Patient's present with a flulike illness with fever, malaise, and

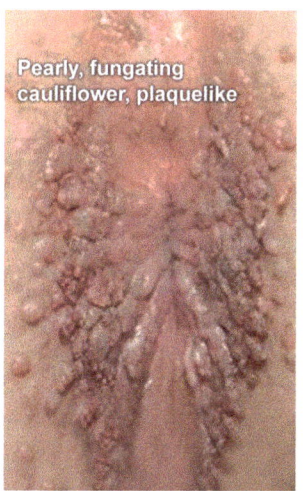

**Fig. 3:** Condylomata acuminata caused by human papilomavirus.
*Source:* https://www.pinterest.co.uk/pin/429812358163393738/.

lymphadenopathy. During the clinical latency stage, HIV is still active but reproduces at a low level. This period can last for 10 years or longer. Patients may not have symptoms but are still infectious. Acquired immunodeficiency syndrome (AIDS) is the sequela of HIV and is diagnosed when the CD4+ cell count drops below 200 cells/mm or when the patient develops an opportunistic infection.

### Treatment

HIV treatment is given as a combination of three drugs:
- Two drugs from nucleoside/nucleotide reverse transcriptase inhibitors (NRTIs) such as lamivudine and emtricitabine. Combination drugs are also available. Truvada is a combination drug of tenofovir and emtricitabine
- Integrase strand transfer inhibitors (INSTI) like raltegravir, protease inhibitors (PI) like ritonavir or a non-nucleoside reverse transcriptase inhibitors (NNRTI) like efavirenz.

Please refer to the CDC chart for treatment of other most common sexually transmitted diseases..

## FURTHER READING

1. https://www.cdc.gov/hiv/basics/whatishiv.html.
2. https://www.uptodate.com/contents/acute-and-early-hiv-infection-treatment?source=search_result&search=HIV&selectedTitle=4~150#H175057212.
3. https://emedicine.medscape.com/article/211316-treatment#d8.
4. https://www.cdc.gov/std/tg2015/2015-wall-chart.pdf.

# CHAPTER 11

# Pediatrics

## CASE STUDY 69: ACUTE APPENDICITIS

### CASE HISTORY

Patient is a 14-year-old male who is seen in the emergency room for abdominal pain. The pain started with a dull periumbilical pain radiating to the right lower quadrant (RLQ). He feels anorexic, nauseated, and vomited twice since morning. Over the past 24 h, he also complained of dysuria and colicky abdominal pain. Abdominal examination shows a positive McBurney's sign, Rovsing's sign, positive psoas sign, and obturator sign. Rectal examination was painful. On examination, his temperature is 102.2°F. Abdominal examination shows some abdominal rigidity. Complete blood count (CBC) shows white blood cell (WBC) count of 14,700/μL$^3$ with left shift, polymorphonuclear neutrophil (PMN) is 90%, urinalysis (UA) is positive for RBCs and leukocytes. Abdominal ultrasound and computed tomography (CT) of abdomen are both negative.

### DIAGNOSIS

Acute appendicitis—most likely this is a pelvic appendicitis. A pelvic CT was ordered, and diagnosis of acute appendicitis confirmed (Fig. 1A).

### DISCUSSION

The incidence of appendicitis is approximately 6% of the general population. Nowadays, unnecessary appendectomies are avoided because of the new imaging techniques. However, there are still some cases in which the classic signs and symptoms are absent, still leading to continued difficulties in diagnosis. Abdominal pain is still the most reliable symptom in the appendicitis. Fever is a relatively late finding unless there are complications or it ruptures.

Appendicitis is the inflammation of the appendix. Obstruction by fecalith, foreign bodies or tumor promotes inflammation and infection, leading to swelling. The distended appendix then touches the peritoneum and irritates it, which presents as the classic acute abdomen typified by involuntary guarding and rebound tenderness. The treatment is appendectomy. If left untreated and the appendix continues to swell, its blood supply can be compromised. The appendix can then infarct and rupture, causing widespread peritonitis, high fever, and septic shock. Therefore, acute appendicitis needs to be treated as a medical emergency. The clinical symptoms of acute appendicitis may vary widely. The symptoms typically start with pain in the umbilicus or the epigastrium, for which the visceral pain of the inflamed appendix is referred. As the inflammation spreads throughout the intestinal wall, the visceral peritoneum irritation localizes the pain to the RLQ. McBurney's point, or one third of the distance from right anterior superior iliac spine (ASIS) to the umbilicus, is the most cited location of pain associated with appendicitis in literature. Other symptoms such as nausea and vomiting may be present. Anorexia, on the other hand, is almost always present.

Although less definitive, the presence of mild leukocytosis along with the presenting symptoms also points to acute appendicitis.

Several clinical examinations and studies are used in aid of diagnosing acute appendicitis. Clinical pain evaluation includes Rovsing's sign, psoas sign, and obturator sign. In Rovsing's sign, deep palpation of the left lower quadrant (LLQ) pushes the visceral contents to the right and causes RLQ pain. Psoas sign is pain elicited by having the patient lying on the left side and either passively extending the hip or actively flexing the hip. This is due to inflammation of the overlying peritoneum and/or the psoas muscle, which may be in contact with the appendix. Obturator sign is documented with internal rotation and flexion of the hip joint. This maneuver puts the obturator externus muscle in contact with the enlarged appendix, thus causing pain. Although supportive, these three techniques to evaluate pain are not diagnostic of appendicitis.

Imaging studies provide better sensitivity and specificity of diagnosing acute appendicitis. Abdominal ultrasound can achieve a sensitivity of 90%, although the results are highly operator-dependent. CT scan with intravenous (IV) contrast has above 95% sensitivity and specificity (Figure 1A shows with contrast and Figure 1B shows without contrast), although a negative result does not rule out the diagnosis. CT scan is now considered the imaging study of choice-not ultra sound. We have to be very careful in patients who are pregnant because nausea and vomiting may be incorrectly linked to pregnancy. We have to remember appendicitis is the most common extrauterine surgical emergency in pregnancy. The fetal mortality rate will be very high if the appendix ruptures and peritonitis sets in. In these cases, ultrasound is the preferred diagnostic tool due to the risk of radiation to the newborn from CT scan. Patients with questionable diagnosis should be observed with serial abdominal examinations to avoid premature surgical interversion or discharge.

For this reason, approximately 20% of appendectomies result in normal appendices.

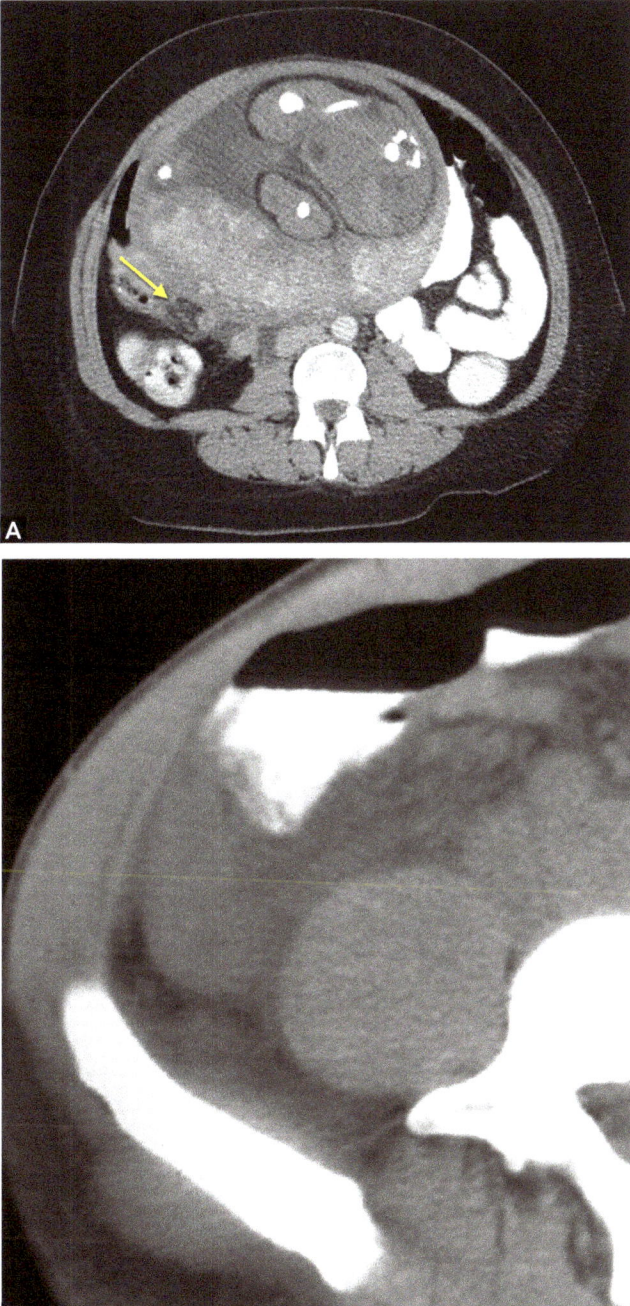

**Figs. 1A and B:** (A) CT abdomen with contrast; (B) CT scan without IV contrast. The contrast shows appendiceal wall changes and periappendiceal fat changes. (CT: computed tomography; IV: intravenous.)

In atypical acute appendicitis, the patient may not present with all the symptoms of typical appendicitis. Clinicians must rely on the patient's history, imaging studies, and clinical experience to make the appropriate diagnosis.

Incidence of acute appendicitis peaks in teenage years to mid-twenties. Important differential diagnoses include ectopic pregnancy, ruptured ovarian cyst, Meckel's diverticulitis, intussusceptions, pelvic inflammatory disease, and other disorders associated with abdominal pain.

## NONOPERATIVE MANAGEMENT

Nonoperative management with antibiotics for uncomplicated appendicitis has shown potential benefits in specific cases. It is recommended if patients meet the following criteria from the study Effectiveness of patient choice in nonoperative vs surgical management of pediatric uncomplicated acute appendicitis.[1]

- Abdominal pain for <48 h
- WBC count ≤18,000/μL
- Normal C-reactive protein
- No appendicolith present on imaging
- Appendix diameter ≤1.1 cm on imaging
- No preoperative concern for rupture based upon clinical findings.

Antibiotic therapy usually includes 1–2 days of broad spectrum IV antibiotics, such as piperacillin–tazobactam, ceftriaxone and metronidazole, or ciprofloxacin and metronidazole. Patients are treated until symptoms resolve and WBC count normalizes. Patients can be given oral antibiotics as outpatient such as ciprofloxacin and metronidazole.

## OPERATIVE MANAGEMENT

Laparoscopic appendectomy is recommended in patients with early appendicitis (appendicitis without perforation or gangrene). Preoperative care should include antibiotic prophylaxis with a single dose of broad spectrum antibiotics such as cefoxitin, or ceftriaxone and metronidazole, IV hydration, and analgesia. Patients with perforated appendix should be continued on IV antibiotics postoperatively until they are afebrile and are able to consume a regular diet. WBC count should be within a normal range before patient is discharged.

### Emergency Room Treatment

Patients need to be NPO (nothing by mouth). IV access, analgesia, and antibiotics.
- *Analgesia*: Fentanyl 1–2 μg/kg IV every 1–4 h
- *Antibiotics*: Ampicillin/sulbactam 3 g IV or piperacillin/tazobactam 3.375 g IV
- Patient care can be divided into four subgroups:

*Group 1*: With classic appendicitis will go for surgical consult and appendectomy.
*Group 2*: Patients suspicious for appendicitis will go for serial imaging and serial examinations.
*Group 3*: High-risk patients like pediatric, geriatric, or pregnant will need surgical consult and follow-up.
*Group 4*: Non-specific abdominal pain. Close follow-up and specific discharge instructions to follow-up with primary care provider or return to the emergency room if the symptoms return.

## REFERENCE

1. Minneci PC, Mahida JB, Lodwick DL, et al. Effectiveness of Patient Choice in Nonoperative vs Surgical Management of Pediatric Uncomplicated Acute Appendicitis. JAMA Surg. 2016;151(5):408-15.

## FURTHER READING

1. Taylor C. Appendicitis: avoiding pitfalls in diagnosis. Medscape. New Haven, USA; 2018.
2. http://en.wikipedia.org/wiki/Appendicitis.
3. Fitzgerald DJ., Panciolli AM. Acute Appendicitis In: Emergency medicine manual. 6th ed. 2004. p. 728-33.
4. https://www.uptodate.com/contents/acute-appendicitis-in-children-management?source=machineLearning&search=appendicitis%20in%20children&selectedTitle=2~150&sectionRank=1&anchor=H3#H12.
5. https://jamanetwork.com/journals/jamasurgery/fullarticle/2475977.

## CASE STUDY 70: CHILD ABUSE

*"If I prevent one child from being abused and one child from drowning, I'll consider myself fortunate."*

—Badar M Zaheer

*(Studies show Child Abuse and Neglect Cost the United States $124 Billion)*

## CASE HISTORY

The patient is a 6-year-old boy accompanied by his mother, who presents to the emergency room with complaints of right leg pain. Mother reported that the patient had fallen down a flight of stairs earlier in the day and has been unable to walk since then, secondary to pain. During the patient encounter, the child remained quiet and mother answered all questions which were asked. Mother asked several questions regarding what the plan was and what tests the doctors were planning on running. The patient was sent for an X-ray of the leg to evaluate for possible fractures.

The results of the lower extremity X-ray demonstrated a transverse fracture of the tibia (Figs. 1A and B). The radiologist also noticed some old healing

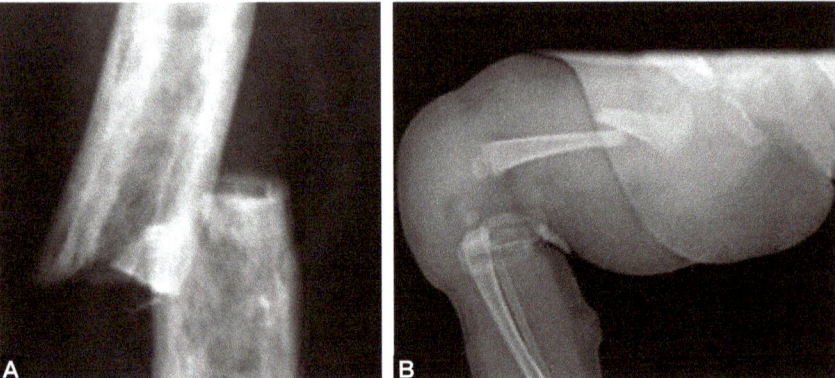

**Figs. 1A and B:** Femur fracture of the 50-day-old infant who also suffered from head injuries.

fractures on the lower extremity and recommended a skeletal survey to check for other healing fractures. When the mother was informed that her son needed to get some more X-rays, she asked why they wanted to expose the child to unnecessary radiation. She denied that her son had suffered any previous trauma, but this poor child suffered a fracture to the base of skull and multiple rib fractures (Figs. 2 and 3).

## DISCUSSION

Current research states that 3% of all children seen in the emergency department for child abuse will return with a secondary maltreatment diagnosis within 1 year.[1] In the United States, there are 3.3 million cases of child abuse/neglect reported annually with an estimated cost of over $100 billion. Child abuse is not limited by socioeconomic level, culture, religion, or education level.

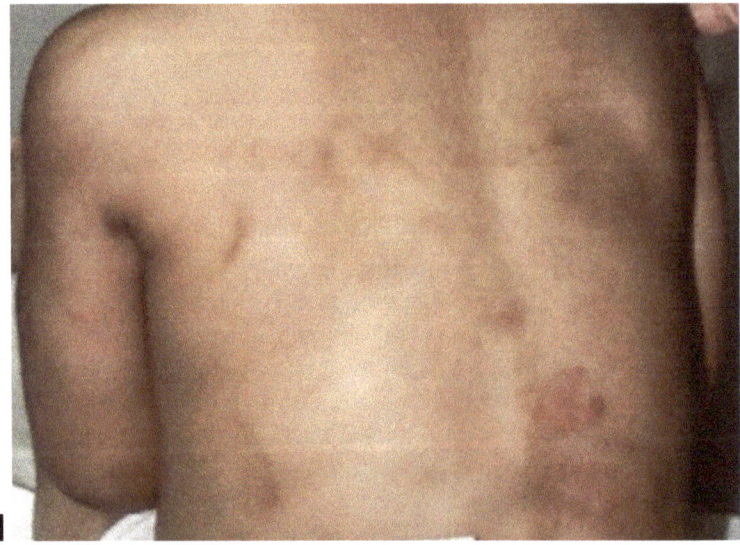

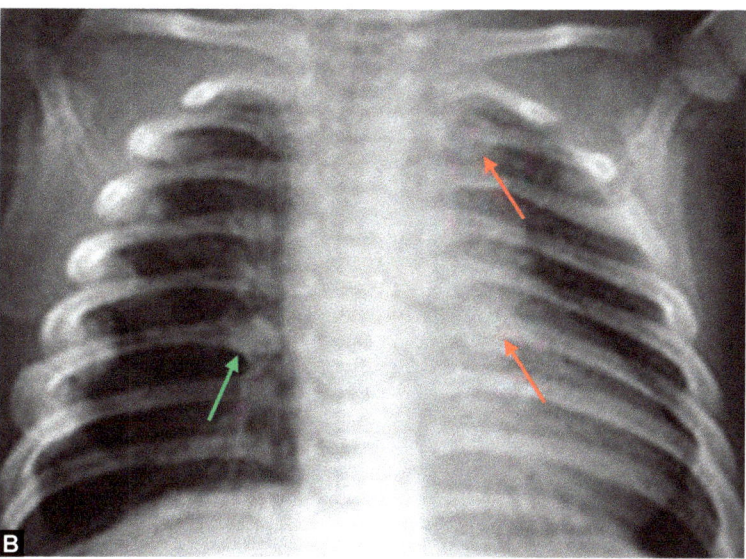

**Figs. 2A and B:** A child suffering from a fracture to the base of skull and multiple rib fractures. (A) Clinical photograph; (B) Chest X-rays
*Source:* Wikipedia.

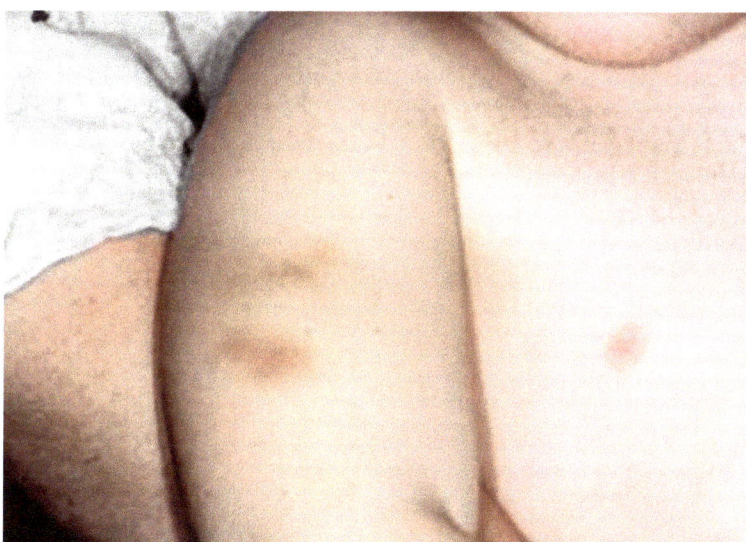

**Fig. 3:** Circumferential fingerprint bruising on the arm of a 6-month-old baby.

The best way to prevent child abuse, according to the Centers for Disease Control and Prevention (CDC), is to stop it before it starts (Fig. 4). As healthcare professionals, we must promote the development of safe and stable relationships between children and their parents/caregivers to prevent abuse before it starts.

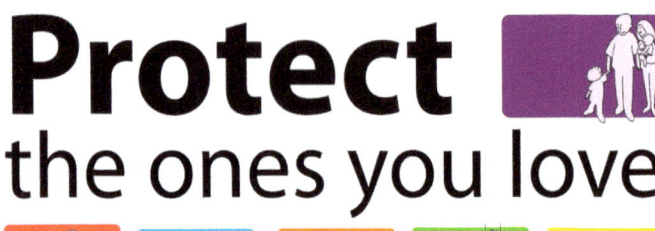
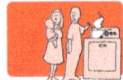 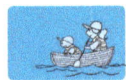 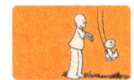 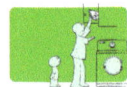 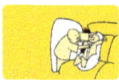

**Fig. 4:** Reporting child abuse.

Unless our governments act to enforce laws to prevent child abuse, the work of doctors will not be enough.

Community education and involvement is essential to prevent child abuse. Free reporting without obligation and without a burden of proof on the witness should be made compulsory. Those who do not report cases should be punishable by law, especially medical professionals, governmental authorities, teachers, school administrators, etc. It is a team effort to prevent this, and a universal responsibility on the shoulders of all human beings.

Evaluation of suspected child abuse starts with a complete history using open ended questions, physical examination, and watching child communications with the caregiver.

## Physical Child Abuse Red Flags

- *Bruises:* Patients younger than 6 years, located on the torso/ear/buttock, pattern of striking object, human bit marks
- *Oral injuries:* Lip or tongue lacerations in non-ambulatory infants, missing or fractured teeth with absent or unlikely history
- *Burns:* Scalds in children <5 years without unintentional spill pattern, scalds from hot water immersion (with sharp line of demarcation and on both sides of body symmetrically), cigarette burns with deep circular pattern
- *Fractures:* Metaphyseal corner fractures, multiple fractures in different stages of healing, long bone fractures in non-ambulatory infants
- Serious injury without explanation.

## MANAGMENT

Suspected child abuse should be evaluated after proper treatment of immediate medical needs have been addresses. Consultation with a multidisciplinary team is advised (social worker, nurse) and reporting to appropriate governmental authorities. Hospitalization may be utilized to treat for extensive injuries or if there is concern about child safety. Other children living in the household should be evaluated for potential abuse.[2]

## PRACTICE PEARLS

Mandated reporting is necessary in many parts of the world, including the United States, United Kingdom, India, Canada, and Australia, to avoid risking your license. The agency to which you must report is different depending on your place of practice—know where you must report!

Barriers to reporting include uncertainty as to what constitutes a "reasonable suspicion," familiarity with patient families, inadequate training, and lack of support from professional societies.

The report of abuse must include the nature of the child's medical condition or injuries, the reasons why abuse or neglect is suspected as the cause of the condition, and the strength of the suspicion.

## REFERENCES

1. Osterweil N. Abused children treated in ED at risk of return. Annual meeting of the pediatric academic societies. Elsevier Global Medical News. May 15, 2012.
2. Narang S. Child abuse: social and medicolegal issues. UpToDate.com; Waltham, MA, USA: September 6, 2017.

## FURTHER READING

1. Child abuse and neglect cost the United States $124 billion. (2012, February 1). Retrieved October 12, 2018, from CDC Home website: https://www.cdc.gov/media/releases/2012/p0201_child_abuse.html.
2. www.cdc.gov/safechild.

## CASE STUDY 71: INTUSSUSCEPTION

## CASE HISTORY

A 5-year-old boy is presents to the emergency department with the chief complaint of abdominal pain colicky in nature associated with vomiting, has fever since morning, and looks dehydrated. He is drawing his legs up to control the pain when he gets abdominal colic. Mother noticed that he is passing currant jelly stools (Fig. 1). Physical examination shows low skin turgor, decreased capillary refill, and tongue slightly dehydrated. Examination of the abdomen

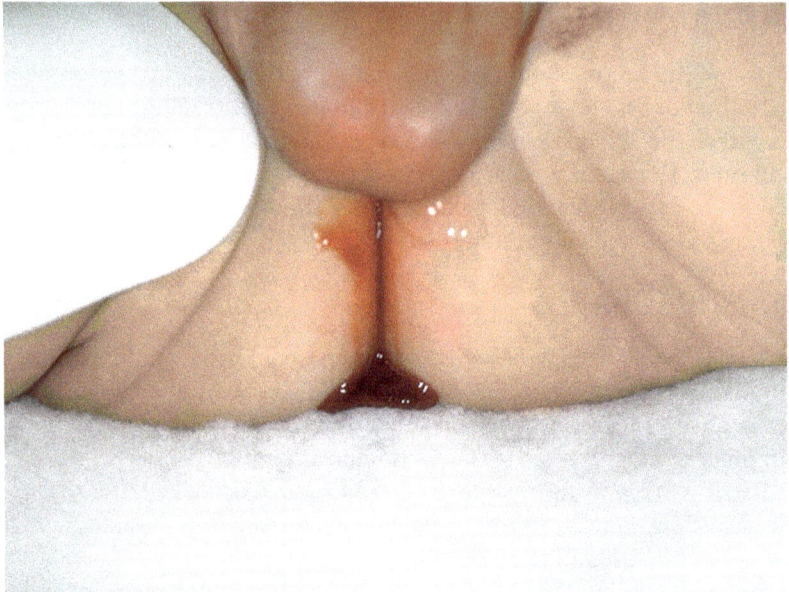

**Fig.1:** Currant jelly stool.
*Source:* www.virtualpediatrichospital.org/.

shows diminished bowel sounds and palpable mass which looks like sausage. Anal examination shows some rectal prolapse like appearance. His vitals are pulse rate of 150 beats/min, respiratory rate 28 breaths/min, and temperature 99.9°F. Diagnostic test includes abdominal X-ray obstructive series which show absence of gas in the right upper quadrant, and ultrasonography shows telescopic bowel.

## DIAGNOSTIC TEST

Diagnostic test includes abdominal X-ray obstructive series which show absence of gas in the right upper quadrant, and ultrasonography shows telescopic bowel (Fig. 2). CT scans are also useful when indicated (Fig. 3).

## DISCUSSION

Intussusception is the most common cause of bowel obstruction in children from 3 months to 6 years of age. It occurs when a portion of the bowel "telescopes" into itself, causing intestinal obstruction. The intestinal obstruction may progress to a segment of the intestine. The condition can progress from intestinal obstruction to necrosis (tissue death) of a segment of the intestine. Initially, blood supply to the intestine is compromised causing edema and inflammation which leads to perforation, peritonitis, shock, and death.

Pediatrics

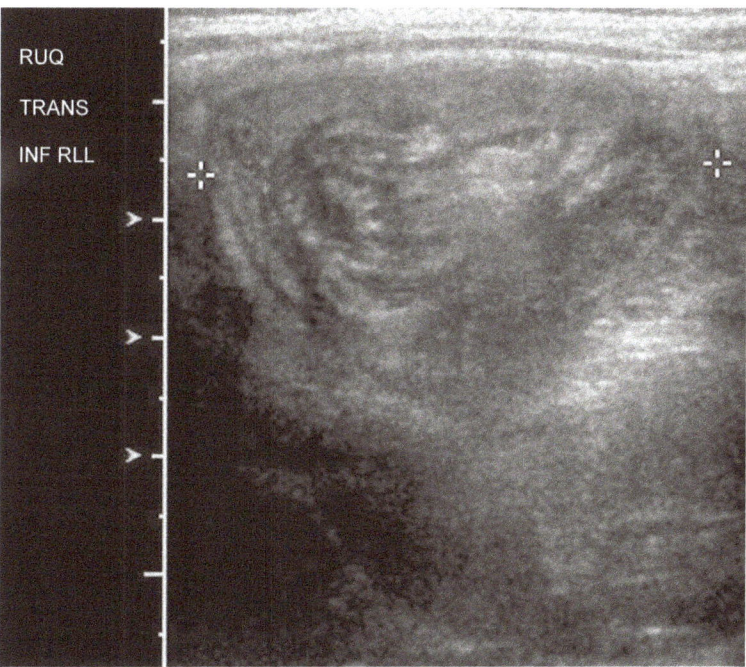

Fig. 2: Ultrasound image of intussusception.
Source: Wikipedia.

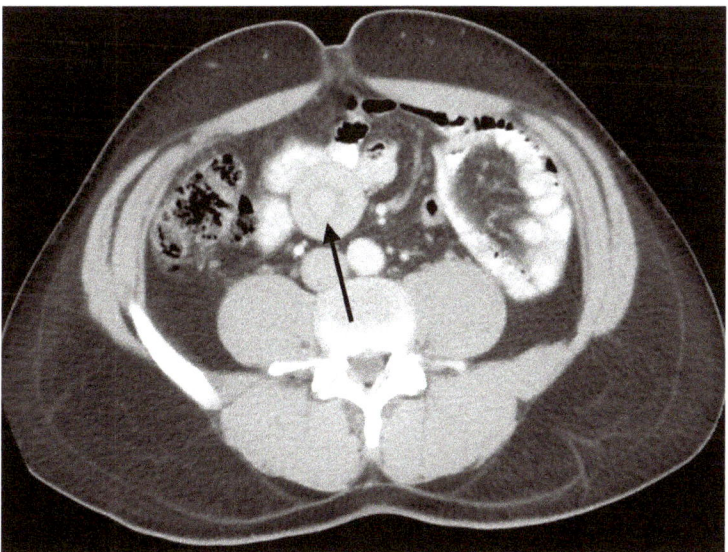

Fig. 3: CT scan of intussuception.
Source: Wikipedia.

Intussusception occurs most often near the ileocecal junction (ileocolic intussusception). The intussusceptum, a proximal segment of bowel, telescopes into the intussuscipiens, a distal segment, dragging associated mesentery with it. The most common lead points for intussusception in children are Meckel diverticulum and hypertrophic Peyer patches (lymphatic tissue) in the ileum.

## Lead Point

A lead point is a lesion or variation in the intestine that is trapped by peristalsis and dragged into a distal segment of the intestine. A Meckel diverticulum, polyp, tumor, hematoma, lymphoid hyperplasia, or vascular malformation can act as a lead point for intussusception.

### ETIOLOGY

- Idiopathic
- Viral infection
- *Cystic fibrosis*: Patients suffering from this disease are more prone to get intussusception because of change in mucosa. Another underlying condition such as hematoma from trauma or following surgery.

### TREATMENT

Management of intussusception through nonoperative and operative procedures is shown in Flowchart 1 and Figure 4.
- *Intravenous fluid:* Measure intake and output of fluid
- Maintain NPO status as ordered
- Insert nasogastric tube, if ordered to decompress stomach.

**Flowchart 1:** Management plan of intussusception.

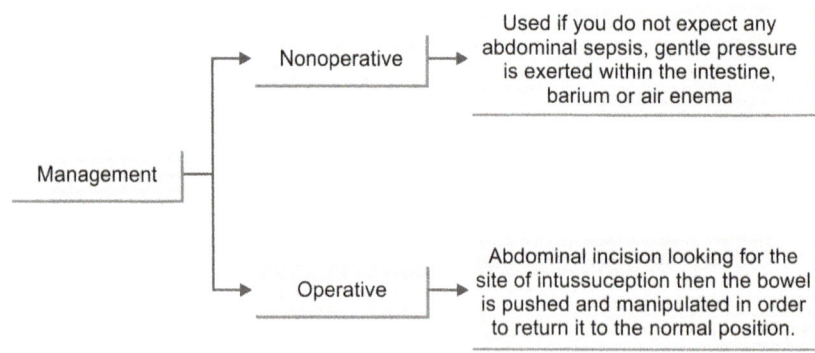

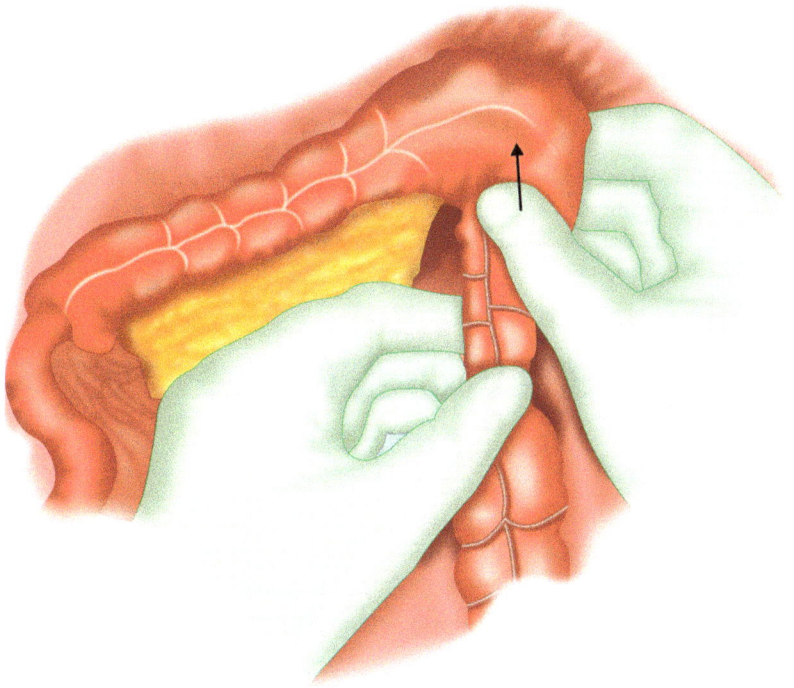

**Fig. 4:** Operative management of intussusception. Technique for reduction of an intussusception in the operating room. The intussusception is being squeezed by the surgeon rather than pulled.[1]

- Continually reassess condition because increased pain and bloody stools may indicate perforation.
- After reduction by hydrostatic enema, monitor vital signs and general condition.
- After successful reduction of an ileocolic intussusception, a temperature higher than 38°C (100.4°F) is often noted because of bacterial translocation or the release of endotoxin or cytokines.
- After reduction, the patient is also at increased risk to develop recurrent intussusception in the near term, possibly because of residual bowel inflammation, which may itself act as a lead point.

Although intussusception is relatively common in pediatrics,[2] significant variability in diagnosis and treatment modalities exists. The management of children after a successful enema reduction is an area that has not been well studied. Now, it is well documented that recurrences of intussusception can be reduced safely with enema techniques with a success rate of up to 95%, and that the incidence of pathologic lead point (PLP) is not increased until the patient has more than one recurrence.[3] There was an association between rotavirus and intussusception and some of the earlier vaccines had to be recalled. Recent vaccines are not supposed to have the same effect.

## REFERENCES

1. Bajaj L, Roback MG. Postreduction management of intussusception in a children's hospital emergency department. Pediatrics. 2003;112:1302-7.
2. Daneman A. Intussusception: issues and controversies related to diagnosis and treatment. Radiol Clin North Am. 1999;34:743.
3. Kitagawa S, Miqdady M. Intussusception in children. UpToDate.com; March 30, 2016.

## CASE STUDY 72: MALROTATION AND VOLVULUS

## CASE HISTORY

A 1-year-old boy with his parents is presented in the emergency department (ED) with abdominal pain. The pain started last night and is associated with bilious vomiting. Today he had a bloody bowel movement. Past medical and surgical history is insignificant. Immunization is up-to-date. Prenatal and postnatal history is unremarkable.

## PHYSICAL EXAMINATION AND LABORATORY VALUES

On examination, mild to moderate distension and diffuse tenderness with guarding of the abdomen noticed.

### Laboratory Tests

Complete blood count (CBC) and electrolytes are within normal limits (WNL). *Stool*: Positive for occult blood. Radiography results are as shown (in Figures 1A and B). Dilated loops of bowel overlying the liver shadow and little gas distal to the obstruction noted.

## DISCUSSION

Malrotation of the gut occurs in approximately 1 in 500 births.[1] The gut rotates itself into the abdominal cavity during development. If this process does not proceed properly, the intestines may be out of their usual locations. The mesentery stalk or the connective tissue that fixes the bowels to the abdominal wall and channels blood vessels and lymphatics may not form properly. The mesentery is usually a broad band that secures its connection. In a malrotated gut, the mesentery may be thin, making the intestines more prone to twist on themselves. In individuals with gut malrotation, the most common

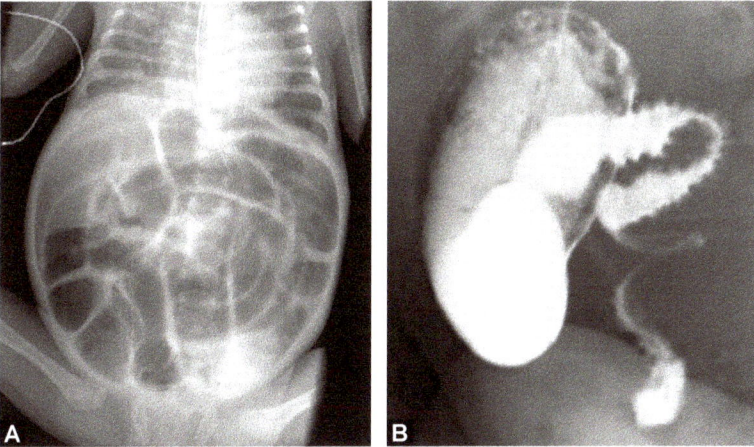

**Figs. 1A and B:** (A) The "coffee bean" sign in which two bubbles are formed around the volvulus; (B) Example of "bird's beak" sign in barium enema study.

form of twisting is midgut volvulus, in which the intestines twist around the superior mesentery artery (Figs. 2A and B).
- Traditionally, intestinal malrotation has been considered primarily a disease of infancy, with 75% of cases presenting before 5 years of age.
- Associated congenital defects: up to 62% of children who have intestinal malrotation have an associated anomaly, including congenital diaphragmatic hernia, congenital heart disease (especially heterotaxy syndrome), omphalocele, gastroschisis, prune belly syndrome, intestinal atresias, esophageal atresia, biliary atresia, Meckel diverticulum, anorectal malformations, and Cornelia de Lange syndrome.

## Midgut Volvulus

Midgut volvulus is commonly seen in the pediatric population due to its congenital etiology. The patient presents with bilious vomiting, abdominal pain, lethargy, crying, and failure to pass stool or gas. Other symptoms such as hematemesis, rectal bleeding, or signs of sepsis suggest perforation or infarction of the bowels.

The gold standard for diagnosing volvulus is an upper gastrointestinal (GI) series, or barium swallow. With the help of oral contrast, abdominal X-ray may show the "coffee bean" sign, which is formed from two air bubbles proximal and distal to the volvulus (Fig. 1A). A barium enema may also be performed, which may show the "bird's beak" sign at the point of volvulus (Fig. 1B).[1] Differential diagnoses include carcinoma or other forms of intestinal obstruction.

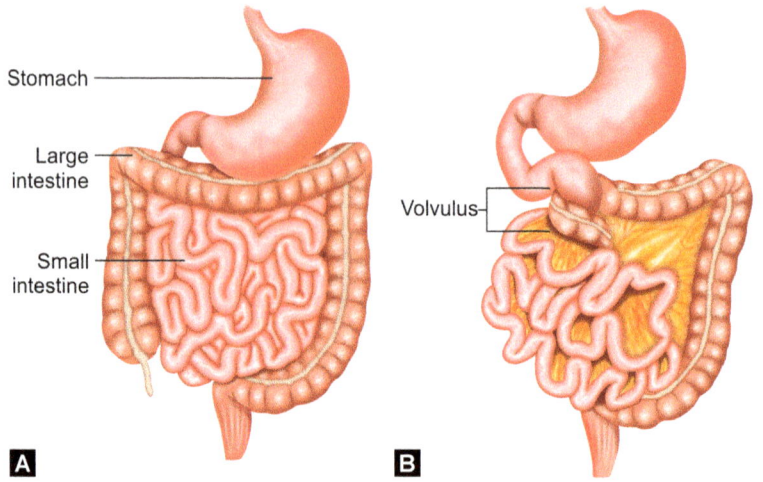

**Figs. 2A and B:** Midgut volvulus. The large intestine twists around the duodenum and superior mesenteric artery, which jeopardizes the entire midgut.

## TREATMENT

The treatment is emergency pediatric surgery. Ladd's procedure is usually performed. After the surgeon untwists the volvulus, he or she frees malformed connecting stalk and fixes the intestines to the abdominal wall. The small intestine is usually fixed to the right side of the abdominal cavity, while the large intestine fixed to the left.[1] Because this is not the normal positioning of the usual anatomy, prophylactic appendectomy is usually done to avoid diagnostic confusion if the patient later suffers from appendicitis. If the surgeon determines a segment of the bowels is necrotic, resection of that segment would be performed.

Many individuals with malrotation do not develop volvulus. In fact, many do not know about their condition until they have either imaging studies or surgeries unrelated to their malrotation.[2]

## REFERENCES

1. Ingoe R, Lange P. The Ladd's procedure for correction of intestinal malrotation with volvulus in children. AORN J. 2007;85(2):300-8.
2. Brandt M. Intestinal malrotation in children. UpToDate.com; Waltham: MA, USA; January 3, 2017.

## FURTHER READING

1. Duggan CP. Intestinal malrotation. [Online]. Available from www.childrenshospital.org/az/Site1181/mainpageS1181P0.html; 2011 [accessed August, 2012].
2. Nemattalla W. Sigmoid volvulus. [Online]. Available from radiopaedia.org/cases/sigmoid-volvulus 2010 [accessed August, 2012].

# CASE STUDY 73: ACUTE LARYNGOTRACHEITIS/CROUP

## CASE HISTORY

A 2-year-old child is brought by her parents for the chief complaint of harsh barking cough, hoarseness of voice, and a mild stridor. The child had upper respiratory tract infection symptoms for the past 3 days with low rate fever, rhinorrhea, and mild cough followed by certain onset of inspiratory stridor (Fig. 1). On examination, her vital signs are stable (Fig. 2), oxygen saturation level is 99% on room air, and chest X-ray shows steeple signs in anteroposterior view of chest (Figs. 3 and 4).

## CLINICAL MANAGEMENT

This includes the following:
- Avoid excessive agitation and crying—this will increase respiratory distress causing hypoxia and oxygen demand
- Humidified oxygen or cool mist can be provided by mask
- Nebulizer treatment with racepinephrine for patients with moderate-to-severe respiratory distress
- Corticosteroids such as dexamethasone.

## DIFFERENTIAL DIAGNOSIS

- Epiglottitis
- Laryngomalacia
- Vocal cord dysfunction

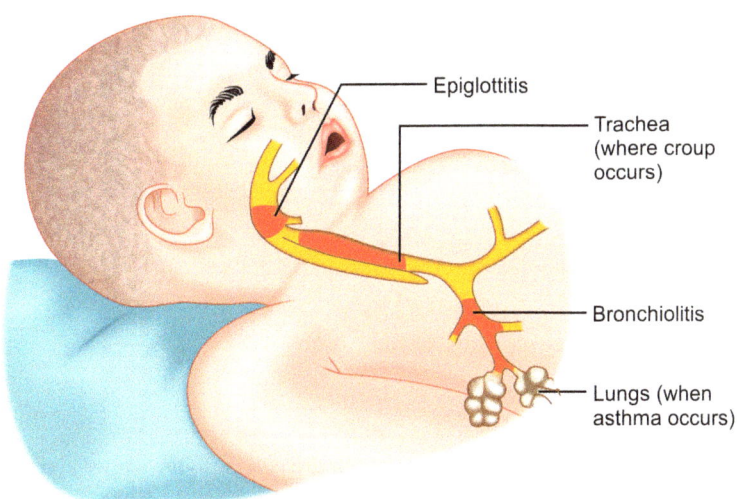

**Fig. 1:** Location of airway obstruction.

- *Spasmodic croup*: Much less common than infectious croup and is thought to be allergic in origin. There are no preceding or associated symptoms such as fever or rhinorrhea. Spasmodic croup resolves within a few hours without specific treatment.

## DISCUSSION

Acute laryngotracheobronchitis (infectious croup) is the most common cause of upper airway obstruction in young children beyond the neonatal period. The majority of cases result from infection with parainfluenza virus, although influenza, adenovirus, and respiratory syncytial virus can also cause croup. Typically, a 1–3-day period of low-grade fever, rhinorrhea, and mild cough is followed by the sudden onset of inspiratory stridor and the characteristic barking cough, often during the night. Hypoxia is unusual, even among patients brought to the emergency department in respiratory distress. Infectious croup is generally a clinical diagnosis (Fig. 1). Subglottic narrowing (the "steeple sign") may or may not be appreciated on an anteroposterior chest radiograph (Figs. 2 to 4). Administration of systemic steroids such as dexamethasone results in significant improvement within hours. For moderate to severe cases, suggested dose is 0.6 mg/kg intravenous (IV)/ intramuscular (IM)/by mouth (PO), max dose is up to 10 mg/daily. Nebulized epinephrine is reserved for the patient with moderate-to-severe respiratory distress.

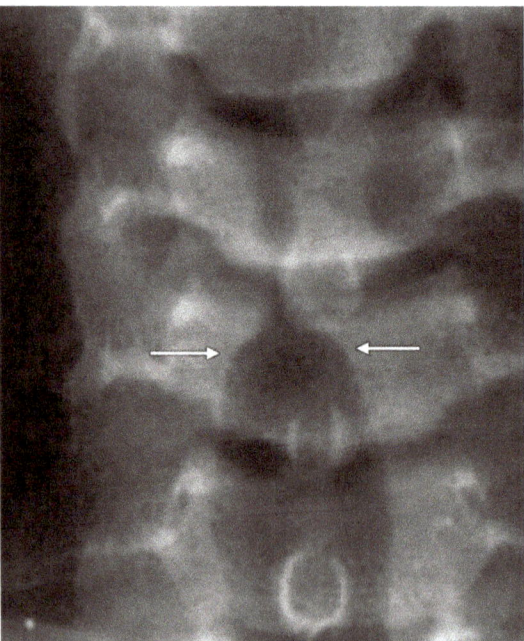

**Fig. 2:** Normal anteroposterior radiograph of upper airway, with the normal appearance of the subglottic region (arrows).

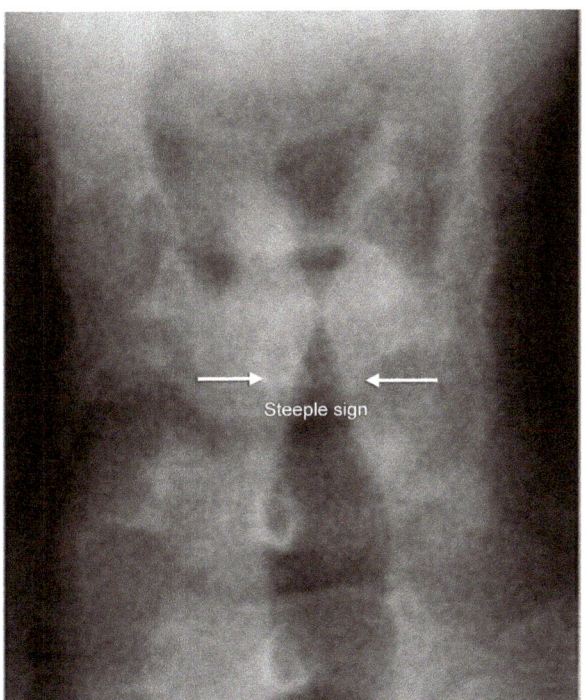

**Fig. 3:** Anteroposterior radiograph of the upper airway of a patient with croup. The subglottic tracheal narrowing produces an inverted V appearance known as "steeple sign" (arrows).

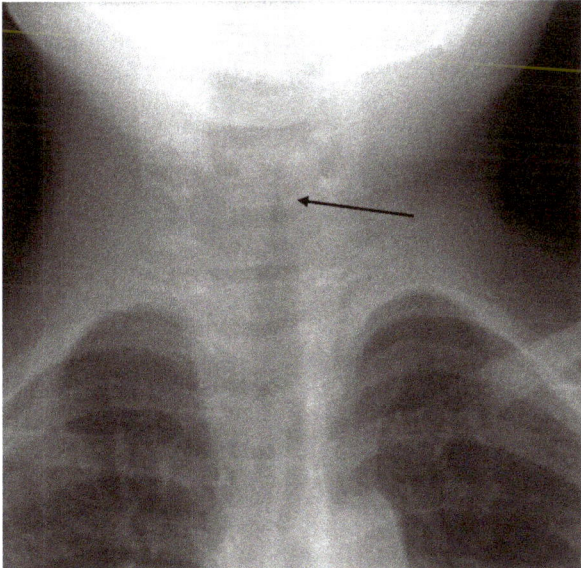

**Fig. 4:** The steeple sign as seen on an AP neck X-ray of a child with croup.
*Source:* Wikipedia.

Croup severity score-Westley croup score:
- Mild croup (Westley croup score of ≤2)—No stridor at rest, a barking cough, hoarse cry, and either no, or only mild, chest wall/subcostal retractions. Can be managed by phone. Treated symptomatically with humidity, fever reduction, and oral fluids.[1]
- Moderate croup (Westley croup score of 3–7)—Stridor at rest, at least mild retractions, may have other symptoms of respiratory distress, but little or no agitation.
- Severe croup (Westley croup score of ≥8)—significant stridor at rest, severe retractions.
- Impending respiratory failure (Westley croup score of ≥12)—characterized by fatigue and listlessness, marked retractions, decreased or absent breath sounds, depressed level of consciousness, tachycardia, cyanosis or pallor.

## REFERENCE

1. Woods C. Croup: approach to management. UpToDate.com; Waltham, MA, USA, August 30, 2017.

## CASE STUDY 74: FEBRILE SEIZURES

### CASE HISTORY

A 2-year-old boy is brought to the emergency department by his mother after she witnessed him having an episode of "full body shaking." The child has had symptoms of an upper respiratory viral infection for the last 2–3 days. She reports that the shaking lasted approximately 5 min, and the child was very sleepy afterward. On physical examination, the patient has vital signs of temperature 102.4°F, pulse rate 79 bpm, respiratory rate 18 breaths/min, and blood pressure 110/65 mm Hg. He is sleepy but arousable, and neurological examination reveals no focal deficits and no meningeal signs. Laboratory studies show a normal complete blood count and electrolytes. Blood glucose level is 100 mg/dL. He is diagnosed with a febrile seizure.

### FEBRILE SEIZURES

Febrile seizures are common in children between the ages of 6 months and 5 years. They often occur with temperatures over 39°C but are not related to the actual temperature, rather to the rate of rise of the temperature. There are two types of febrile seizures: simple and complex (Table 1). A simple febrile seizure is one which <15 min, does not recur within 24 h, is generalized and occurs in children <6 years of age with no underlying neurological disorders. If any of these conditions are not met, then it is categorized as a complex febrile seizure.

Table 1: Comparison between simple febrile seizure and complex febrile seizure.[1]

| Simple febrile seizure | Complex febrile seizure |
|---|---|
| Lasts <15 min | Lasts 15 min or longer |
| Occurs once in a 24-h period—generalized | Occurs more than once in a 24-h period—focal |
| No previous neurologic problems | Patient has known neurologic problems, such as cerebral palsy |

The children should have additional workup including computed tomography or lumbar puncture and possible hospital admission for observation. Any child with a toxic appearance, meningeal signs, an abnormality on neurologic examination or underlying brain abnormality should not be assumed to have a febrile seizure. Any child who is found to have meningitis during workup should have the seizure attributed to the infection, not to the fever.

## DIFFERENTIAL DIAGNOSIS OF SEIZURES IN CHILDREN

- Fever
- Epidural and subdural infections
- Meningitis or encephalitis
- Epidural hematoma
- Sepsis or bacteremia
- Epilepsy.

## MANAGEMENT

The basis of management of a child who has had a febrile seizure is antipyretic therapy, both during the current illness, as well as during future febrile illnesses. Anticonvulsant therapy is not recommended for children who have experienced febrile seizures, even if they have occurred more than once. Anticonvulsants have serious risks and there is no evidence that children who are given anticonvulsants after the first febrile seizure are at any decreased risk from having another one. It is important to educate parents and caregivers on fever prevention and seizure safety.

## PROGNOSIS

One third of children with a febrile seizure will have another seizure during a subsequent febrile event. Risk factors for recurrent episodes include younger age, family history of febrile seizures, short duration of the fever and a relatively low fever at the initiation of the seizure. There is a small increase in the risk of epilepsy in later life in children who have had a febrile seizure. This risk is greatest in those with a family history of epilepsy, complex febrile seizures, and any developmental abnormality.

## REFERENCE

1. Millar JS. Evaluation and treatment of the child with febrile seizure. Am Fam Physician. 2006;73(10):1761-4. [Online]. Available from http://www.aafp.org/afp/2006/0515/p1761 html. [accessed 2012].

## CASE STUDY 75: NEAR DROWNING

*"Look before you leap"*
*"I was much further out than you thought, and not waving but drowning"*
*"Drown not thyself to save a drowning man"*

Coast guards are not in place in many developing countries, which leads to the deaths of many children and young adult. These deaths are preventable by the government implementing laws and its citizens respecting the laws. If there are no guards present, then swimming should not be permissible.

—Badar M Zaheer

## CASE HISTORY

A 4-year-old boy is brought to the emergency room by ambulance after being found in a backyard pool. The boy had been playing in the backyard unsupervised and fell into the pool. On arrival, he is intubated and vital signs are temperature of 95°F, pulse rate 35 bpm, respiratory rate 16 breaths/min (mechanically), and blood pressure 70/40 mm Hg. His Glasgow coma score (GCS) is 9.

## DISCUSSION

### Clinical Presentation

*There are two types of drowning:* Dry drowning and wet drowning (Figs. 1 to 4). Dry drowning is caused by laryngospasm, which then causes hypoxemia and neurological insult. This accounts for up to 20% of submersion injuries. Wet drowning is due to the aspiration of water into the lungs causing a washout of surfactant, diminished alveolar gas exchange, atelectasis, and a ventilation–perfusion mismatch. This leads to noncardiac pulmonary edema with moderate to severe aspiration. Physical examination may reveal clear lungs, wheezes, rhonchi or rales, and mental status may range from normal to comatose. Hypothermia can be seen even in warm water submersions.

### Diagnosis

The diagnosis of drowning is usually obvious, but it is important to look for other injuries. Spinal cord injuries can occur with diving or surfing injuries or boating accidents. Other conditions, including syncope, hypoglycemia, underlying heart disease such as myocardial infarction or dysrhythmias, have been linked to drowning. Laboratory testing may reveal metabolic

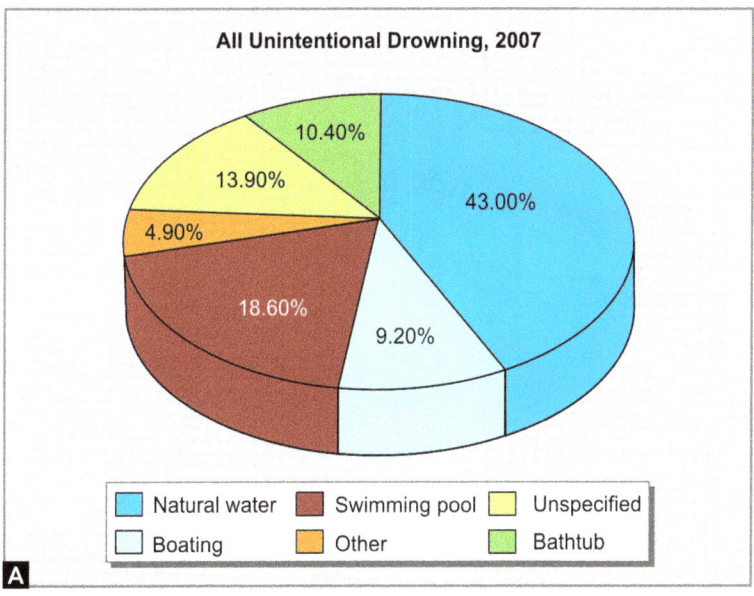

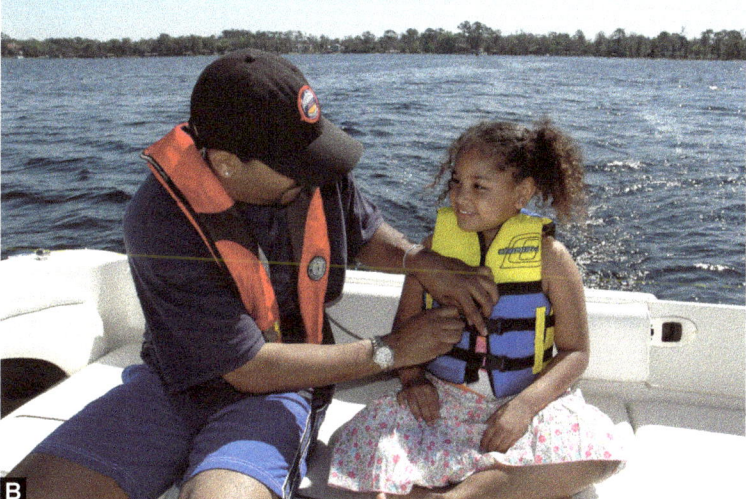

**Figs. 1A and B:** Drowning happens quickly—learn how to reduce your risk. About 10 people die every day from unintentional drowning. Of these, 2 are children 14 or younger. Learning the risks and taking safety precautions are proven ways to prevent drowning injuries and deaths.

acidosis and electrolyte abnormalities. There is associated renal injury from the hypoxemia. You may also see hemoglobinuria or myoglobinuria.

Massive hemolysis can occur with large volumes of aspiration of fresh water, but disseminated intravascular coagulation (DIC) is rare. Necessary tests include a chest X-ray and arterial blood gas analysis. The chest X-ray often shows generalized pulmonary edema or perihilar infiltrates or it may be normal. The arterial blood gas is necessary because chest radiograph

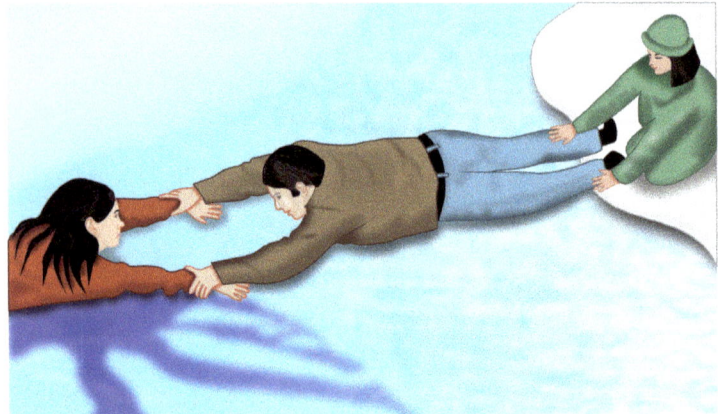

**Fig. 2:** If a person falls through ice, and there is more than one person on solid ground, form a chain of bodies from a secure location out to the fallen person.

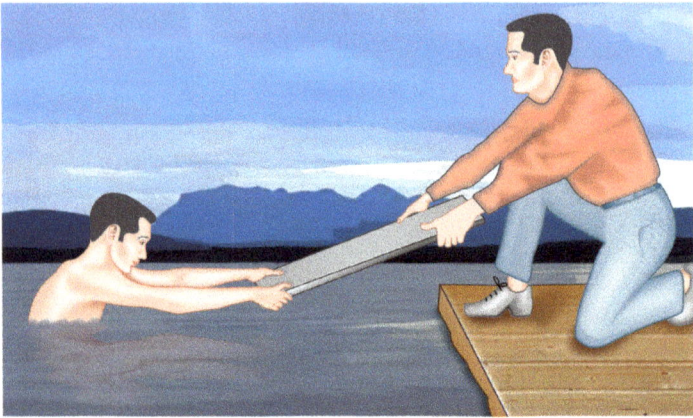

**Fig. 3:** If the victim is in deep or dangerous water, but there is a dock to stand on, try a reaching assist with a long, sturdy object.

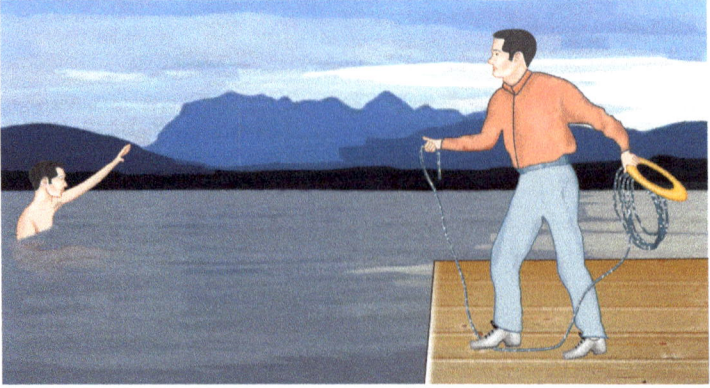

**Fig. 4:** If the water is too deep or dangerous to enter or if the victim is too far out to reach with a long object, a throwing assist may be wisest.

findings often do not correlate with arterial $pO_2$ and oxygen saturation, and metabolic acidosis must be assessed.

## Pulmonary Treatment

The first step is assessing airway, ventilation, and oxygenation status along with cervical spine stabilization in the scenario of diving accidents, multiple trauma, or unknown mechanisms. If hypothermia is present, the patient should be given warmed intravenous normal saline and warming adjuncts such as overhead warmers or heating blankets. Core temperature must be monitored closely. Victims can then be divided into two categories based on their GCS. Patients with a GCS of $\geq 14$ should be given supplemental $O_2$ to maintain saturation level above 95%. They may be discharged home after being observed for 4-6 h as long as pulmonary and neurological examinations and $O_2$ saturation levels return to normal. If the patient still requires oxygen or has an abnormal examination after 4-6 h, they should be admitted. Patients with a GCS <14 should also be given supplemental $O_2$, and intubation with mechanical ventilation should be considered if $PaO_2$ cannot be maintained above 60 mm Hg in adults or 80 mm Hg in children despite high flow oxygen. Pediatric victims of fresh water drowning can sometimes develop dilutional hyponatremia and seizures. These can be controlled by correcting the electrolyte abnormality. The development of pneumonia is rare, so prophylactic antibiotics are not indicated as part of treatment.

## Neurologic Treatment

"Brain resuscitation" using mannitol, loop diuretics, hypertonic saline, fluid resuscitation, mechanical hyperventilation, controlled hypothermia, barbiturate coma, and intracranial pressure monitoring have been attempted but have shown no benefit. Asystole outside of the hospital is a poor prognostic sign in pediatric warm water submersion injuries, but there have been reports of neurologic recovery in these situations. If submersion and transfer time were both short, the patient should undergo vigorous attempts at resuscitation. Continuous vasopressor infusion may be necessary in the postresuscitation phase, and consideration should be given for withholding resuscitation efforts in patients with prolonged submersion and transport time. There have been reports of full neurologic recovery in near drowning cases in adults and children even after asystole in icy water submersions. Hypothermic victims of cold water drowning in cardiac arrest should undergo prolonged and aggressive resuscitation until they are normothermic and not viable.

## ARTICLE

## Injury Death in Children Ages One to Four

Time (5/18, Rochman) reports, "Drowning is the leading cause of injury death in children ages 1-4 years, according to a Centers for Disease Control and Prevention (CDC) report released Thursday." While, "drowning rates in the US have declined, children between the ages of 1 and 4 years have the highest rate of both fatal and nonfatal drowning with 50% of fatal incidents occurring in swimming pools." The report is based on, "death certificate data from the National Vital Statistics System and injury data from the National Electronic Injury Surveillance System—All Injury Program (NEISS-AIP) for the years 2005–2009."

HealthDay (5/18, Reinberg) reports, "Males are victims four times as often as females". In the years covered, "more than 3,800 people of all ages drowned annually nationwide."

WebMD (5/18, Nierenberg) reports, "Children under 4 years accounted for nearly 53% of emergency visits for drowning-related injuries, while children aged 5–14 years were responsible for almost 18% of them."

## Take Action to Reduce Risks

Learn to swim. Formal swimming lessons can reduce the risk of drowning by as much as 88% among young children aged 1–4 years, who are at greatest risk of drowning. However, even when children have had formal swimming lessons, constant, careful supervision when in the water, and barriers to prevent unsupervised access are necessary to prevent drowning.

Closely watch swimmers in or around the water. Designate a responsible adult who can swim and knows cardiopulmonary resuscitation (CPR) to watch swimmers in or around water—even when lifeguards are present. That adult should not be involved in any other distracting activity (such as reading, or talking on the phone) while watching children.

Learn CPR. In the time it might take for lifeguards or paramedics to arrive, your CPR skills could save someone's life.

Fence it off. Barriers to pool access should be used to help prevent young children from gaining access to the pool area without caregivers' awareness when they are not supposed to be swimming. Pool fences should completely separate the house and play area from the pool, be ≥4-ft high, and have self-closing and self-latching gates that open outward, with latches that are out of the reach of children.

- Use the buddy system. Regardless of your age, always swim with a buddy.
- Look for lifeguards. Select swimming sites that have lifeguards whenever possible.
- Heed warning flags. Know the meaning of and obey warnings represented by colored beach flags which may vary from one beach to another.
- Know the terrain. Be aware of and avoid drop-offs and hidden obstacles in natural water sites. Always enter water feet first.
- Avoid rip currents. Watch for dangerous waves and signs of rip currents, like water that is discolored and choppy, foamy, or filled with debris and moving in a channel away from shore. If you are caught in a rip current,

swim parallel to shore; once free of the current, swim diagonally toward shore. More information about rip currents.
- Use approved life jackets. Do not use air-filled or foam toys, such as "water wings," "noodles," or inner-tubes, in place of life jackets. These toys are not designed to keep swimmers safe.
- Avoid alcohol. Avoid drinking alcohol before or during swimming, boating, or water skiing. Do not drink alcohol while supervising children.
- Do not hyperventilate. Swimmers should never hyperventilate before swimming underwater or try to hold their breath for long periods of time.
- This can cause them to pass out (sometimes called "shallow water blackout") and drown.

CHAPTER **12**

# Obstetrics and Gynecology

## CASE STUDY 76: TOXIC SHOCK SYNDROME

### CASE HISTORY

A 30-year-old female is brought to emergency room (ER) for feeling exhausted, tired, weak, nauseous, and vomiting for 3 days and has a fever of 103°F with body aches. On physical examination, patient has a blood pressure (BP) of 60/40 mm Hg. She is toxic looking, lethargic, and confused. Diffuse rash noticed (Figs. 1A and B). On heart examination, she is tachycardic. Lungs have crackles on the bilateral bases. The rest of the examination is normal. Resuscitative measures are taken immediately. Intravenous (IV) fluids started with 0.9% normal saline (NS) bolus through 18G cannulae in each arm in the antecubital vein. After fluid resuscitation, blood cultures are drawn and IV methicillin and nafcillin are started (Flowchart 1 and Box 1). After the bolus, BP improved, and the patient is now more alert, coherent, and widely awake.

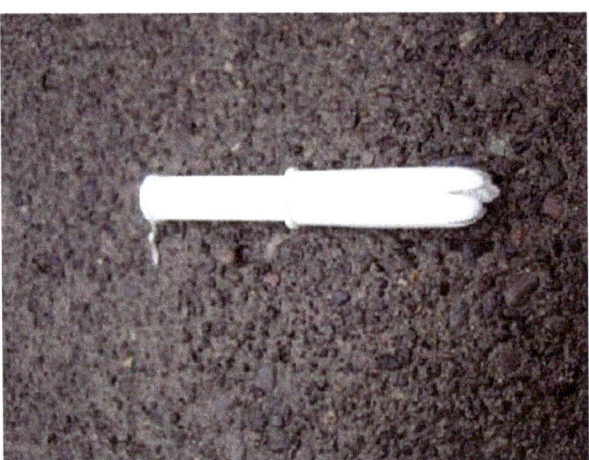

**Fig. 1A :** Forgotten tampon.

# Obstetrics and Gynecology

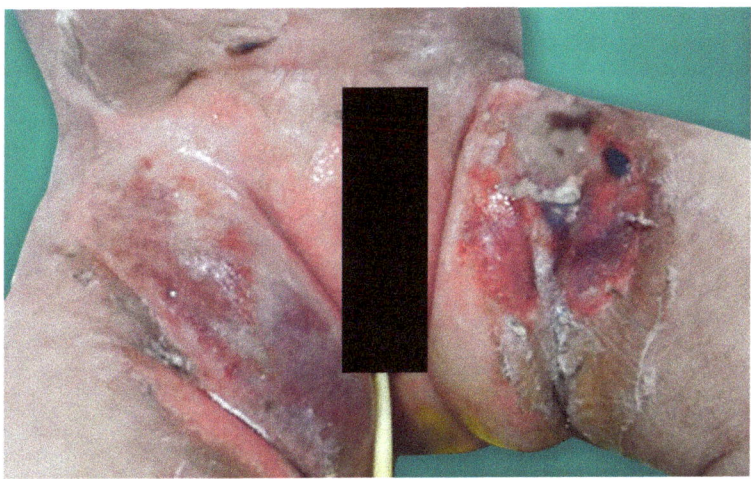

**Fig. 1B:** Typical rash of toxic shock syndrome.
*Courtesy:* Stephanie Williford Chief Executive Officer, EB Medicine, Atlanta Georgia, USA.

**Flowchart 1:** Goals of treatment.

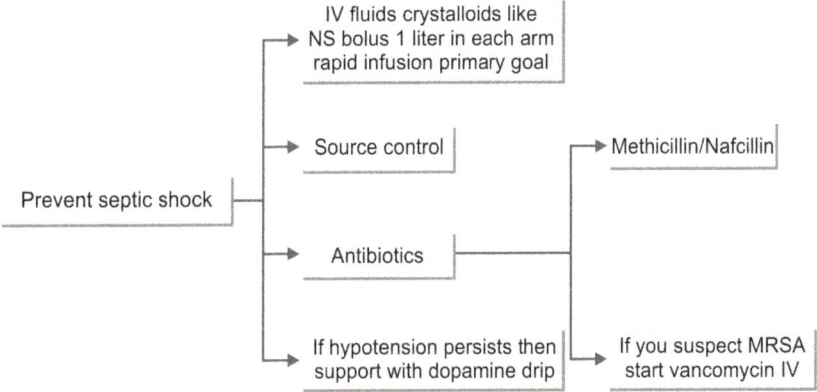

(IV: intravenous; NS: normal saline; MRSA: methicillin-resistant *Staphylococcus aureus*.)

**Box 1:** Toxic shock syndrome: case definition.

- Fever >38.9°C
- Diffuse macular erythroderma
- Desquamation 1–2 weeks after onset of illness, especially on palms and soles
- Hypotension (systolic blood pressure less than fifth percentile)
- Involvement of three or more organ systems
  - Gastrointestinal (vomiting or diarrhea)

*(Contd...)*

*( Contd...)*

> **Box 1:** Toxic shock syndrome: case definition.
>
> - Muscular (severe myalgia or CPK greater than two times normal)
> - Mucous membranes (vaginal, oropharyngeal, or conjunctival hyperemia)
> - Renal (BUN or creatinine greater than two times normal)
> - Hepatic (total bilirubin, SGOT, or SGPT greater than two times normal)
> - Hematologic (platelets <100,000)
> - Central nervous system (altered mental status without focal neurologic signs)
> - Negative results on the following tests
>   - Throat, CSF cultures
>   - Serologic tests for rocky mountain spotted fever or measles.

(CPK: creatine phosphokinase; BUN: blood urea nitrogen; SGOT: serum glutamic–oxaloacetic transaminase; SGPT: serum glutamic–pyruvic transaminase; CSF: cerebrospinal fluid).

## DISCUSSION

### Treatment Plan

Treatment plan is discussed in Flowchart 1. But the empiric treatment remains clindamycin plus vancomycin. The main goal for treating toxic shock syndrome (TSS) is to prevent septic shock. Early introduction of IV fluids and antibiotics are necessary.

TSS is most often caused by *Staphylococcus aureus,* more specifically by the exotoxin, TSS toxin-1 (TSST-1). It most often affects women, with one report detailing TSS cases between 1979 and 1996 showing 96% occurring among women.

## FURTHER READING

1. Hajjeh RA, Reingold A, Weil A, et al. Toxic shock syndrome in the United States: surveillance update, 1979 1996. Emerg Infect Dis. 1999;5:807. https://www.uptodate.com/contents/staphylococcal-toxic-shock-syndrome/abstract/15
2. Chu, V. Staphylococcal toxic shock syndrome. In Melin JA (Ed), UpToDate; 2018. Retrieved September 25, 2018 from https://www.uptodate.com/contents/staphylococcal-toxic-shock-syndrome

## CASE STUDY 77: PLACENTA PREVIA

### CASE HISTORY

A 32-year-old gravida 6, parity 5 (G6P5) female is presented to the emergency room (ER) with painless vaginal bleeding. This started early in the morning of presentation. It is profuse and very bright red in color (Fig. 1). Patient had some spotting a month ago after intercourse. On examination in the ER, vitals included temperature 99°F, pulse rate 80 bpm, blood pressure 110/60 mm Hg. Fetal heart rate monitor shows 140–150 bpm.

# Obstetrics and Gynecology

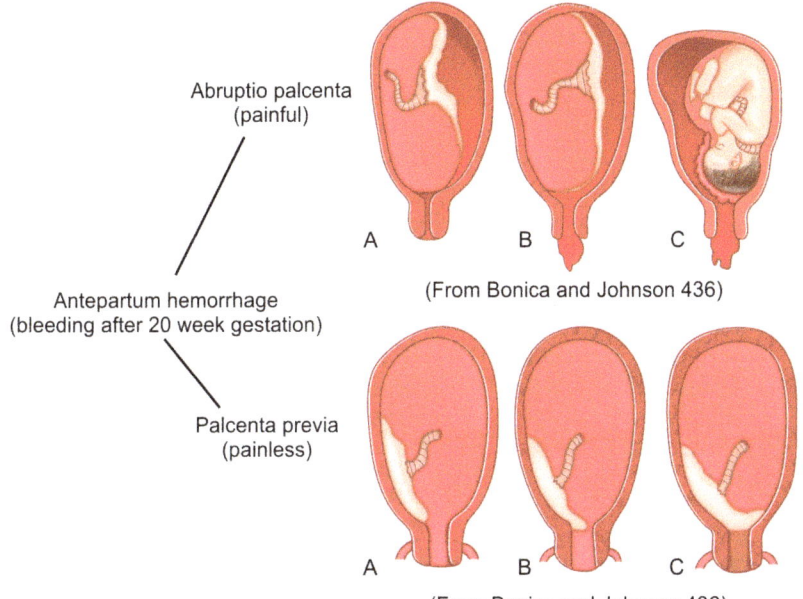

Fig. 1: Types of placenta.

## DISCUSSION

Placenta previa is defined as the implantation of the placenta over the cervical os. There are three types: (1) total, (2) partial, and (3) marginal.

## MANAGEMENT

- Please do not do any digital or speculum examination when you have a patient who presents with antepartum painless vaginal bleeding.
- Always suspect placenta previa and rule it out with a transabdominal ultrasound. A transabdominal ultrasound will not always be able to detect the location of the placenta. In such cases, a transvaginal ultrasound is necessary by an experienced physician.
- The first episode of vaginal bleeding does not cause sufficient concern to necessitate emergent delivery. In such cases, with a preterm gestation in placenta previa, patients are usually observed on bed rest. This is done with the expectation that time may be gained for fetal maturity. Amniocentesis is done to establish fetal lung maturity.
- If fetal lungs are immature, prescribe corticosteroids to encourage surfactant development.
- If the fetal lungs appear to be mature (beyond 32 weeks or based on clinical information), then delivery by cesarean (C)-section will be scheduled.
- It is advised that women with placenta previa after 20 weeks of gestation (earlier if they have experienced vaginal bleeding) to avoid any sexual

activity that may lead to orgasm and to avoid moderate and strenuous exercise or standing for long periods of time.

## CAUTION

Digital examination should not be performed prior to ultrasound.

Avoid medical malpractice by avoiding digital cervical examination as this procedure may cause placental rupture and potentially lethal hemorrhage.

## FURTHER READING

1. Lockwood C, Russo-Stieglitz K. Placenta previa: Management. In: Melin JA, editors. UpToDate; 2018. Retrieved September 25, 2018, from https://www.uptodate.com/contents/placenta-previa-management
2. Toy E. Case files obstetrics and gynecology, 3rd ed. McGraw-Hill Education / Medical 2009; 2009. ISBN: 978-0-07-160581-6.

# CASE STUDY 78: ECTOPIC PREGNANCY

## CASE HISTORY

The patient is a 26-year-old gravida 3, parity 4 (Gravida 4. parity 3. G4P3) female with history of past ectopic pregnancy (EP) who presents to the emergency room with severe right-sided abdominal pain for 3 days. The pain is 10/10, sharp, and localized to the right lower abdomen without radiation. She reports associated nausea, but no vomiting. Tylenol did not relieve the pain. Patient denies any light headedness or loss of consciousness. She states that this pain feels exactly as the pain she had with her previous EP which she believes was located on the left side. Patient denies vaginal bleeding or discharge. She did not take a pregnancy test at home, but she is sexually active with her husband and is not currently using birth control because she wishes to become pregnant. No history of sexually transmitted diseases (STDs) in the past is noted. Last menstrual period (LMP) was approximately 6 weeks ago. No significant past medical history is noted. Surgical history is significant for two cesarean (C)-sections and laparoscopic removal of the EP with preservation of the uterine tubes. Patient does not drink, smoke, or use any recreational drugs. On physical examination, patient is afebrile with blood pressure of 100/70 mm Hg, pulse rate 120 bpm, respiratory rate 20 breaths/min, and saturation is 99% on room air. On abdominal examination, patient is severely tender to light palpation in the right lower quadrant. No rebound tenderness, or percussion tenderness, but positive Rovsing sign noticed. Urine pregnancy test is positive. IV fluids, Zofran, and pain medications are started.[1] Two large bore intravenous (IV) lines are placed. Pelvic examination was positive for cervical motion tenderness (CMT), but no evidence of vaginal bleeding or discharge was found. Transvaginal ultrasound revealed a large sac-like structure on the right adnexa. Ultrasound revealed only gestational sac. Beta-human chorionic gonadotropin (β-hCG) was 3,000 mIU/mL. Obstetrician/gynecologist (ob/gyn) was consulted for further management of likely EP. Further ob/gyn transvaginal ultrasound confirmed EP on the right side measuring 4 × 5 cm (Fig. 1). Patient was taken to the operating room (OR) for laparoscopic removal.

## DISCUSSION

In 20% of cases, ectopic pregnancies are ruptured at the time of presentation (Fig. 2). Risk factors for EP include history of pelvic inflammatory disease

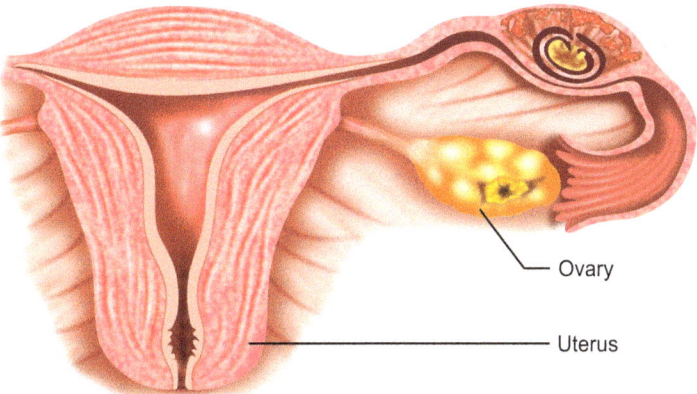

**Fig. 1:** Ectopic pregnancy.

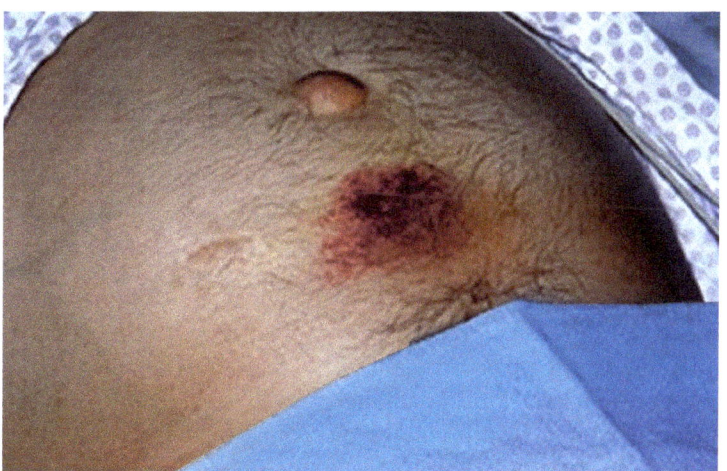

**Fig. 2:** Cullen sign—sign of ruptured ectopic.
*Courtesy:* Herbert L Fred, MD, Houston, Texas, USA and Hendrik A van Dijk, Houston, Texas, USA.

(PID), surgical procedure of the fallopian tubes including tubal ligations, previous EP, intrauterine device (IUD) use, assisted reproductive technologies, abdominal pain, vaginal bleeding, and amenorrhea. Only 90% of women with EP complain of abdominal pain, 80% have vaginal bleeding, and 70% have a history of amenorrhea. Pain is described as sudden, lateral, extreme, and diffuse. Vaginal bleeding is usually light. Heavy bleeding is common with abortion or other complications of pregnancy.

Abdominal examination shows signs of localized or diffuse tenderness with or without peritoneal signs. Pelvic examination findings may be normal, but most often shows CMT and adnexal tenderness, with or without a mass. The patient may possibly have an enlarged uterus. Fetal heart tones are rarely audible.

In order to make a diagnosis, transvaginal ultrasound is the test of choice. A progesterone level of 5 ng/mL or lower with an empty uterus is highly suggestive of EP, but it cannot be used to exclude EP. A high β-hCG level >6,000 mIU/mL with empty uterus is suggestive of EP. If hCG is low and <1,000 mIU/mL, then the pregnancy may be intrauterine or ectopic, but not able to be visualized on ultrasound. In 2 days, a repeat β-hCG must be performed in these situations.

The emergency department management depends on vital signs, physical examination findings, and symptoms. Two large bore IV lines are started in case rapid infusion of crystalloids and/or packed red blood cells (pRBCs) are needed. Urine pregnancy test should always be obtained first. If identified, ob/gyn consultation is necessary for further workup.

Blood is typically drawn for complete blood count (CBC), blood type, Rhesus (Rh) factor, β-hCG, and serum electrolytes. For unstable patients, the diagnostic workup includes transvaginal ultrasound. Patients with indeterminate ultrasound and hCG <1,000 mIU/mL can be discharged with ectopic precautions and follow-up in 2 days.

The vast majority (70%) of tubal pregnancies occur in the ampullary portion of the fallopian tube, with the remainder about equally between fimbrial and isthmus. A very small proportion occurs in the interstitial portion.

Risk factors for EP include previous EP, tubal pathology and/or surgery, in utero Diethylstilbestrol (DES) exposure, previous genital infections (including PID, salpingitis, chlamydia, gonorrhea), smoking, In vitro fertilization (IVF), vaginal douching, and young age at the first sexual encounter.

## CAUTION

Unless the medical team is very vigilant and maintains a high index of suspicion, it is easy to miss ectopic pregnancies.

Anytime a woman of reproductive age comes in with abdominal pain, be sure to perform a urine hCG test to rule out/rule in pregnancy. If positive, perform an ultrasound to view the uterus, fallopian tubes, and peritoneum. Delays in diagnosis and treatment will affect future fertility and may result in a medical malpractice suit.

## REFERENCE

1. Dunn RJ, Dilley S, Brookes JG, et al. The emergency medicine manual. [Online]. Available from www.emergencymedicinemanual.com/; 2013 [accessed September, 2013].

CHAPTER 13

# Ear, Nose and Throat Emergencies

## CASE STUDY 79: EPISTAXIS

*"Not every epistaxis is just a bloody nose."*

—Badar M Zaheer

### CASE HISTORY

A 10-year-old boy comes in emergency department (ED) for recurrent nosebleeds. He has a history of allergies and has been taking fluticasone propionate (a nasal spray) regularly to control his sinusitis. He presents to the ED overnight when the father can no longer control the bleeding on his own. The physician locates a source near the anterior nare, but the bleeding does not stop after administering cotton swabs moistened with lidocaine several times. Finally, the bleeding is stopped after administering silver nitrate. Patient is instructed to follow-up with an ENT physician in 3 days.

### DISCUSSION

The key of managing epistaxis is to determine whether the bleeding is anterior or posterior. Usually posterior bleeding is identified by lack of visualization of anterior source, bleeding from both nares, or drainage into posterior pharynx after controlling anterior source (Flowcharts 1 and 2). The majority are anterior bleeds which come from Kiesselbach's plexus (Fig. 1). These patients are usually children or young adults. Risk factors include trauma, epistaxis digitorum, winter syndrome, allergies, irritants such as cocaine or nasal sprays, and pregnancy. Posterior bleeding accounts for only 10% and is usually present in the elderly. Anatomically, these bleeds are arterial in nature. Etiologies include coagulopathy, atherosclerosis, neoplasm, and questionable hypertension.

Anterior epistaxis can be treated with anterior packing balloons, but some patients are uncomfortable with this option. Alternative treatment can be fashioned from available materials in the ER. An absorbable hemostatic

Ear, Nose and Throat Emergencies

**Flowchart 1:** Management of epistaxis.

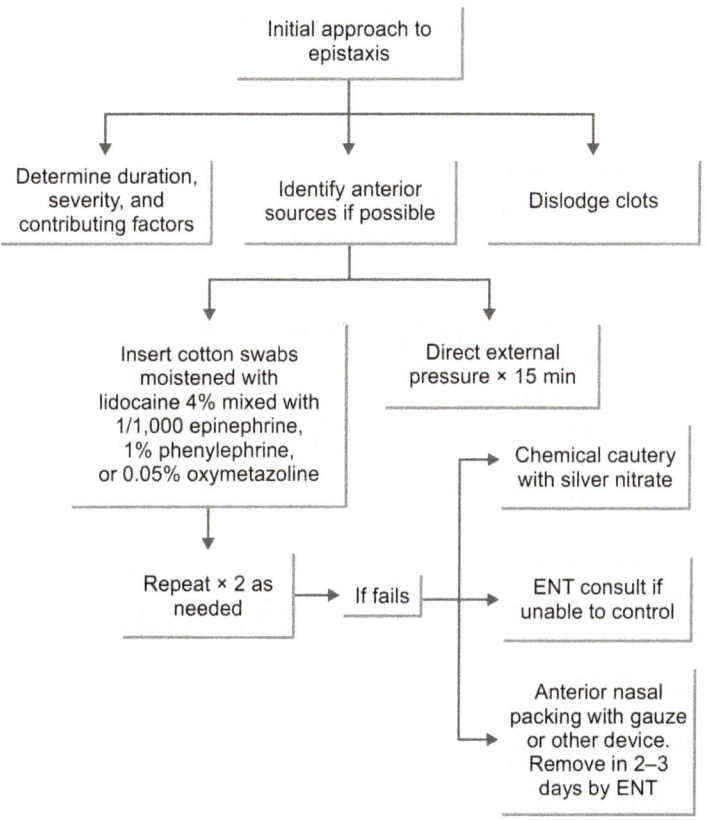

**Flowchart 2:** Management of posterior epistaxis.

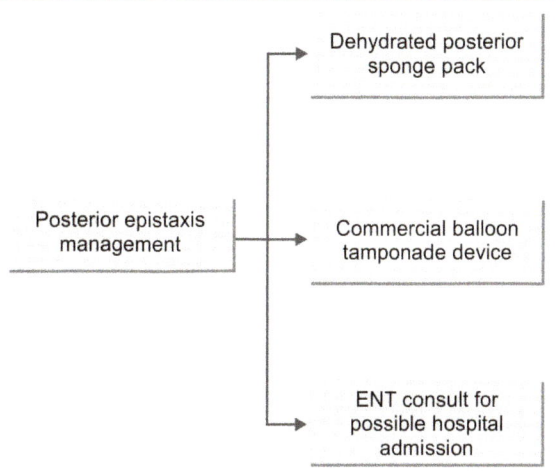

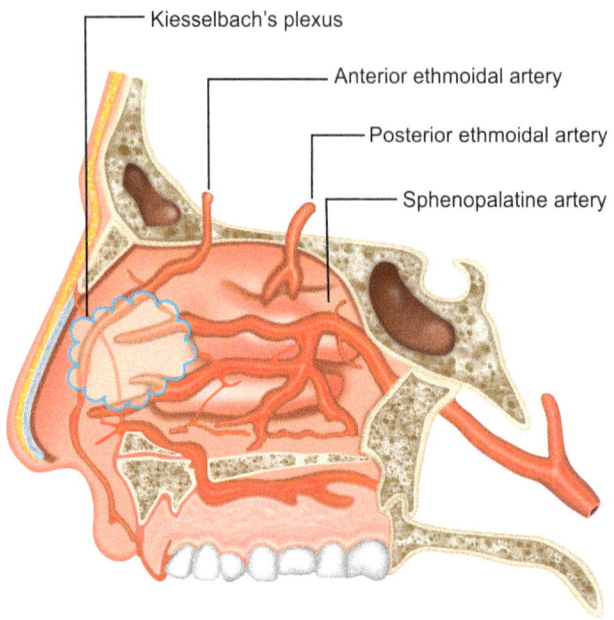

**Fig. 1:** Nasal vascular anatomy.
*Source:* Goralnick E. Posterior epistaxis nasal pack. [Online]. Available from emedicine.medscape.com/article/80545-overview; 2012 [accessed September, 2013].

sponge can be coated with bacitracin, inserted into the nare, and affixed to the septum using tissue adhesive. Tongue depressors can be taped together two third from the distal end and used to provide compression.

Alternatively, a rhino rocket may be used, which is a nasal packing with applicator for epistaxis management. After application of nasal saline drops, the packing expands, controlling the bleeding (Fig. 2).

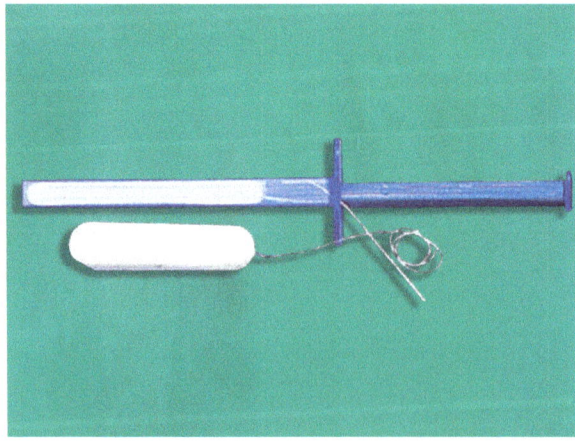

**Fig. 2:** Rhino Rocket applicator and packing.

Nasal cautery may also be used. After local anesthetic is sprayed in the nostril, cautery is used to control source of bleeding (Fig. 3).

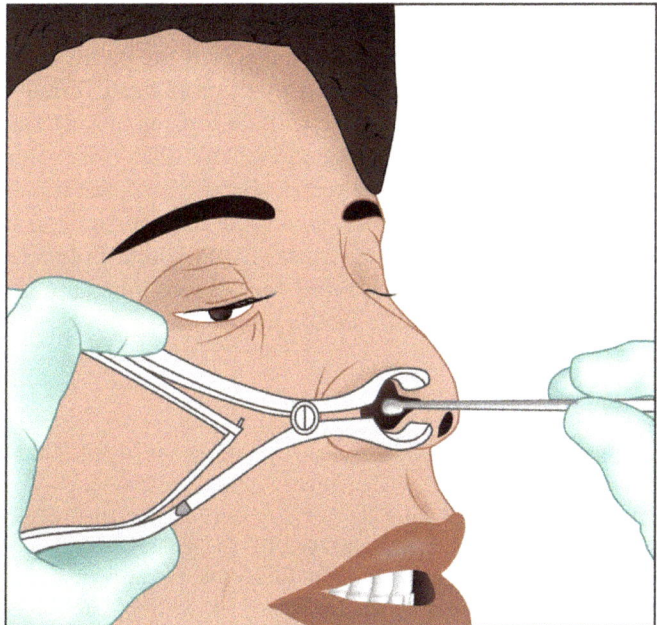

**Fig. 3:** Nasal cautery.
*Source:* https://aneskey.com/wp-content/uploads/2016/ 08/B9780323079099000271_f27-03-9780323079099.jpg.

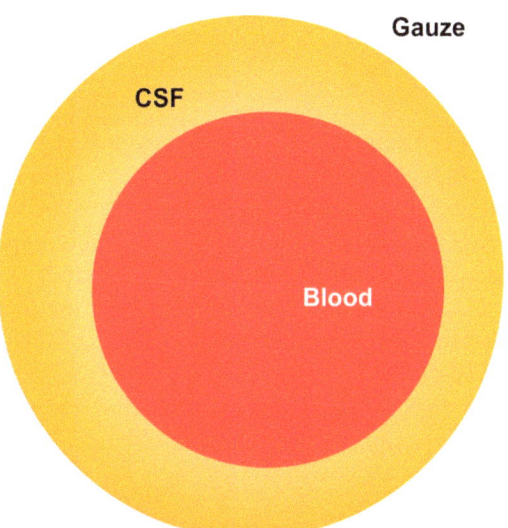

**Fig. 4:** A positive halo sign on the background of tissue paper.
*Courtesy:* Dr. Badar M Zaheer, Chicago, USA.

Complications of nasal packing include dislodgment of the pack, recurrent bleeding including septal hematomas, abscesses, neurogenic syncope, pressure necrosis, sinusitis, and toxic shock syndrome. If pack is placed, use antibiotic prophylaxis such as cephalexin 250–500 mg PO q 6 h or amoxicillin/clavulanate 250/150 mg PO q 8 h. However, if the patient is allergic to penicillin, you may use clindamycin or trimethoprim or sulfamethoxazole. It is also important to consider comorbid CSF rhinorrhea (Fig. 4). Clues which should raise a clinician's level of suspicion for this diagnosis include unilateral nasal discharge and loss of the sense of smell; however, the absence of these signs and symptoms does not rule out CSF rhinorrhea. A positive "halo sign" can be found if the blood has mixed with another fluid such as CSF, tears, or saliva. If a CSF leak is suspected, high-resolution computed tomography (CT) and CT cisternography should be obtained.

## FURTHER READING

1. Glaspy J. Ear, nose and sinus emergencies. In: Emergency medicine manual. 6th ed. McGraw-Hill Professional; (December 11, 2003). p. 728-33.
2. Kucik CJ, Clenney T. Management of epistaxis. Am Fam Physician. 2005;71(2):305-11. Available from www.aafp.org/afp/2005/0115/p305.pdf.
3. Viduchich R, Blanda M, Gerson L. Posterior epistaxis: clinical features and acute complications. Ann Emerg Med. 1995;25(5):592-6. http://download.journals.elsevierhealth.com/pdfs/journals/0196-0644/ PIIS0196064495701699.pdf.

## CASE STUDY 80: NASAL FRACTURES

### CASE HISTORY

A 13-year-old girl is presented to the emergency department (ED) with swelling, tenderness, crepitus, and nose deformity. On examination, vital signs are stable. X-ray of the nasal bone shows fracture of the nasal bones. ENT examination shows collection of bluish-filled sacs and grape-like cluster on the left nasal side. Patient is initially treated with ice pack and ibuprofen and then referred to ENT department. She returns with worsening pain, difficulty in breathing, and drainage from the site of the bluish-filled sac. Patient has an abscess at the site of the septal hematoma, which is drained with incision and drainage. Pain significantly decreases after the procedure and patient is discharged with a 7-day course of antibiotics.

### DISCUSSION

This patient has a fracture of the nasal bones with the complication of a septal hematoma as indicated by the bluish-filled sac in the left nasal side (Fig. 1).

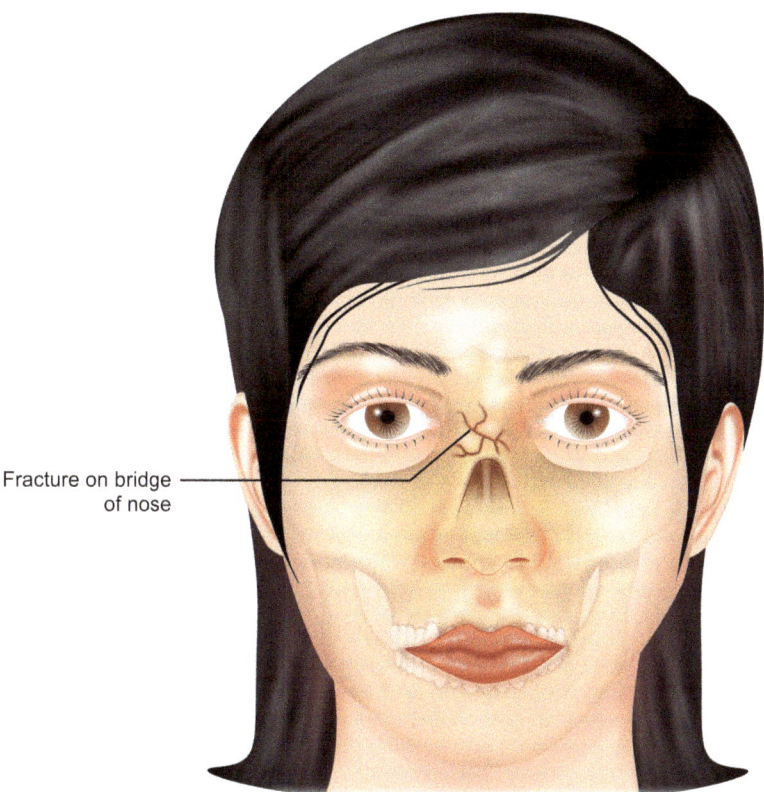

**Fig. 1:** Nasal fracture.
*Source:* Vorvick LJ. Nasal fracture. [Online]. Available from www.nlm.nih.gov/medlineplus/ency/imagepages/8873.htm; 2011 [accessed September, 2012].

Treatment is generally conservative with ice packs, ibuprofen, nasal packing if necessary and referral to ENT.[1] Despite conservative treatment, the patient presented with difficulty in breathing and swelling of the left nasal septum suggestive of a superimposed infection on the left nasal septal hematoma. Incision and drainage is performed with lidocaine nasal spray, which is used to anesthetize the wound area. Prophylactic antibiotics are prescribed as indicated.

Nasal fracture is a clinical diagnosis if the injury mechanism, swelling, tenderness, crepitus, gross deformity, and periorbital ecchymosis are seen.[2] Other symptoms include epistaxis, rhinitis, nasal vestibular stenosis, and airway obstruction. Radiological study is usually not required in the ED.

Follow-up should be done in 2–5 days for reassessment. The nose should be evaluated for a septal hematoma because if left untreated, it may result in abscess formation or necrosis of the nasal septum. A septal hematoma is a collection of blood beneath the perichondrium. It may appear as a bluish, fluid-filled sac on nasal septum. Treatment is with local incision and drainage followed by anterior nasal packing. If a cribriform plate injury is suspected, computed tomography scans should be performed followed by immediate neurological consultation.

## REFERENCES

1. Blaker S. Nasal injuries. 2008. [Online]. Available from www.slideshare.net/pdhpemag/nasal-injuries-presentation-583816. [Accessed September, 2012].
2. Glaspy JN. Nasal fractures. In: Emergency medicine manual. 6th ed. New York: McGraw Hill; 2004. p. 732.

# CASE STUDY 81: NASAL FOREIGN BODIES

## CASE HISTORY

A 6-year-old girl is brought to the clinic by her parents. The parents found unilateral, foul smelling purulent discharge from her nose. Her younger sister said she was playing with beads and inserted one in her nose. Child complains of difficulty breathing from one nostril and feels something in the nose. Child complains of irritation and pain upon assessment.

## DIAGNOSIS

Nasal foreign body.

## MANAGEMENT

Topical anesthesia is given, which is followed by removal of the foreign body with a probe.

Do not attempt to search the nose with cotton swab or other tools for risk of pushing object further in.

## DISCUSSION

Patients with nasal foreign bodies usually present with unilateral nasal obstruction, foul rhinorrhea, or persistent unilateral epistaxis. Topical vasoconstrictors and anesthesia should be used, and the foreign body should then be removed. Hooked probes, balloon-tipped, or suction catheters and/or forceps are the standard tools used to remove the foreign body (Fig. 1). For pediatric patients, the nonaffected nostril should be occluded with a finger and positive air pressure should be applied to the patient's mouth. For any unsuccessful removal, an ENT consultation should be sought and may necessitate the use of balloon-catheter removal.

Ear, Nose and Throat Emergencies

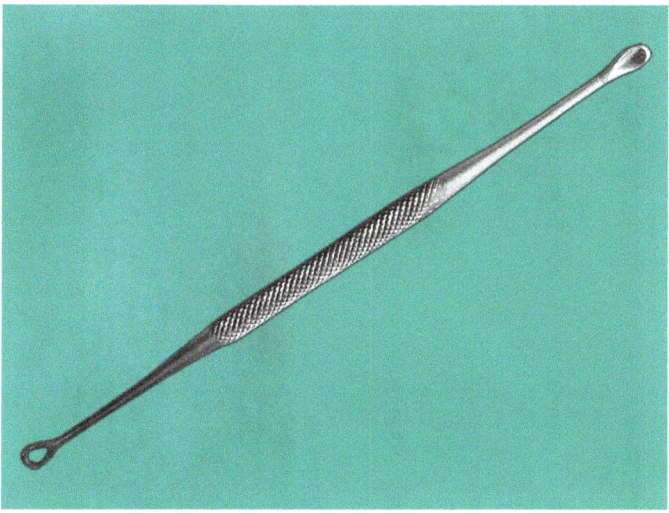

**Fig. 1:** Nasal foreign body removal hook used in ENT practice.
*Source:* Reprinted with permission from entinstruments.blogspot.com.

## CASE STUDY 82: RETROPHARYNGEAL ABSCESS

### CASE HISTORY

A 40-year-old male is presented to the emergency department (ED) at 2 AM with symptoms of sore throat, difficulty in swallowing, and trismus. Patient initially had a sore throat and difficulty in swallowing over the past 2 weeks but is now getting worse. He can no longer open his jaw and he continues to have high fevers at home up to 104°F. On presentation to the ED, the patient is ill-appearing. Vitals are temperature 39.5°C, blood pressure 100/70 mm Hg, pulse rate 120 bpm, respiratory rate 18 bpm, and $O_2$ saturation level 100%. Computed tomography (CT) scan of neck is done and reveals paravertebral abscess. Physical examination shows tender cervical lymphadenopathy, neck swelling, and torticollis. Movement of the trachea or larynx side to side (tracheal "rock") is painful.

### DISCUSSION

Retropharyngeal abscesses occur anterior to the prevertebral space and posterior to the pharynx (Fig. 1). These generally occur in children <4 years of age but may occur in adults as well.

Symptoms include pain, dysphagia, dyspnea, fever, muffled voice, stridor, and neck stiffness. Patients typically present in a supine position with slight

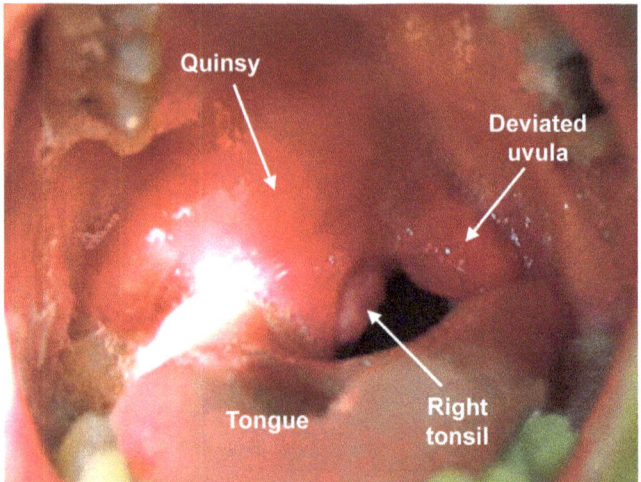

**Fig. 1:** Peritonsillar abscess, quinsy is inflammation of the throat, particularly in the peritonsillar area.
*Source:* Available from http://1.bp.blogspot.com/-ETI_7tws-Mk/T00p3R3zCFI/AAAAAAAAC78/8NYql1YWkk0/s1600/quinsy1.jpg.

neck extension to improve dyspnea. Physical findings include tender cervical lymphadenopathy, neck swelling, torticollis, pharyngeal erythema, and edema. Swelling of retropharyngeal space and thickening of the prevertebral space may be evident on X-ray of lateral soft tissue of the neck (Fig. 2). Further evaluation to define the abscess as well differentiation from cellulitis can be done by CT scan. Complications of retropharyngeal abscess include mediastinitis.

Due to the anatomic and pathophysiologic differences, retropharyngeal abscess is more localized in children than adults.

## Differential Diagnosis

X-ray of the neck, lateral soft tissue, will show thickening in the prevertebral space. CT scan of the neck, with enhanced intravenous (IV) contrast, will help to differentiate between cellulitis and abscess. It also helps us to define the extent of the infections. Cultures taken from the abscess are usually polymicrobial and include aerobic and anaerobic organisms.

## Management

Management should initially focus on airway management. ENT consultation should be obtained for drainage. Antibiotics should be started. Regime for adults may include clindamycin 600–900 mg intravenously (IV) q 8 h or ampicillin–sulbactam 3 g IV q 6 h.

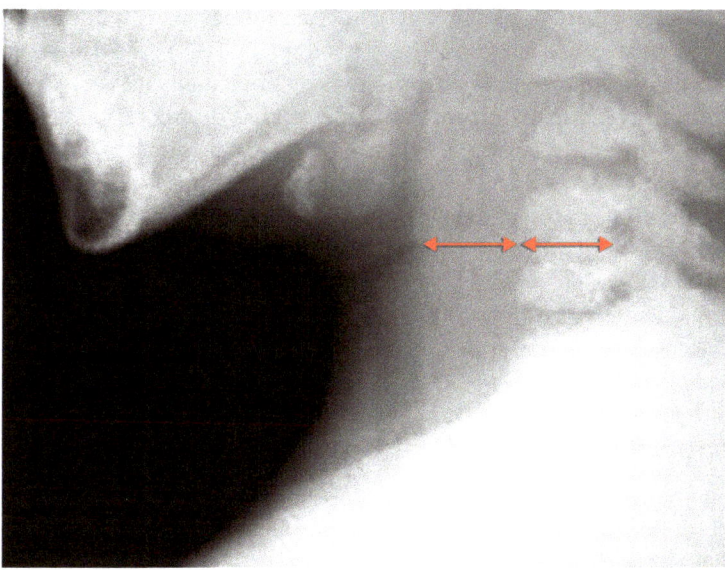

**Fig. 2:** Retropharyngeal abscess.
*Source:* Acevedo JL. Pediatric retropharyngeal abscess. [Online]. Available from reference.medscape.com/features/slideshow/pediatric-respiratory; 2011 [accessed September, 2012].

## CASE STUDY 83: FOREIGN BODY/COIN INGESTION

### CASE HISTORY

A 3-year-old girl is presented to the emergency department after swallowing a coin. Her mother saw her take the coin off the floor but was unable to reach her in time before the coin was ingested. She is certain it is a coin and not a battery because she saw the copper color of a penny. The mother does not note any signs of difficulty in breathing or swallowing. The girl appears to be normal, but the mother is concerned that the coin will "get stuck." Vitals are unremarkable including the child being afebrile. On examination, there are no signs of respiratory distress. There is some mild erythema present in the throat. Abdominal examination does not reveal any peritoneal signs. An X-ray is taken and reveals that the coin is now in the child's stomach. Serial abdominal examinations are done, and the child is discharged home with close follow-up by the primary care physician.

### DISCUSSION

The majority of foreign body ingestions occur in children; however, they may occur at any age.[1] In adults, foreign body ingestions rate is higher in inmates, toothless adults, and psychiatric patients. The foreign body tends to get stuck at sites of narrowing throughout the gastrointestinal (GI) tract. However, once past the pylorus of the stomach, problems do not usually occur.

Symptoms of ingestion may include anxiety, retrosternal discomfort, retching, vomiting, dysphagia, coughing, choking, aspiration, and difficulty in swallowing secretions. Physical examination should include the upper airway. Findings in the pediatric population that are supportive of a foreign body ingestion include red throat, palatal abrasion, temperature elevation, and peritoneal signs. Either X-ray or laryngoscopy or endoscopy may be used. Be aware that only radiopaque objects will be evident on X-ray. The differentials should include dysphagia, esophageal carcinoma, and GI reflux.

## Management

Management should include either aspiration of the foreign body or suction of secretions. Abdominal examinations should be monitored closely to watch for signs of perforation. Serial abdominal X-rays may monitor progress of the foreign body through the GI tract. If the type of foreign body is known, treatment can be geared toward the individual type of foreign body. With food, conservation treatment is safe when the patient is able to manage his or her own secretions. If there is no passage after 12 h, then intervention is deemed necessary. Intervention may include lower esophageal sphincter relaxation with glucagon, nitroglycerin or nifedipine, or endoscopy. Avoid proteolytic enzymes as they may cause esophageal perforation. GI consultation will usually be required in the presence of impaction.

For coins, 33% of children will be asymptomatic if the coin is in the esophagus.[2] X-ray is recommended. If in the esophagus, the coin will be in the frontal plane. If in the trachea, the coin will be in the sagittal plane (Fig. 1). If present in the esophagus, the foreign body is generally considered impacted. If lodged in the esophagus, endoscopy is required. If the coin is in the stomach, it will almost always pass on its own.

Battery ingestion is always an emergency situation. Emergent imaging and endoscopy is required except in cases of asymptomatic button batteries that have already passed the esophagus. Button batteries can be conservatively managed unless they are lodged in a fixed location. Burns may occur within 4 h, and perforation may occur within 6 h. About the size of a nickel, 20 mm, 3-V lithium coin cells are the most hazardous as they are large enough to get stuck and burn faster. If a mercury-containing battery has opened, be sure to monitor blood and mercury levels.[3]

Sharp object ingestion management is controversial. An X-ray should be performed to determine location. If longer than 5 cm and wider than 2 cm, it is unlikely that the object will pass the stomach. Pointed objects may cause perforation especially at the ileocecal valve.

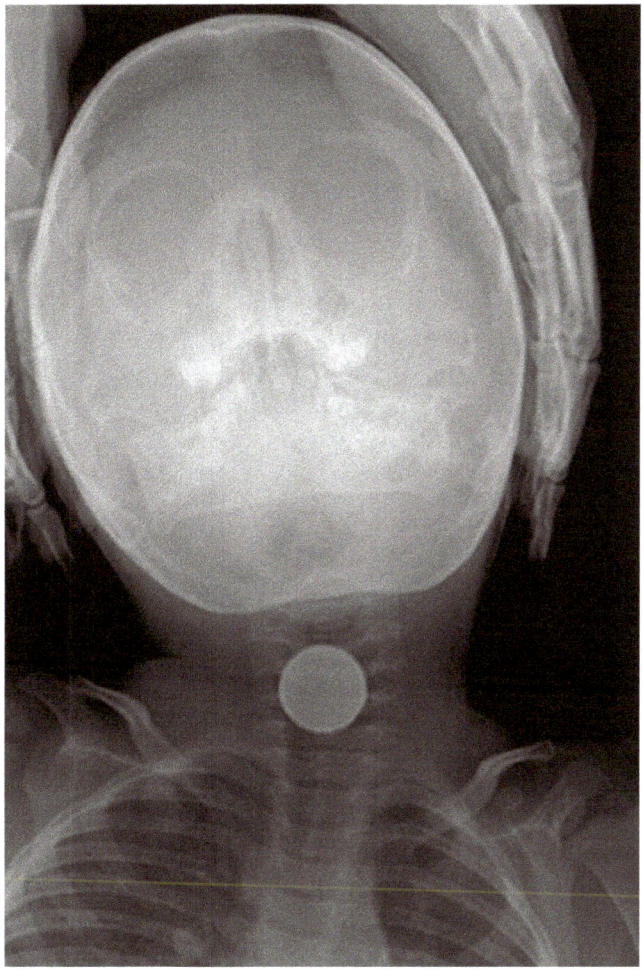

**Fig. 1:** Frontal view of esophageal button (disk) battery; note distinctive double-circle appearance, useful to differentiate a button battery from a coin.
*Source:* Available from emedicine.medscape.com/article/801821-treatment#a1126.

Cocaine ingestion is also a consideration. Multiple small bags are often swallowed for drug concealment. Full bowel irrigation has been used successfully but is not always required. Be careful to monitor vital signs in case the bags burst. Endoscopy should not be performed due to risk of bag rupture. Surgical intervention is safer.

## REFERENCES

1. Baines P. Swallowed foreign bodies. In: Emergency medicine manual. 6th ed. New York: McGraw Hill; 2004. p. 209-11.

2. Conners GP. Pediatric foreign body ingestion. [Online] Available from emedicine.medscape.com/article/801821-treatment#a1126; 2011 [accessed September, 2012].
3. Litovitz TL, Whitaker N, Clark L, White NC, Marsolek M. Emerging battery-ingestion hazard: clinical implications. Pediatrics. 2010;125(6):1168-77.

# CHAPTER 14

# Hematology/Oncology

## CASE STUDY 84: NEUTROPENIC FEVER

### CASE HISTORY

A 40-year-old woman with history of non-Hodgkin's lymphoma is presented to the emergency department (ED) with fever. Patient has no complaints except occasional weakness and fever this morning while at home. She has not traveled anywhere recently and has been careful to avoid sick contacts. In the ED, she is febrile at temperature 38.4°C, and her other vitals are blood pressure 140/70 mm Hg, pulse rate 95 bpm, respiratory rate 18 breaths/min, and $O_2$ saturation level 96% on room air. Her venous catheter site is without erythema or swelling. Lungs have scattered rhonchi throughout. Remainder of examination is unremarkable. Chest X-ray (CXR) shows no evidence of infiltrate. Absolute neutrophil count (ANC) of 450 cells/mL is revealed. What should be considered in this case?

### DISCUSSION

Neutropenic fever is defined as a single fever >38.3°C or a sustained fever >38°C in a person with neutropenia. Neutropenia is defined as having an ANC <500 cells/mL. This is a medical emergency with a high-risk of death with ANC <100. The potential for death within hours may occur and rapid action is crucial. Because patients without neutrophils are unable to mount a response, there are usually minimal symptoms with a high-risk of rapid deterioration. Because the magnitude of the neutrophilic response is blunted in these patients, fever may be the earliest and only sign of infection. Patients also on steroids may not mount a febrile response and in fact may become hypothermic and hypotensive. Deterioration may be unexplained in these patients. The fever may be due to viral or bacterial causes. It is vital to recognize neutropenic fever and empirically treat promptly in order to avoid progression to sepsis and possibly death. International guidelines advocate the administration of empiric antibacterial therapy within 60 min of presentation (or as early as possible) in all patients with suspected neutropenic fever.

## DIFFERENTIAL DIAGNOSIS AND WORKUP

The differential diagnosis for sources of infection includes the central venous catheter site, skin, mouth, sinuses, chest or lung, abdomen, perianal region, and central nervous system (brain abscess, encephalitis, meningitis). Take cultures from all lumens, skin and line sites, sputum, urine, and stool for bacterial, fungal, and viral cultures. As mentioned previously, the patient may have an absence of the usual evidence of infection since neutrophils are required to mount a response, and thus it is vital that empiric antibiotics be initiated within 60 min of presentation. For example, the patient may lack evidence of an infiltrate on CXR with suspected pneumonia.

A complete workup should be performed after history, physical, and initiation of empiric antibiotics and requires a complete blood count, chemistry, liver panel, coagulation panel, urine analysis, blood culture, and sputum culture.

### Emergency Room Care and Disposition

- Antibiotics should be started within 60 min empirically
- Start IV fluids to maintain hemodynamics to prevent the patient from going to septic shock
- Catheter removal for catheter related infections.

Central venous catheter removal for infections caused by *Staphylococcus aureus*, *Pseudomonas aeruginosa*, *Candida* spp., or rapidly growing nontuberculous mycobacteria.

Empiric antibiotic therapy should be initiated. In the case of persistent or recurrent fever, antifungal agents should be tried.

## FURTHER READING

1. John Ma O, Cline DM, Tintinalli JE, et al. Emergency medicine manual. 6th ed. New York: McGraw Hill; 2004. p. 662.
2. Bow E, Wingard J. (2018). Overview of neutropenic fever syndromes. In: Melin JA (Ed.), UpToDate. Retrieved October 2, 2018 from https://www.uptodate.com/contents/overview-of-neutropenic-fever-syndromes.

## CASE STUDY 85: TUMOR LYSIS SYNDROME

### CASE HISTORY

A 45-year-old woman is presented to the emergency department (ED) after her first round of chemotherapy for her newly diagnosed chronic myelogenous leukemia (CML). Patient reports increasing lethargy, muscle cramps, and nausea/vomiting since her chemotherapy. Fluids and ondansetron tablets are started. Laboratory tests reveal values of potassium 5.5 mEq/L and serum creatinine 1.8 mg/L. Patient is presumed to be at high risk of tumor lysis syndrome. Aggressive fluid hydration is started, and uric acid, phosphate, and calcium levels are ordered.

## DISCUSSION

Acute tumor lysis syndrome is a group of metabolic disturbances as a result of the death of rapidly growing tumors. This typically occurs within hours to days after chemotherapy or radiation.[1] Furthermore, this typically occurs after chemotherapy for hematologic malignancies including acute leukemias or high-grade non-Hodgkin's lymphomas. There is increased risk with increased bulk of tumor, and hyperuricemia or renal impairment before chemotherapy. Other risk factors include lactate dehydrogenase levels (>1,500 U/L), advanced disease with abdominal involvement, preexisting renal dysfunction, post-treatment renal failure, acidic urine, preexisting volume depletion, and a young age.

Features of acute tumor lysis syndrome include hyperuricemia, high blood lactate level, hyperkalemia, hyperphosphatemia, hypocalcemia secondary to hyperphosphatemia, acute renal failure, cardiac dysrhythmias, neuromuscular symptoms, lactic acidosis, and metabolic acidosis. These metabolic abnormalities may result in muscle cramps, tetany, confusion or convulsions, and even sudden death. The major causes of death in patients with clinical tumor lysis syndrome are hemorrhage and acute kidney injury.

## MANAGEMENT

### Identifying Patients

Management should focus on prevention by identifying high-risk patients. In order to preserve renal function, it is important to recognize renal complications early. Chemotherapy should be delayed until metabolic abnormalities are corrected.

### Hydration

Hydration is crucial with rate as high as 4–5 L/day in order to maintain urine volumes of 2–3 L/day. Of note, IV hydration is potentially dangerous in fluid overload states, including congestive heart failure and acute kidney injury. In these settings, close monitoring of vital signs and urine output is crucial. Hydration is also important before chemotherapy or radiation therapy.

### *Hemodialysis*

In extreme cases, hemodialysis may be considered. Hemodialysis should be done if serum potassium is 6 mEq/L, serum uric acid is 10 mg/dL, serum creatinine is 10 mg/dL, serum phosphorus is 10 mg/dL, or rapidly rising, with symptomatic hypocalcemia, or if there is a need to reduce volume overload.

## Reducing Uric Acid Levels

There are multiple ways to reduce uric acid levels. Allopurinol may be used but may not affect levels until 48–72 h. Rasburicase is rarely used in the ED. Urine may be alkalinized (pharmacologically with probenecid or non-pharmacologically with citrus fruits, vegetables, and legumes), but this is used with caution. Overall, patients have a good prognosis in the absence of renal failure.

## REFERENCE

1. Marx JA, Hockberger RS, Walls RM, et al. Selected oncologic emergencies. In: Marx: Rosen's emergency medicine concepts and clinical practice. 7th ed. Philadelphia, PA: Mosby Elsevier; 2009.

# CASE STUDY 86: SUPERIOR VENA CAVA SYNDROME

## CASE HISTORY

A 62-year-old male is presented to the emergency department with left upper extremity and neck swelling, cough, shortness of breath, and weight loss for the past several weeks. Cough is productive and sometimes blood streaked. Shortness of breath is exertional and mildly alleviated by his albuterol inhaler. Past history is significant for chronic obstructive pulmonary disease and smoking one pack/day since the age of 17 years. On physical examination, vitals are unremarkable. Remainder of examination is significant for facial fullness, left arm enlargement, and distended superficial veins on the chest wall. Chest reveals expiratory wheezing throughout and decreased breath sounds in the left upper lung field.

## DISCUSSION

Superior vena cava (SVC) syndrome results from any condition that leads to obstruction of blood flow through the SVC and is commonly caused by malignancy, especially lung cancer and lymphoma.[1] Approximately 2–4% of patients with lung cancer develop SVC syndrome, although the incidence is higher in small cell lung cancer. The cause is usually due to masses in the middle or extrinsic mediastinum, right paratracheal or precarinal lymph nodes, and tumors extending from the right upper lobe bronchus.

## SYMPTOMS

Symptoms typically include facial or neck swelling, arm swelling, dyspnea, cough, and dilated chest veins (Fig. 1). Other symptoms may include chest pain, dysphagia, hoarseness, headache, confusion, dizziness, or syncope. Red flag signs are stridor suggestive of laryngeal edema and confusion and obtundation suggestive of cerebral edema. SVC syndrome is only a medical emergency when signs of laryngeal or bronchial or cerebral edema are present, so these are important signs to look for.

## DIAGNOSIS

The diagnosis is initially based on clinical signs and symptoms and then confirmed by imaging, such as plain film or ultrasound. Further clarification requires biopsy and further imaging, such as CT. Treatment is based on specific malignancy including staging. Eighty-four percent of people will have an abnormal chest X-ray with possible mediastinal widening and pleural effusion. However, computed tomography scan of chest with contrast is the best possible way to look for enlarged paratracheal lymph nodes as well as lung or pleural abnormalities. Venography should be done if there are plans to place a stent.

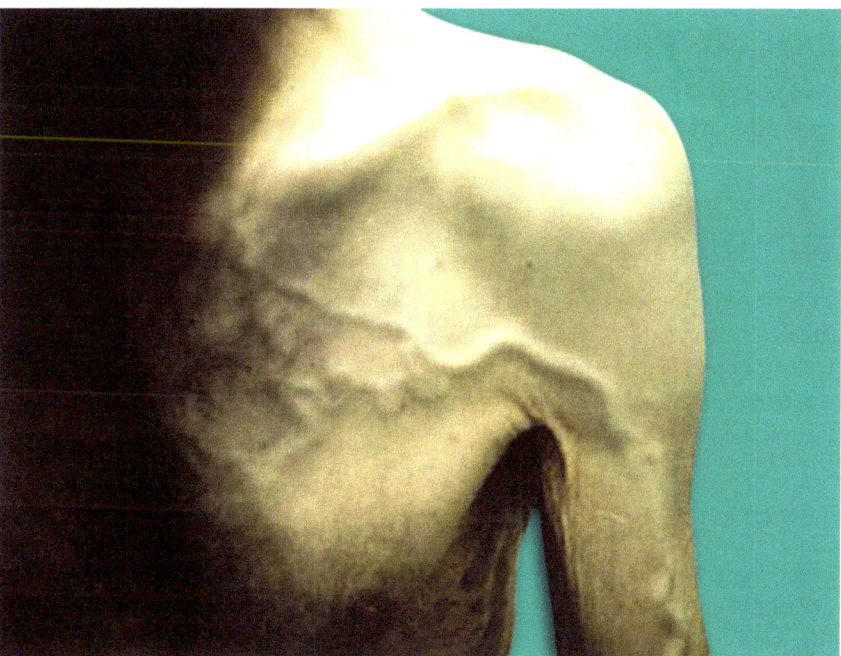

**Fig. 1:** A person suffering from superior vena cava syndrome having distended veins in the upper chest and arms.

## MANAGEMENT

Management is mostly geared toward symptomatic relief. This includes oxygen support, minimizing hydrostatic pressure in the upper torso by fluid restriction, head elevation, and diuretics as well as protecting the airway as necessary. For cerebral edema, consider decreasing intracranial pressure by standard measures. Steroids are controversial but may be considered as a temporary measure to reduce edema. Definitive therapy includes radiation therapy or chemotherapy to treat malignancy. Endovascular stenting by an interventional radiologist may have immediate relief or within 24–72 h. This restores venous return in cases with chemotherapy or radiotherapy resistant tumors.[2]

## REFERENCES

1. Ugras-Rey S, Watson M. Selected oncologic emergencies, Chapter 121. In: Marx JA, Hockberger RS, Walls RM, editors. Rosen's emergency medicine concepts and clinical practice. 7th ed. Philadelphia, PA: Mosby Elsevier; 2009.
2. Wan JF, Bezjak A. Superior vena cava syndrome. Emerg Med Clin North Am. 2009;27(2):243-55.

# CASE STUDY 87: VON WILLEBRAND DISEASE

## CASE HISTORY

Two girls with known von Willebrand disease are presented to the emergency department after a motor vehicle accident. They are currently stable but bleeding is still a major concern.

## ETIOLOGY

This disease is a genetic inherited deficiency in von Willebrand factor causing defective primary hemostasis between the platelets and the blood vessel walls. There are three major categories of von Willebrand deficiency: Type 1 is partial quantitative deficiency, type 2 is qualitative deficiency, and type 3 is total deficiency.[1]

## TREATMENT

Bleeding is a major concern in patients with von Willebrand disease as they are unable to form clots to stop major sites of bleeding (Figs. 1A and B). The first step in treating a trauma patient with this disease is to administer 10 units of cryoprecipitate as well as fresh frozen plasma as these contain functional von Willebrand factor and will thus allow the patient to stop bleeding.

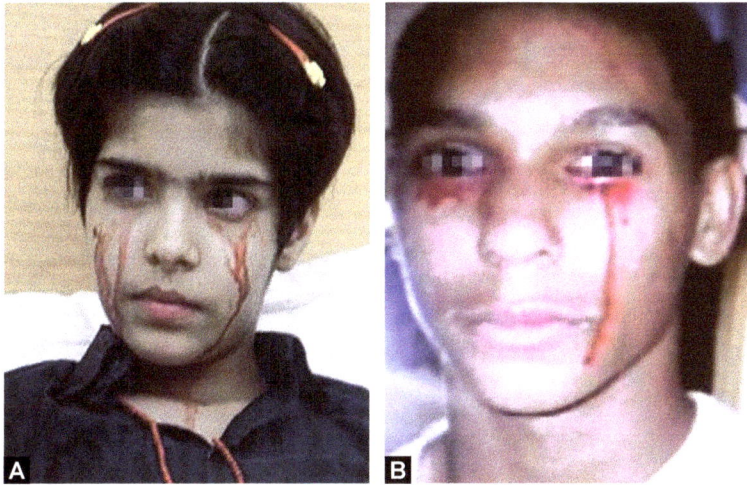

**Figs. 1A and B:** Girls suffering from von Willebrand disease having bleeding from eyes.

These treatments are usually reserved for trauma scenarios because of the high risk associated with foreign blood product transfusion.

## REFERENCE

1. Pollak ES. von Willebrand disease. [Online]. Available from emedicine.medscape.com/article/206996-overview; 2012 [accessed September, 2012].

# CHAPTER 15

# Trauma in Extremes of Age

## CASE STUDY 88: TRAUMA IN ELDERLY

*"Respecting your parents and elders is a universal commandment in every religion."*

—Badar M Zaheer

### CASE HISTORY

A 70-year-old female is presented to the emergency department (ED) after a fall. The patient was walking out to her car when she slipped and fell on the driveway with an outstretched hand. A neighbor stepped out just in time to see the fall and immediately dialed emergency, for emergency medical help. The neighbor reported that she stopped most of the fall with her hand, but she did strike her head on the pavement. However, she never lost consciousness. On presentation to the ED, the patient is slightly drowsy but responsive to commands as well as alert and oriented. Primary survey does not reveal any abnormalities and vitals are unremarkable. Remainder of examination reveals that the patient is unable to move her left wrist, but distal capillary refill is <2 s and sensation is intact. Ecchymosis is present on the patient's left forehead. History is significant for high blood pressure, diabetes, and atrial fibrillation for which the patient takes Coumadin, atenolol, and metformin. X-ray of the left wrist, chest X-ray (CXR), and computed tomography (CT) head are ordered. Patient is found to have both a Colles and small subdural hematoma in the left frontal lobe. Fresh frozen plasma (FFP) is ordered and neurosurgical consultation is obtained. What other steps in management should be taken? What special considerations should be taken into account in the elderly population?

### DISCUSSION

#### Overview
- Less likely to be injured than younger individuals
- More likely to have fatality

- Possible for 80% to return to pre-existing state
- Must take pre-existing disease into account
- Leading causes of death from injury:
  - *Falls*: Most common cause of unintentional injury. Keep in mind that minor mechanism of injury may cause serious harm especially when anticoagulation is on board
  - *Motor vehicle accidents*: Be aware that as patients age, they have worsening daylight acuity, glare resistance, and night vision
  - *Burns*: Be aware of limited mobility. They may worsen burn risk and severity of burns.

## Airway

- Elderly patients have limited cardiopulmonary reserve and therefore the threshold for intubation should be lower
- Considerations:
  - Dentition
  - Nasopharyngeal fragility
  - Macroglossia
  - Microstomia
  - *Cervical arthritis*: Higher risk for cord injury from undue manipulation.

## Breathing and Ventilation

- Supplemental oxygen placement; be careful with chronic $CO_2$ retainers
- Lifelong exposure to environmental toxins and possibly tobacco smoke
- Chest injuries have higher mortality rate
- Rib fractures and pulmonary contusions are common but poorly tolerated.

## Circulation

- Progressive loss of cardiac function with aging
- Predisposition to re-entry dysrhythmias, diastolic dysfunction from myocardial stiffness
- Reduced creatinine clearance makes elderly patients more susceptible to kidney injury from hypovolemia, medications, and other nephrotoxins.

### Evaluation and Management

- Do not assume "normal" vital signs are "normal." A patient may have relative hypotension compared to their baseline but have a "normal" blood pressure
- Onset of abnormal vital signs such as hypotension may be delayed
- Patients with hypotension and metabolic acidosis have very high mortality rate, especially in the setting of brain injury
- Optimal hemoglobin level is controversial, generally higher than 10 g/dL is accepted for patients who are >65 years old

- Important to identify any possible sites of bleeding early using focused abdominal sonography for trauma (FAST) or diagnostic peritoneal lavage (DPL) due to limited cardiopulmonary reserve
- Be careful not to miss bleeding in the retroperitoneum.

## Disability

- Brain and spinal cord injuries
- Decreased brain weight with replacement by cerebrospinal fluid (CSF) and more tightly adhered dura; decreased risk of contusion, but increased risk of parasagittal bridging vein rupture due to stretching. Also allows more blood to be collected before symptoms are apparent
- Loss of water and protein making the intervertebral disks more compressible. Higher risk of spine and spinal cord injury
- Osteoarthritis causes canal stenosis, segmental instability, and kyphotic deformity may complicate management; increased risk of central cord compression. It may need magnetic resonance imaging (MRI) evaluation; makes fracture diagnosis more difficult
- Much higher risk of subdural hematomas.

## Exposure and Environment

- Consider that elderly individuals have decreased ability to regulate their thermal temperature
- Decrease dermal barrier against bacteria
- Impaired wound healing.

## Musculoskeletal

- Increased risk of fracture to long bones
- Most common areas of fracture are proximal femur, hip, humerus, and wrist.

## SPECIAL CONSIDERATIONS[1]

- Drug interactions
- Beta-blockade may cause peripheral vasoconstriction and hypotension
- Nonsteroidal anti-inflammatory drugs (NSAIDs) or anticoagulants may contribute to blood loss
- Steroids may reduce immune response
- Diuretics may lead to dehydration.

## REFERENCE

1. Alexander BH, Rivara FP, Wolf ME. The cost and frequency of hospitalization for fall-related injuries in older adults. Am J Public Health. 1992;82:1020-3.

## FURTHER READING

1. DeGoede KM, Ashton-Miller JA, Schutlz AB. Fall-related upper body injuries in the older adult: a review of the biochemical issues. J Biomech. 2003;36:1043-53.
2. Oreskovich MR, Howard JD, Copass MK, et al. Geriatric trauma: Injury patterns and outcome. J Trauma. 1984;24:565-72.

## CASE STUDY 89: PELVIC FRACTURE

## CASE HISTORY

A 31-year-old male is presented to the trauma bay after a motor vehicle accident (MVA). The patient was a restrained driver when his vehicle was T-boned on the driver's side by another car. When patient arrives by emergency medical services (EMS), he is alert and oriented to person, place, and time with cervical-spine collar in place. Vitals are temperature 37.5°C, blood pressure (BP) 100/70 mm Hg, pulse rate 110 bpm, respiratory rate 25 breaths/min, and $O_2$ saturation level of 98% on room air. Primary survey reveals intact airway, breathing, and circulation. On secondary survey, patient has tenderness on his right hip, with evidence of bony instability when anterior pressure is applied. A right lateral compression fracture is suspected. Hip binder is placed, a bolus of normal saline is started and patient is sent for further imaging. What imaging should be ordered? What should be considered in the management of pelvic fractures?

## APPROACH TO PELVIC FRACTURES

When evaluating pelvic fractures, an understanding of the mechanism of injury is very important. The damage done during a small fall versus an MVA at 90 mph will be very different. Symptoms of pelvic injuries are often nonspecific, and any pain from the midthigh to the midabdomen should raise concern. Due to the risk of massive blood loss with pelvic injuries, it is very important that the pelvis is never rocked during the physical examination. Every time the pelvis is rocked, the patient may lose up to 2 units of blood. When examining the pelvis, grab the iliac crests and push in. Any movement suggests bony instability. If the patient is awake and alert with no pain or tenderness on examination, a pelvic X-ray is not necessary. The gold standard for viewing a pelvic fracture is a 3D reconstructed computed tomography (CT) scan which gives an excellent understanding and can also diagnose the presence of retroperitoneal hemorrhage.

## CLASSIFICATIONS OF PELVIC FRACTURES

### Lateral Compression Pelvic Fractures

These are caused by lateral impact from a T-bone MVA. The impact causes pelvis to shorten and implode, and the force is applied through back of sacrum so the ligaments stay intact. These generally do not bleed, therefore if a patient has hypotension with a lateral compression pelvic fracture, you should search elsewhere for an intra-abdominal bleed or blunt aortic injury (Figs. 1A to C).

## Anterior Pressure Compression Fracture

These are caused by a head-on MVA or head-on blunt force such as during horseback riding causing the pelvis to explode. There is pure ligamentous rupture resulting in lots of bleeding requiring an average transfusion of 5–6 units in 24 h (Figs. 2A, C and 3).

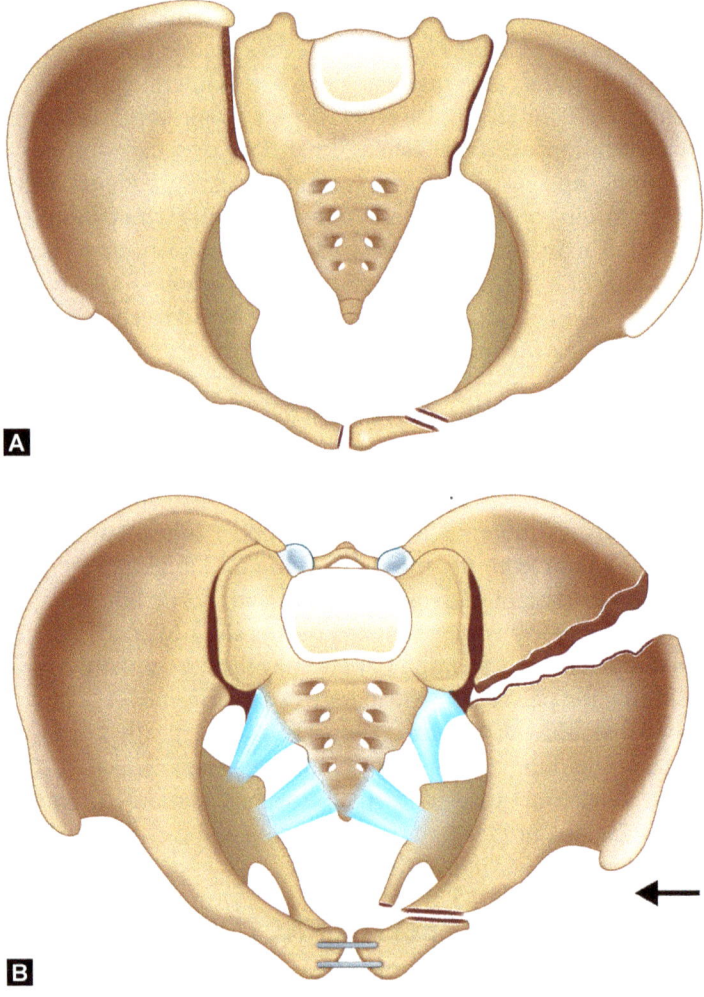

**Figs. 1A and B:** (A) Sacral compression Fx on side of impact; (B) Iliac wing fracture on side of impact.

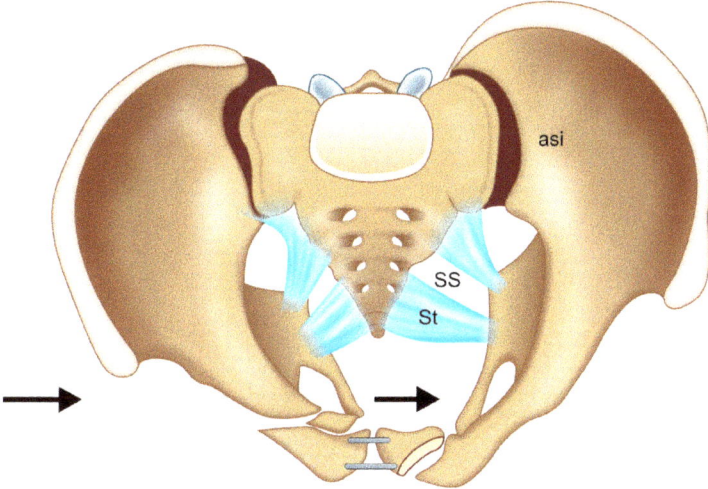

**Fig. 1C:** Lateral compression (LC) type 1 or 1 fracture and contralateral anteroposterior compression fracture.

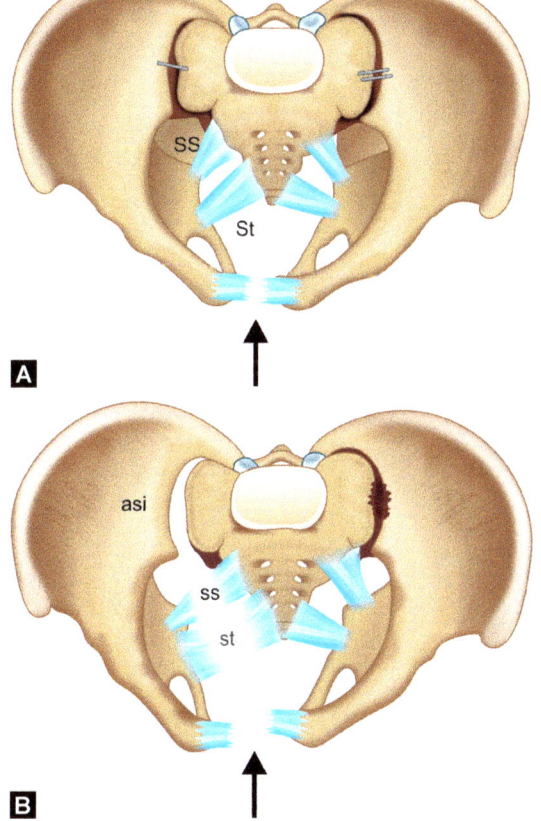

**Figs. 2A and B:** (A) Pubic rami or ligament disruption; slight widening of symphysis; (B) Iliac wings rotated externally "hinging" at SI joint posterior aspect; open book.

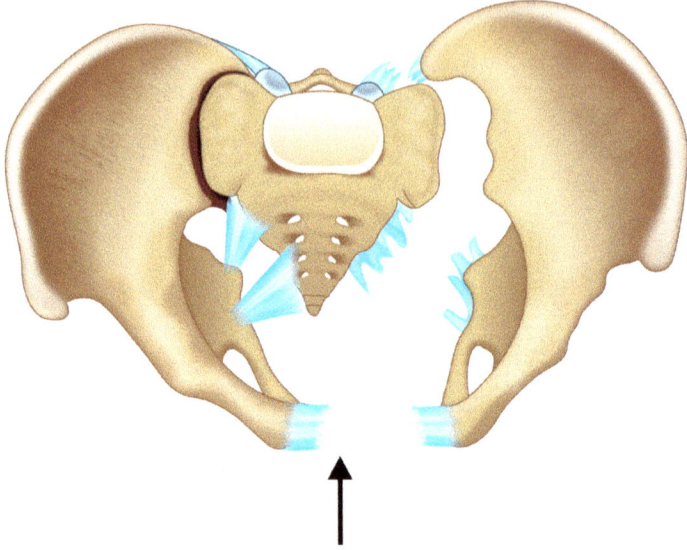

**Fig. 2C:** Complete disruption of sacroiliac ligaments; unstable.

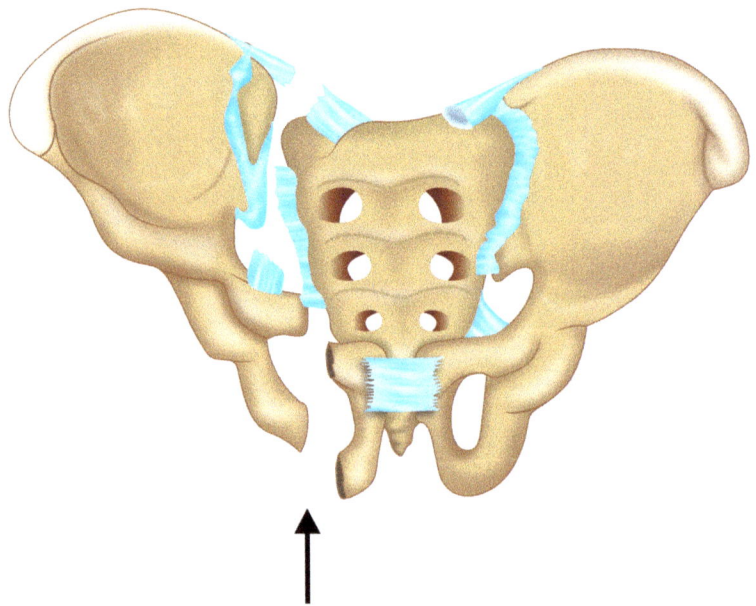

**Fig. 3:** Full from heights; *anterior*: both pubic ramus fracture; *posterior*: Sacroiliac (SI) complex or sacral Fracture.

## Vertical Shear

These result from a fall from a height or head-on motorcycle accident with legs outstretched and are often visually impressive. The diagnosis can be made on physical examination, if one iliac crest is higher than the other. These fractures usually have minimal bleeding.

## TREATMENT OF PELVIC FRACTURES

Any patient with a significant pelvic fracture should be intubated because they may decompensate quickly. You should also have blood ready for transfusion as significant bleeding is often present. A brief lower extremity neurologic assessment should be performed in order to obtain a baseline and assessment of the injury. Other sites of bleeding, such as the abdomen and thorax, should also be excluded. The best method of resuscitation of a patient with a pelvic fracture is giving blood, platelets, and fresh frozen plasma early, and later lactated Ringer's solution and normal saline. Factor VII can also be used to help normalize the international normalized ratio and stop the bleeding. The dose should be 100 µg/kg of body weight for severe bleeding.

Open pelvic fractures can cause exsanguinating hemorrhage. To stop the bleeding, pack the hole and push hard. It is okay to make the opening bigger to get the packing in. Vicryl mesh and fibrin glue can also be used followed by the towels and gauze. Angiography is required early for open fractures but laparotomy is not required early on. Immediately call for operating room and orthopedics simultaneously (or transfer if needed). Do not explore the wound in emergency department.

Bleeding can not necessarily be predicted based on fracture pattern because lots of low-grade injuries and lateral compression fractures do bleed. The low-grade injuries do suggest that you should look elsewhere, but you must be aware that the fracture is also a possible source of the bleeding. It is especially important to be aware that, in older adults, lateral compression fractures often bleed and are highly lethal. At some point, everyone with a pelvic fracture needs an abdominal CT even with a negative FAST scan.

### Controlling Pelvic Hemorrhage

The goal for controlling pelvic hemorrhage is stabilizing the clot via external compression and reduction of the pelvic fragments. This can be done through any of the following methods:

*Bedsheet*: Place a bedsheet on a gurney, place the patient on the sheet, and crisscross and tie the sheet over the patient (Fig. 4).

*Medical antishock trousers*: The method uses a pelvic splint which provides pressure. If the abdominal part is used, you must also use lower extremity part as well. This raises the BP by increasing systemic vascular resistance. The major complication is that it also increases abdominal pressure which may precipitate abdominal compartment syndrome. However, it is still very effective at treating bleeding.

*External fixation*: This can be rapidly applied and may be definitive. It can also disrupt the view on CT and may increase displacement of certain elements.

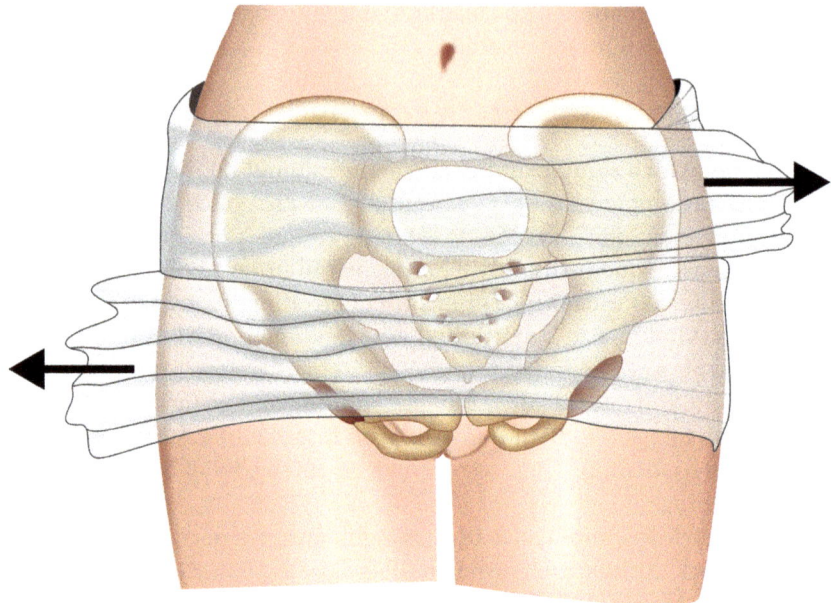

**Fig. 4:** Bedsheet/binder used to control bleeding.

*Binder*: These are placed on the trochanters. It is a Velcro apparatus that makes everything simpler and is very effective to the point that it will fix the displacement.

*Angiography*: This is an excellent test to achieve hemostasis and is both diagnostic and therapeutic; however, it does take time to set up. The use of angiography varies by institution so it helps to have an algorithm in place for indications at your institution.

## COMMON ACCOMPANYING INJURIES

Pelvic fractures frequently occur along with other injuries due to the severity of the mechanisms of injury that cause pelvic fractures. Urethral injuries are common comorbidities. These require a retrograde urethrogram for evaluation before a Foley catheter can be safely inserted. If the urethrogram shows a urethral injury that contraindicated the use of a Foley catheter, a suprapubic tube should be used. Bladder ruptures can also be seen with pelvic fractures and usually indicated by gross hematuria. A CT cystogram is diagnostic.

## OUTCOME

The morbidity of pelvic fractures is often high, but mortality is low due to the institution of good multidisciplinary approaches. However, these results are time dependent. All aspects must be managed simultaneously, not by a step-by-step approach.

## FURTHER READING

1. Cullinane DC, Schiller HJ, Zielinski MD, et al. Eastern association for the surgery of trauma practice management guidelines for hemorrhage in pelvic fracture–update and systematic review. J Trauma. 2011;71(6):1850-1868.
2. Young JW, Resnik CS. Fracture of the pelvis: current concepts of classification. AJR 1990;155:1169-1175.

## CASE STUDY 90: COMPARTMENT SYNDROME

## CASE HISTORY

A 32-year-old man's right leg is trapped beneath his overturned car for nearly 2 h before he is extricated. On arrival in the emergency room, his right lower leg is cool, mottled, insensate, and motionless. Despite normal vital signs, pulses cannot be palpated below the femoral vessel and the muscles of the lower extremity are firm and hard. During the initial assessment of this patient, which of the following is most likely to improve the chances for limb salvage?

## DISCUSSION

Compartment syndrome causes generalized painful swelling and increases pressure which deprives the muscle and nerves of oxygen and nutrients. This may lead to neurologic deficit, muscle necrosis, ischemic contracture, infection, delayed healing, and possible amputation. Common sites for compartment syndrome include lower leg, forearm, foot, gluteal region, and thigh. Injuries such as tibial and forearm fracture, crush injury to muscle, burns, excessive exercise, prolonged external pressure to an extremity, and use of extremity immobilization devices, such as dressing or casts, may increase the risk for compartment syndrome. Early diagnosis is essential as a treatment.

## SIGNS AND SYMPTOMS

These include increased or severe pain, asymmetry, palpable tenderness, altered sensation, weak or nonpalpable pulses and pain on passive stretch. Pressure measurement >30–45 mm Hg indicates decreased blood flow, which may result in muscle damage.

## MANAGEMENT

Fasciotomy is a surgical procedure where the fascia is cut to relieve tension or pressure. Compartment syndrome is one of the conditions where the

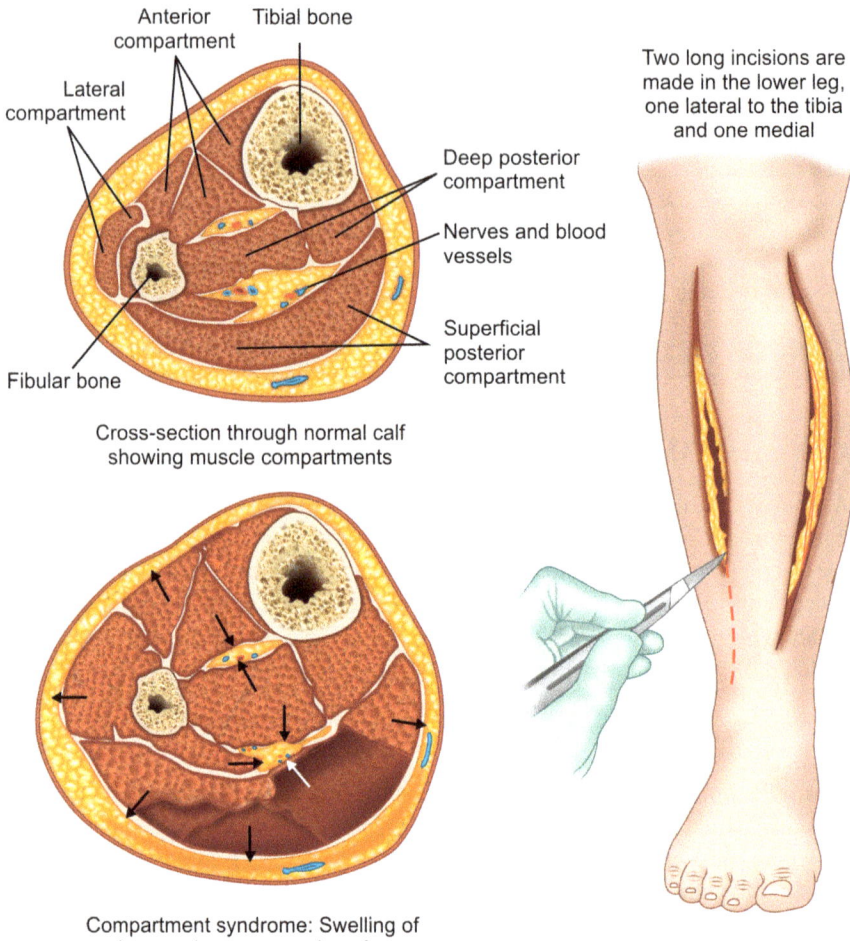

**Fig. 1:** Compartment syndrome with fasciotomy procedure.
*Source:* Nucleus Medical Media. Compartment syndrome with fasciotomy procedure—medical illustration, human anatomy drawing. [Online]. Available from catalog.nucleusinc.com/generateexhibit.php?ID=173. [Accessed September, 2012].

fasciotomy is indicated. Patient is monitored for 30 min, and if no change is observed in that time period, then fasciotomy is urgent (Fig. 1). Delay in the treatment may result in myoglobinuria and as a result decrease in renal function occurs.

CHAPTER 16

# Infectious Diseases

## CASE STUDY 91: MENINGOCOCCEMIA

### CASE HISTORY

A 19-year-old college student who lives in a dormitory is presented to the emergency department (ED) with the chief complaint of fever, chills, rigor, throat pain, joint pain, and muscle aches. He denies foreign travel. He presents with maculopapular rash, petechiae and purpuric spots. Upon examination, the patient has a temperature of 104°F (40°C). A blood culture, complete blood count (CBC), and skin biopsy are ordered by the ED doctor with the assumption that the rash may be meningococcemia.

### DIFFERENTIAL DIAGNOSIS

Any ill appearing or toxic looking patient with a petechial rash and associated symptoms ranging from pharyngitis to meningitis to bacteremia will make you think this is a potentially fatal infectious disease. The differential diagnosis includes:
- Rocky mountain spotted fever
- Gonococcemia
- Bacterial endocarditis
- Toxic shock syndrome (TSS)
- Vasculitis
- Disseminated intravascular coagulation (DIC).

### DISCUSSION

Meningococcemia is caused by *Neisseria meningitidis* in the blood leading to a wide range of symptoms (Figs. 1 to 4). This is the leading cause of bacterial meningitis in children and young adults in the United States, and the second most common cause of community-acquired adult bacterial meningitis. Patients present with fever, headache, decreased sensorium, neck rigidity,

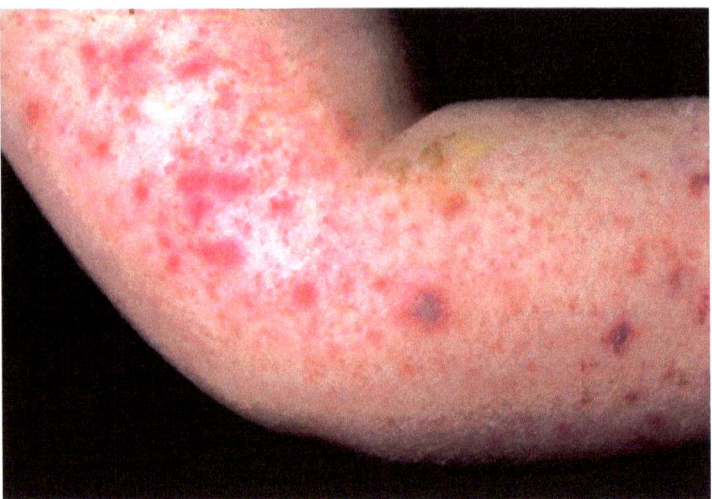

**Fig. 1:** Meningococcemia.
*Courtesy:* Logical Images, Inc. 2009, Rochester, New York, USA.

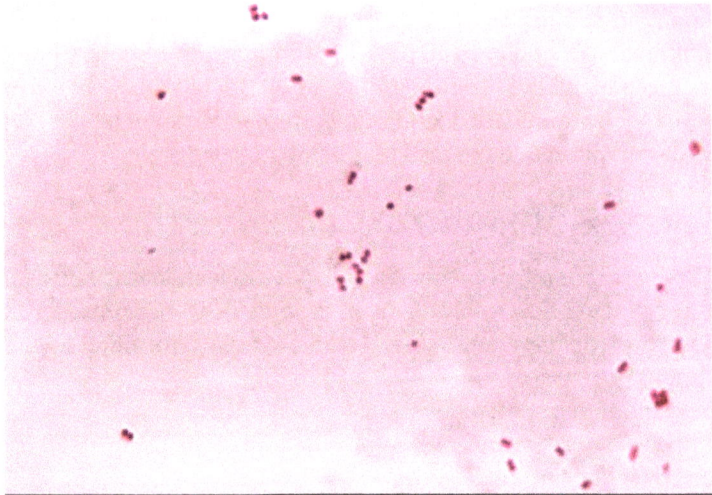

**Fig. 2:** Gram-negative *Neisseria meningitidis* diplococcal bacteria, 1,150×.
*Source:* Available online at http://www.cdc.gov/meningococcal/index.html.

rash, and hypotension. If meningococcemia is suspected, treatment should be started promptly.[1] Early treatment usually results in good outcomes. If the patient is in shock, has DIC or kidney failure, the prognosis is not as positive. *Neisseria meningitidis* can also cause a hemorrhage into the adrenal gland, leading to adrenal gland failure, known as Waterhouse–Friderichsen syndrome (WFS). WFS is considered the most severe form of meningococcal sepsis and can contribute to hypotension.

# Infectious Diseases

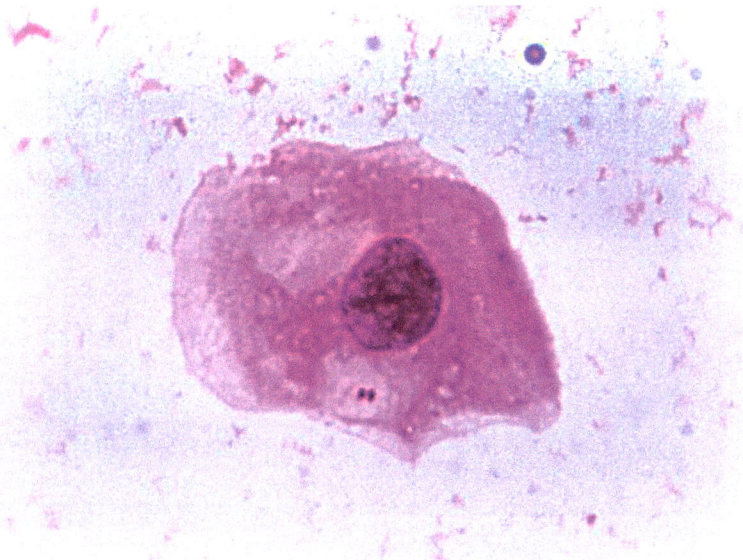

**Fig. 3:** *Neisseria meningitidis*; photomicrograph, 1,125×.
*Source:* Available online at http://www.cdc.gov/meningococcal/index.html.

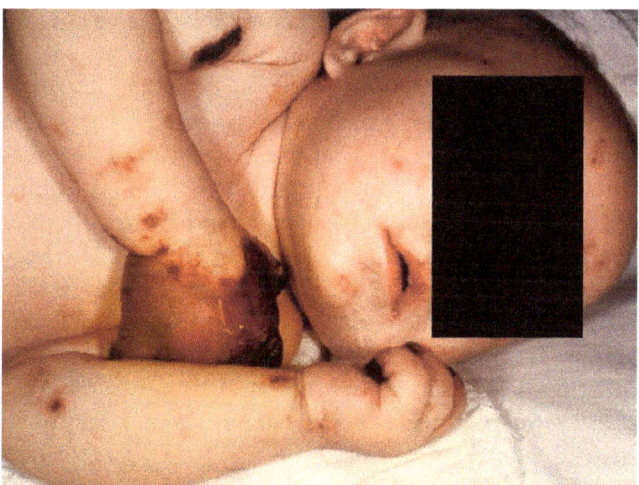

**Fig. 4:** A 4-month-old girl with gangrene of hands secondary to meningococcemia-induced arterial occlusions.
*Source:* Available online at http://www.cdc.gov/meningococcal/index.html.

Meningococcal disease[2] is important to recognize and treat quickly as severe complications can rapidly arise, as in the high-profile 2004 case of "miracle baby born in Charlotte" (Fig. 5). Within 30 min of the first appearance of a petechial rash, her entire body was swollen, purple, and her limbs

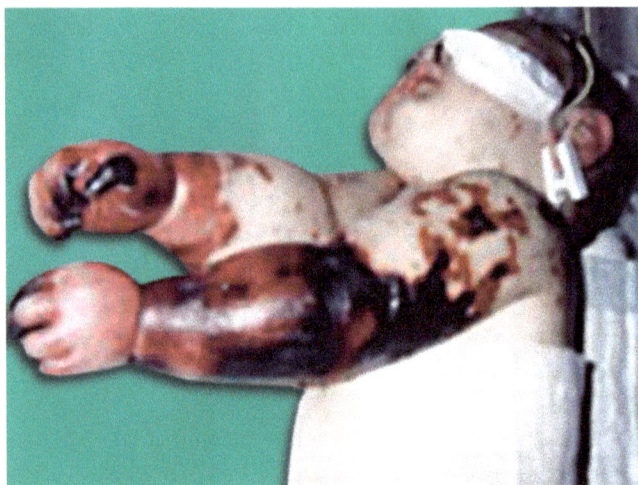

**Fig. 5:** "Miracle baby" Charlotte Cleverley–Bisman, with peripheral complications of meningococcal disease.
*Source:* wikimedia.org.

were blackening. She required resuscitation twice in the first day and ultimately all four limbs were amputated as a result of gangrene. Her parents decided to use her publicity to raise awareness about the speed of this disease and to encourage research of the development of vaccines.

When dealing with patients with meningococcemia, 24 h of airborne isolation is often ordered until the patient is stable and some antibiotics have been able to work in their system. Dexamethasone and antibiotics are often given intravenously. The addition of dexamethasone as an adjunct in bacterial meningitis cases has shown effectiveness in reducing the mortality rate and hearing loss for patients in developing countries.[1] The same benefits have been seen less in populations heavily affected by human immunodeficiency virus (HIV). The patient may also receive fluids, treatment for hypotension, or other symptoms associated with the disease.

ED Treatment and Disposition:
- Give ceftriaxone 2 g IV and vancomycin 1 g IV empirically pending blood cultures/CSF cultures and skin culture
- Patient needs to be hospitalized under infectious disease consult for anticipated complications like WFS.

## PROPHYLAXIS, PREVENTION AND TREATMENT OF CONTACTS

The most effective way to prevent this dreadful, fatal disease is to complete the recommended vaccine schedule. Twenty-four hours isolation followed by treating the contacts with prophylactic antibiotics.

If one member of a household has the disease, prophylactic antibiotics are often given to the rest of the family for prevention purposes, typically either rifampin twice daily for 2 days or a single 500 mg dose of ciprofloxacin. Also, a vaccine exists that protects against some variations of *Meningococcus* (not all). This vaccine is recommended for children and anyone moving into a dormitory. The vaccine is often given 3 weeks before the student leaves for college. Additionally, current CDC recommendations include administering the vaccine prior to travel to endemic areas, such as sub-Saharan Africa, and especially Saudi Arabia during the Hajj and Umrah pilgrimage.

## REFERENCES

1. Cooper DD, Seupaul RA. Is adjunctive dexamethasone beneficial in patients with bacterial meningitis?. Ann Emerg Med. 2012;59(3):225-6.
2. Centers for Disease Control and Prevention. Meningococcal disease. [Online]. Available at http://www.cdc.gov/meningococcal/index.html; 2013.

CHAPTER 17

# Renal Emergencies

## CASE STUDY 92: NEPHROLITHIASIS/RENAL COLIC

### CASE HISTORY

A 45-year-old male presents with flank abdominal pain for 1 day. Pain started suddenly in his right side and then began to radiate to his right groin. Pain is sharp, 9/10, and waxes and wanes. No nausea, vomiting, or diarrhea is noticed. Patient denies having a pain like this in the past or ever having kidney stones. He does report that he thinks his father did have a stone at one time. Patient denies any abdominal surgeries including appendectomy. He has no known medical problems. On physical examination, vitals are significant for mildly elevated pulse and blood pressure. On further examination, patient is nontender with normal external genital examination. Computed tomography (CT) of abdomen/pelvis is ordered and is found to have evidence of a stone in the right ureter. No evidence of hydronephrosis or other obstructing signs are found. Patient is discharged with pain medication with instructions to increase fluid intake and follow-up with primary care physician (PCP).

### DISCUSSION

Patient is a male presenting with right-sided abdominal pain. Differential diagnosis includes appendicitis, testicular torsion, hernia, and nephrolithiasis. Physical examination did not reveal any signs of torsion or hernia and therefore CT was done to further rule out appendicitis and nephrolithiasis. Patient had evidence of a small stone that would most likely pass on its own, and therefore no further intervention was needed.

### Ureterolithiasis Discussion

*Tamsulosin for Ureteral Stones in the Emergency Department: A Randomized, Controlled Trial*
- Renal colic, stones that are lodged in distal ureter.

- The main factors affecting the retention of ureteral calculi are:
  - Ureteral muscle spasm
  - Submucosal edema
  - Pain and infection
- $\alpha 1$ receptors are predominant in the ureteral smooth muscle.
- Blockade of these $\alpha$-adrenergic receptors would decrease ureteral peristaltic amplitude and frequency.
- Decreasing intraureteral pressure and allowing increased fluid transport to occur.

*Tamsulosin:*
- Selective $\alpha 1A$ and $\alpha 1D$ adrenoreceptor blocker
- Initial treatment of patients with lower urinary tract symptoms, such as benign prostatic hyperplasia (BPH)
- Use of tamsulosin or other selective adrenoreceptor blockers and standardized pain control regimen in patients with distal ureterolithiasis.

*Interventions* (Fig. 1):
- The treatment group received tamsulosin hydrochloride 0.4 mg by mouth daily for 10 days + standard analgesic therapy
- All subjects also received standard discharge instructions for renal colic and were given a urine strainer and instructions on straining their urine and collecting debris.
- All patients were instructed to follow-up with the hospital's on-call urologist in 10–14 days.

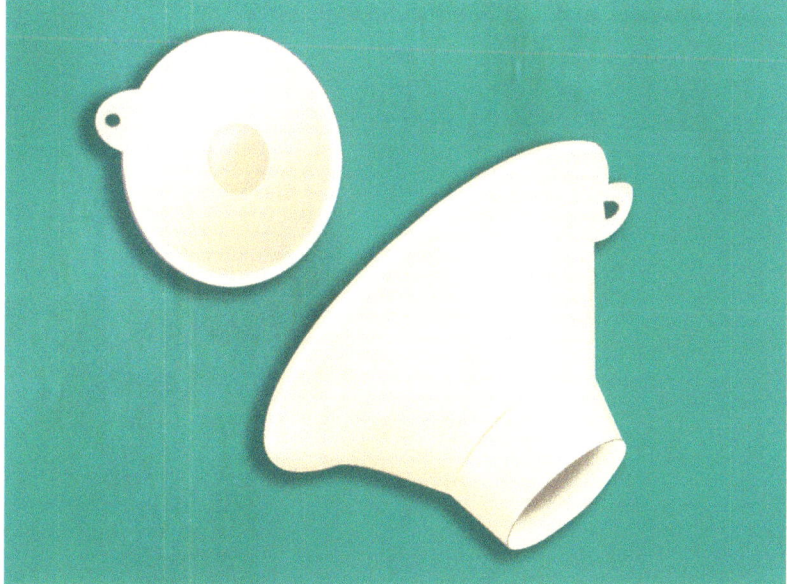

**Fig. 1:** Sieve used to check urine for passed stones.

*Primary outcome:*
- Successful spontaneous ureteral stone expulsion at 14 days (Fig. 2).

*Secondary outcomes:* Below mentioned are the secondary outcomes.
- Time to stone passage
- Self-reported pain scores
- Number of colicky pain episodes
- Number of unscheduled return to ED/primary care visits
- Number of days of missed work/usual function
- Amount of analgesic used
- Adverse events
- All outcomes were evaluated at the 2-, 5-, and 14-day telephone follow-up sessions for patient information (Flowchart 1).

See related article on preventing kidney stones.

## Stay Hydrated

Staying hydrated is not as simple as just drinking water. Other things to consider include:
- Do not overdo it. Avoid drinking more than eight 8-oz glasses of water a day. More water than this can change the balance of particles in your body called electrolytes. This can be harmful and sometimes happens in endurance athletes, such as marathon runners, who drink too much water when losing a lot of sweat. In such circumstances, a mixture of water, electrolytes, and a small amount of sugar can be used. Examples are chicken broth, coconut water, Pedialyte, or use of oral rehydration salts. Artificial sweeteners should be avoided because they have the opposite effect, making it more difficult to rehydrate.

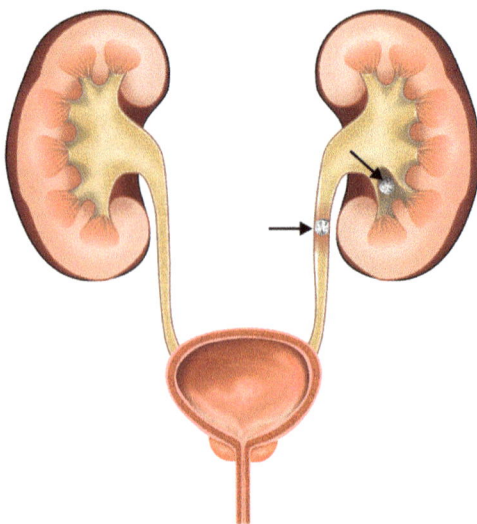

**Fig. 2:** Successful spontaneous ureteral stone expulsion.

**Flowchart 1:** Follow-up case study with tamsulosin.

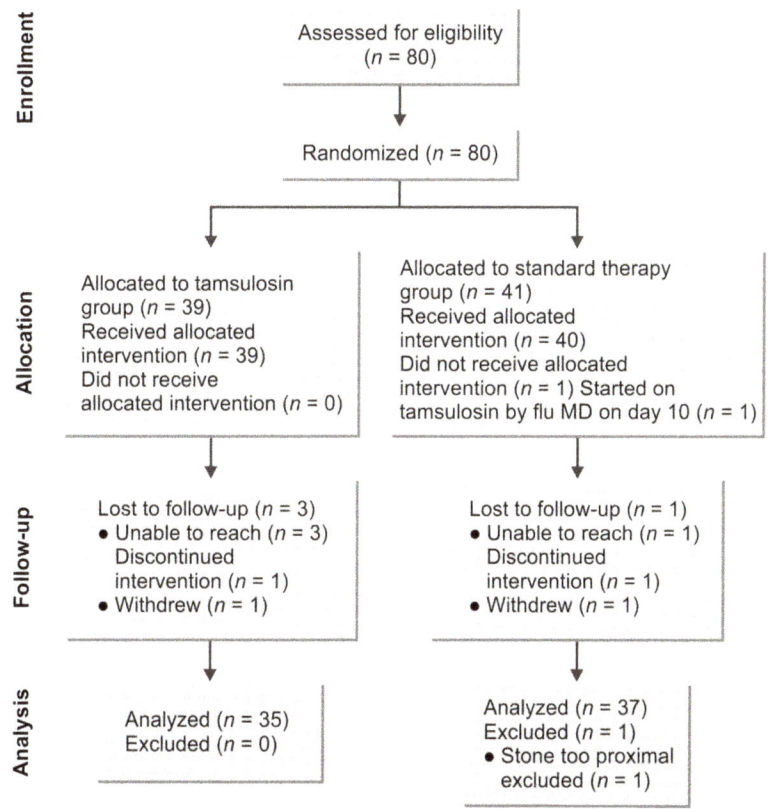

*Source:* Preventing kidney stones with diet and nutrition. Am Fam Physician. 2011;84(11): 1243-4.

- Avoid sugary drinks, such as fruit drinks and sports drinks, because they add calories and change the acid–base balance of the urine.
- For most kidney stones (Flowchart 2 and Fig. 3), urine should be less acidic. One way to make the urine less acidic is to add citrate to drinking water. Lemon and lime juices are great sources of citrate.
- You can also breathe in moisture to stay hydrated by using humidifiers and steam.
- Be aware that obesity increases the risk of dehydration. The more extra weight someone carries, the more important hydration becomes.

## TYPES OF STONES, DIAGNOSIS, AND TREATMENT

- The appearance, density, and location of a stone on CT may suggest its composition.
- Calcium-containing stones are radiopaque, including calcium oxalate and calcium phosphate stones, most struvite (triple phosphate) stones, and pure calcium phosphate stones.

**Flowchart 2:** Types of stones.

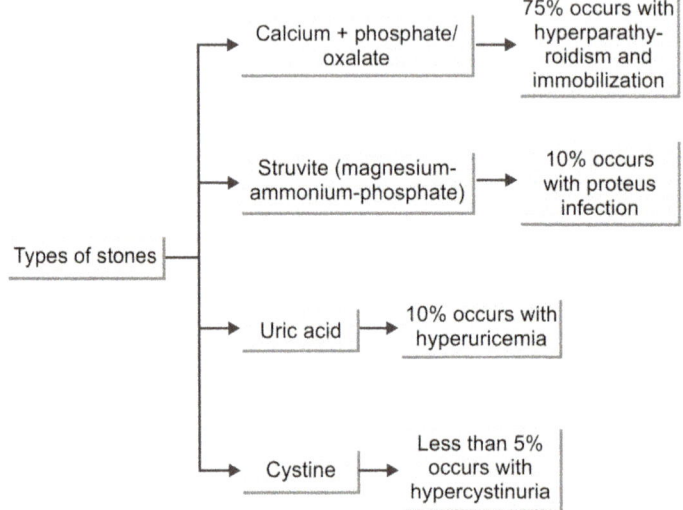

*Courtesy:* Badar M Zaheer, MD, Chicago, USA.

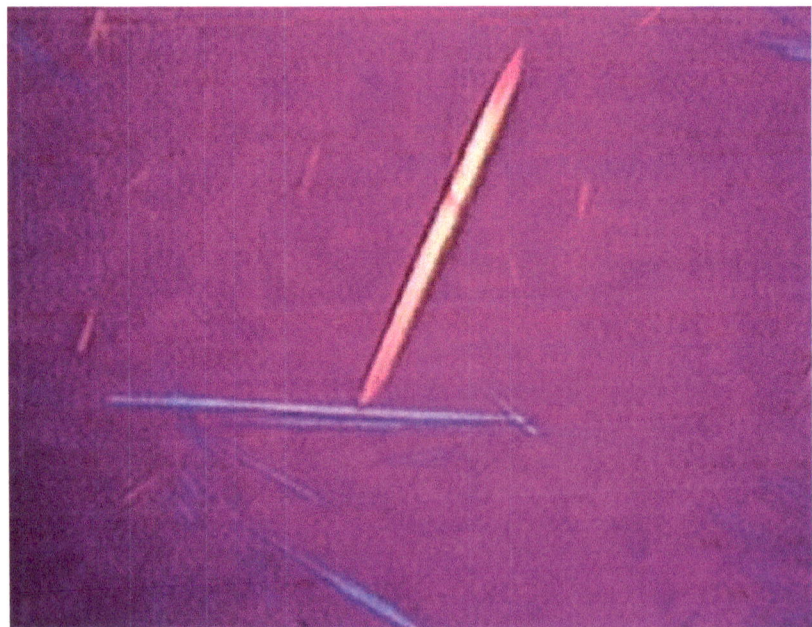

**Fig. 3:** These spiked rods are uric acid crystals photographed under polarized light. Increased uric acid blood levels and formation of uric acid crystals in the joints are associated with gout.
*Source:* ADAM Health Solutions, Ebix, Inc. Uric acid crystals [Online]. Available from www.nlm.nih.gov/medlineplus/ency/imagepages/1222.htm; 2012 [accessed August, 2012].

- Radiolucent stones include uric acid stones, cystine stones, indinavir stones, and pure matrix stones.
- Calcium stones:
  - Small stones can be safely ignored and treated with hydration until the stone is naturally excreted.
  - Larger stones may be treated with extracorporeal shock wave lithotripsy (ESWL) or percutaneous nephrostomy.
- Struvite stones
  - Usually large, staghorn calculi resulting from infection
  - Must be treated surgically and removed completely, including small fragments, which can act as a nidus for future infection and/or stone formation
- Uric acid stones
  - Result from low urinary pH, thus treatment with hydration and urine alkalization is typically sufficient to promote excretion
- Cystine stones
  - Difficult to treat
  - Hydration and alkalization are first-line.

Treatment recommendation based on stone size and location

- Uncomplicated ureteral stones < 10 mm = offer observation, if distal stone of similar size, recommend medical expulsion therapy (MET) with a-blockers (Strong recommendation, evidence Level B).
- Symptomatic, total lower pole stone < 10 mm, recommend shockwave lithotripsy (SWL) or uretoscopy (URS) (Strong recommendation, evidence Level B).
- Symptomatic, total non-lower pole stone burden < 20 mm, recommend SWL or URS (Strong recommendation, evidence Level B).
- Symptomatic, total stone burden >20 mm, recommend percutaneous nephrolithotomy (PCNL) as first-line therapy (Strong recommendation, evidence Level C).

Please use the following citation for the above information:

Assimos, D., & Krambeck, A. (2016). Surgical Management of Stones: AUA/Endourology Society Guideline. Retrieved October 5, 2018, from American Urological Association website: <https://www.auanet.org/guidelines/stone-disease-surgical-(2016)>

## FURTHER READING

1. Curhan GC, Aronson MD, Preminger GM. Diagnosis and acute management of suspected nephrolithiasis in adults. UpToDate.com; 2017.
2. Ferre RM, Wasielewski JN, Strout TD, et al. Tamsulosin for ureteral stones in the emergency department: a randomized, controlled trial. Ann Emerg Med 2009;54(3):432-9, 439.e1-2.
3. Knipe H, Jones J. Urolithiasis. Radiopaedia.org; 2018.
4. Kohlstadt I, Frassetto L. Treatment and prevention of kidney stones: an update. Am Fam Physician 2011;84(11):1243-4.

# CHAPTER 18

# Medical Errors

## CASE STUDY 93: LABORATORY ERROR

*"More people are killed each year by medical errors than by traffic accidents"*
Source: NHTSA.gov

—Badar M Zaheer

## INTRODUCTION

The following case presentation is of a patient who was initially presented with profound electrolyte abnormalities that were later found to be laboratory error.

Patient safety can be greatly influenced by the presence of laboratory errors. There is a large focus on improving patient safety in the healthcare field right now including analyzing various performance measures to determine how to meet higher standards in patient safety.[1]

## CASE HISTORY

A 64-year-old man is presented to the emergency department (ED) at 16:30 hours with 3 days of abdominal pain and 1 day of vomiting. He had also developed significant pallor and diaphoresis.

His past medical history included type 2 diabetes mellitus, hypertension (HTN), and dyslipidemia. He had no history of tobacco, alcohol, or recreational drug use. His medications included glipizide 10 mg twice a day (bid), Lipitor 20 mg daily, cyclobenzaprine three times a day as often as needed (tid prn), metformin 1,000 mg bid, lisinopril 40 mg bid, and Coreg 12.5 mg bid.

On examination, he was found to be hypotensive with blood pressure of 71/42 mm Hg and pulse rate of 84 bpm, respiratory rate 22 breaths/min, temperature 98.3°F, and oxygen saturation 98% on room air. Physical examination showed lethargic patient in moderate to severe distress. Skin examination was positive for pallor and diaphoresis, and abdominal examination was consistent with distension and ascites. Musculoskeletal examination showed an erythematous and ulcerated left great toe with yellow drainage. The remainder of the physical examination was within normal limits.

The patient was given a 1 L bolus of 0.9% normal saline starting at 16:35 hours and ending at 17:45 hours. Complete blood count (CBC) and basic metabolic panel (BMP) were drawn and showed numerous critical values. Although he did not look severely anemic, his hemoglobin level was 4.8 g/dL, had a hematocrit value of 14.2%, and thrombocytopenic with a platelet count of $45 \times 103/\mu L$, as per laboratory report which is unbelievable. The most shocking findings were his comprehensive metabolic panel (CMP) significant for potassium of 1.7 mEq/L chloride of 127 mEq/L, bicarbonate of 7 mEq/L, blood urea nitrogen (BUN) of 36.9 mg/dL, creatinine of 3.0 mg/dL, anion gap of 8, calcium of 3 mg/dL, magnesium of 0.6 mg/dL, and glucose of 150 mg/dL. Blood pressure had improved to 100/54 mm Hg after a normal saline bolus. Electrocardiogram was done at 17:22 hours and showed normal sinus rhythm.

Due to the concern for sepsis, the patient was given intravenous (IV) Rocephin 2 g at 17:30 hours. A second bolus of 0.9% normal saline was started at 17:45 hours along with IV Flagyl 500 mg at 17:50 hours and 20 mEq/L of potassium chloride (KCl) IV at 17:55 hours for potassium replacement. The patient was transferred by medical force to another institution at 18:25 hours.

On arrival to the second institution, laboratory tests were repeated. CBC showed a hemoglobin level of 12.2 g/dL, hematocrit value of 33.5%, and reticulocyte count of 0.6%. CMP showed a chloride of 99 mEq/L, potassium of 4.7 mEq/L, bicarbonate of 20 mEq/L, BUN of 89 mg/dL, creatinine of 2.49 mg/dL, calcium of 7.6 mg/dL, magnesium of 1.6 mg/dL, glucose of 330 mg/dL, and lactic acid of 1.6 mg/dL.

## DISCUSSION

The patient in this case is presented to the ED in shock and was subsequently found to have several severe electrolyte abnormalities. After transfer to an outside institution, his laboratory tests were found to be much closer to normal limits. The patient was only given 20 mEq/L of KCl for replacement and potassium was found to have risen from 1.7 to 4.7 mEq/L. There should not have been a rise of that magnitude from that amount of KCl replacement. Additionally, his magnesium was found to have risen from 0.6 to 1.6 mg/dL, although no replacement doses had been given. It is clear that the first set of results were likely due to laboratory error.

The lesson to be learned from this case is the importance of being aware of the possibility of laboratory error. In this particular patient, all of the measured values were significantly abnormal, making it more likely to be a laboratory error. Additionally, this patient is presented with no symptoms and no electrocardiography (ECG) evidence of hypokalemia or hypomagnesemia,

**Table 1:** Confused drugs and results of error.

| Confused drugs | Results of error |
|---|---|
| Novolin, Novolog, and Novolin 70/30 | Hypoglycemia and poor control of diabetes |
| Clonidine vs Klonopin | Hypotension, loss of seizure control |
| Ambisome, Abelcet, Amphocin (Fungizone) | Respiratory arrest, renal failure |
| Metformin vs metronidazole | Hypoglycemia or untreated infection |
| Vinblastine vs Vincristine | Due to differences in dosages this error has resulted in fatalities |
| Tramadol, trazodone, toradol | Failure of pain control, change in psychiatric state |
| Coumadin, Avandia, Cardura | Coagulation complications |
| Hydromorphone vs morphine | Opioid overdose due to hydromorphone's higher potency |
| Celebrex, Cerebyx, Celexa | Alterations in mental status, failure of pain control, failure of seizure control |

*Courtesy:* Dr. Badar M Zaheer, Chicago, USA.

yet laboratory results showed a profound deficiency.[2] This would be very unlikely.

Being aware of these potential errors can be lifesaving to patients. This patient was given 20 mEq/L of KCl before arriving at the transferred institution. Had this patient been given additional doses of potassium, he could have been at risk for the effects of hyperkalemia including torsades de pointes and cardiac arrest.[3] Additionally, on repeating magnesium measurement, it was found to be near normal. Had this patient been given magnesium replacement initially, he could have been at risk for cardiotoxic effects.[4] Also, imagine if we had given blood transfusion, depending on the laboratory findings. It could have been a serious health risk and caused unnecessary complications from transfusion.

With 1-in-3 hospital patients accidentally harmed every year in the United States (Campaign Zero), it is important to find any ways possible to reduce errors. Using a "cognitive break" during diagnosis can help prevent errors (Table 1). This means to take a break from mental, visual, and auditory stimulation for 1–2 min and then think clearly before making a decision.

## REFERENCES

1. Howanitz PJ. Errors in laboratory medicine: practical lessons to improve patient care. Arch Pathol Lab Med. 2005;129(10):1252-61.
2. Brace RA, Anderson DK, Chen WT, et al. Local effects of hypokalemia on coronary resistance and myocardial contractile force. Am J Physiol. 1974;227(3):590-7.
3. Levinsky NG. Management of emergencies. VI. Hyperkalemia. N Engl J Med. 1966;274(19):1076-7.

4. Cholst IN, Steinberg SF, Tropper PJ, et al. The influence of hypermagnesemia on serum calcium and parathyroid hormone levels in human subjects. N Engl J Med. 1984;310(19):1221-5.

## FURTHER READING

1. Campaign Zero. [Online]. Available from campaignzero.org; 2011 [accessed Sept. 2013].
2. Jaben M. To reduce medical errors, take a cognitive pause. Emergency Physicians Monthly. [Online]. Available from www.epmonthly.com/features/current-features/to-reduce-medical-errors-take-a-cognitive-pause; 2013 [accessed Sept. 2013].

# CHAPTER 19

# Water and Electrolyte Imbalance

## CASE STUDY 94: HYPOKALEMIA

### CASE HISTORY

A 76-year-old female has been experiencing severe diarrhea and vomiting for the past 3 days. She is generally in good health otherwise with only mild hypertension and hyperlipidemia, which are well controlled with hydrochlorothiazide (HCTZ) and atorvastatin, respectively. After 2 days of vomiting and diarrhea, she began feeling fatigued with muscle weakness and soreness. On the third day, she became weaker and felt multiple palpitations (among other symptoms), as depicted in Figure 1. She called emergency services and was transported to the emergency department promptly. Upon arrival, she appeared hypovolemic and dehydrated with pale conjunctiva and prominent skin turgor abnormality. She was started on intravenous (IV) normal saline, an electrocardiogram (ECG) was performed, and routine laboratory tests were drawn. The ECG showed flat T-wave with an additional small wave following it and occasional premature ventricular contractions (PVCs). Her laboratory reports returned with a serum potassium level of 2.4 mEq/L. IV normal saline was continued, and IV $K^+$ was given for 2 h. Over the next 2 days, she was given oral $K^+$ supplementation and IV fluid hydration. Her diarrhea and vomiting subsided, along with all of her prior symptoms. On the third day of hospitalization, she was discharged and her HCTZ was restarted.

### CASE DISCUSSION

This patient developed hypokalemia due to several mechanisms: (1) diarrhea and vomiting, and (2) HCTZ diuretic use. The combination of the two makes it more likely to result in significant hypokalemia. Potassium is very important to the impulses necessary for proper muscle contraction. Therefore, abnormalities in potassium levels may lead to various muscle-related problems, including weakness, soreness, and palpitations. She presented with the classic ECG finding of flattened T-wave as well as a U-wave (Fig. 2). Since she

Water and Electrolyte Imbalance

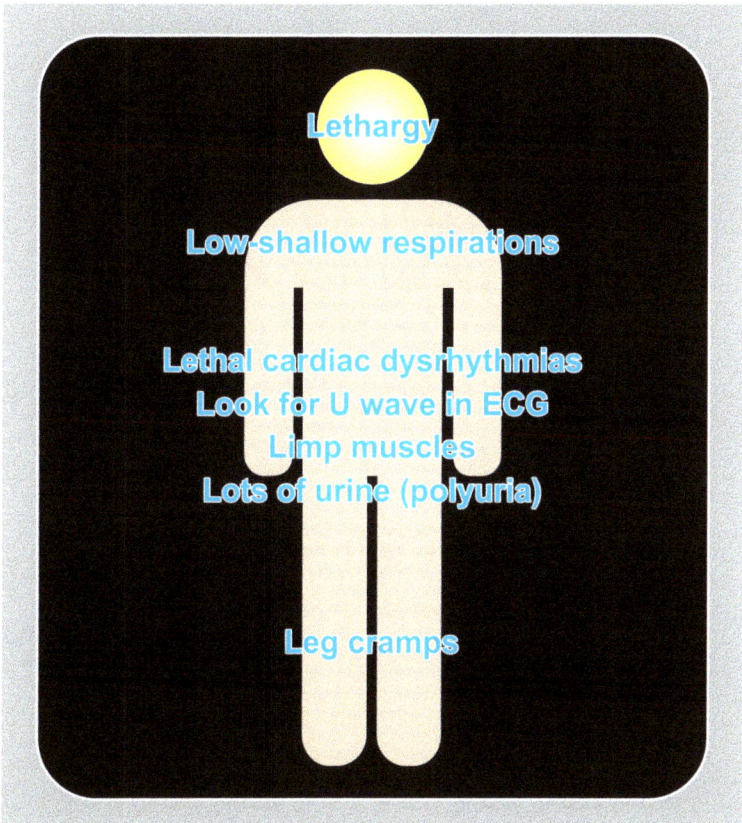

**Fig. 1:** 7 Ls to remember: symptoms of hypokalemia.
*Courtesy:* Dr. Badar M Zaheer, Chicago, USA.

was presenting with severely low potassium and cardiac arrhythmias (i.e., PVCs), potassium repletion was initially performed via IV infusion and then was switched to oral. If the vomiting and diarrhea remained intractable, IV supplementation could have been continued until the vomiting and diarrhea subsides.

## HYPOKALEMIA DISCUSSION

### General

Serum potassium levels are normally in the range of 3.5–5.0 mEq/L, and therefore hypokalemia is defined as a concentration of <3.5 mEq/L (*Source*: 5MinuteConsult). Although hypokalemia can occur in any individual, the frequency increases with age, likely due to a higher use of diuretics and a poor diet (*Source*: Medscape). Furthermore, there are suggestions that hypokalemia is more prevalent in African-Americans and women. High risk groups

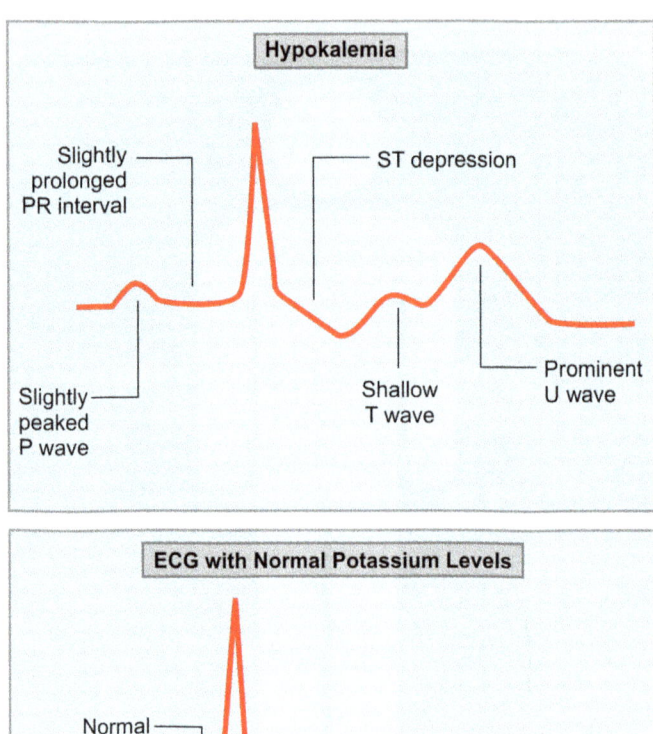

**Fig. 2:** ECG changes.
*Courtesy:* Dr. Badar M Zaheer, Chicago, USA

include person with eating disorder, alcoholism, acquired immunodeficiency syndrome (AIDS), and those who have had bariatric surgery.

## Pathophysiology and Causes

There are three mechanisms that can result in hypokalemia (*Source*: Medscape and 5MinuteConsult): (1) deficient intake, (2) increased excretion, and (3) shift from extracellular to intracellular space. Isolated dietary deficiency is relatively uncommon but can occur in anorexia nervosa, alcoholism, elderly people with very poor dietary intake, and those with prolonged total parenteral nutrition (TPN) with inadequate potassium supplementation. Increased excretion is the most common cause of hypokalemia overall. This can occur from increased sodium delivery to the renal collecting ducts, such as with diuretics (i.e., more sodium to exchange for potassium), mineralocorticoid excess (i.e., primary or secondary hyperaldosteronism), diarrhea, vomiting, nasogastric suction, laxative abuse, bulimia, and metabolic alkalosis (i.e., fewer hydrogen ions to exchange for potassium). The final mechanism is a potassium shift from the extracellular to intracellular space, which often accompanies the increased excretion mechanism. Since the total body potassium is not changed with these potassium shifts, episodes are often transient and self-limited. These intracellular shifts can occur due to alkalosis, insulin excess (endogenous or exogenous), and β-adrenergic stimulation (acute stress or pharmacologically induced).

## Assessment

Hypokalemic patients often have no symptoms and are found incidentally with routine laboratory tests. This is generally true with mild hypokalemia in the range of 3.0–3.5 mEq/L (*Source*: 5MinuteConsult). When symptoms are present, they generally affect the variety of muscles in the body (*Source*: Medscape and 5MinuteConsult). Neuromuscular problems involve skeletal muscles and result in variable weakness ranging from mild to severe with rhabdomyolysis and/or respiratory arrest. Smooth muscle effects can cause hypomotility, constipation, and ileus. Lastly, and most life-threatening, cardiac muscle effects can cause hypotension, arrhythmias, and cardiac arrest. These symptoms are nonspecific and do not aid in determining the cause. For the most part, the physical examination is unrevealing as well. Muscle weakness or flaccid paralysis may be present, as well as depressed or absent reflexes. Vital signs are generally normal with occasional tachycardia or tachypnea due to muscle weakness and/or volume depletion. Although relatively nonspecific, hypertension may point toward primary hyperaldosteronism or renal artery stenosis and relative hypotension may suggest laxative use, diuretic use, excessive diarrhea and/or vomiting, or bulimia. With the symptoms and physical examination findings of moderate value in determining the cause of hypokalemia, it is important to obtain a solid patient history and to employ a diagnostic algorithm including various laboratory tests.[1] Urine tests, including potassium, sodium, and osmolarity, are very important in attempting to determine the mechanism for the hypokalemia. These can all be done quickly with a spot test and the values should be analyzed together. First, a low urine potassium (<20 mEq/L) in the setting of hypokalemia would suggest an inadequate intake, shift to intracellular space, or gastrointestinal loss, and therefore the patient should be asked about vomiting, laxatives, diet, TPN, insulin use, and bicarbonate supplements/medications. Conversely, a high urine potassium (>40 mEq/L) suggests renal loss, in which one should evaluate the patient's medications, acid–base balance, magnesium level, and blood pressure. These can help to distinguish between diuretic use, vomiting with alkalosis, mineralocorticoid excess, renal tubular acidosis, and renal artery stenosis. If urine sodium is low (<20 mEq/L) in the presence of high-urine potassium, then secondary hyperaldosteronism would be suggested. Additionally, the urine osmolarity should be considered since a highly concentrated urine (>700 mom/L) will lead to a misleading absolute value of potassium and sodium. In other words, the value of the electrolyte in the urine will appear higher simply due to the fact that there is less urine volume to dilute it. Although more difficult, if one wants a more accurate measurement of urine electrolytes, a 24-h electrolyte value can be obtained. Serum electrolyte values should be obtained as well. Low sodium, for example, may suggest the use of a thiazide diuretic as the inciting cause. A low bicarbonate level may suggest renal tubular acidosis, diarrhea, or the use of carbonic anhydrase inhibitors, while high bicarbonate level could be due to hyperaldosteronism (primary or secondary), including that due to vomiting or diuretic use. Magnesium is an important electrolyte for potassium regulation. A low magnesium can cause hypokalemia that is refractive to treatment unless the magnesium abnormality is corrected first. Most commonly hypokalemia is due to diuretics or gastrointestinal losses, but this must be confirmed. Further testing for specific causes may include serum renin, aldosterone, and cortisol, urine aldosterone and cortisol, pituitary or adrenal imaging, renal angiography, or enzyme assay for 17-β-hydroxylase deficiency. Besides determining the cause of the hypokalemia, it is also important to assess for possible severe side effects that may result. Since cardiac and skeletal muscles can be affected, an ECG and creatine kinase (CK) values should be determined. Possible ECG abnormalities may include atrial or ventricular tachyarrhythmia, flattened T-wave, or presence of a U-wave, while increased CK result in muscle breakdown or frank rhabdomyolysis.

## Treatment

Treatment for hypokalemia is dependent upon the underlying cause. For all hypokalemic patients, there are some common goals: decrease further potassium losses, replenish lost potassium stores, monitor for potential toxicities, and determine the underlying cause and prevent further hypokalemic episodes. As previously stated, monitoring for toxicity includes ECG and serum CK levels. Initially, anything causing possible potassium losses should be discontinued or addressed, including discontinuing laxative and diuretics or change to potassium-sparing diuretics, treat any diarrhea or vomiting, and control hyperglycemia. Next, potassium repletion should be done to correct the hypokalemia. As a general rule, for each 1 mEq/L decrease in potassium, there is a potassium deficit of roughly 200–400 mEq. This can either overestimate or underestimate the true potassium deficit, and therefore the serum potassium should be checked again after supplementation. The preferred form of supplementation would be an oral form of potassium since it is readily absorbed, and large quantities can be given safely. If gastrointestinal upset occurs or if the patient is vomiting, an enteral form may be used. IV potassium supplementation is less well-tolerated and therefore should be given much slower (<10 mEq/h) and monitored for local reaction due to venous irritation. Glucose supplementation should be monitored carefully since it can increase insulin production leading to more transcellular shifting of potassium into the cells resulting in lower serum potassium levels. Additionally, if the patient is acidotic, the potassium should be repleted before the acidosis is corrected. This is due to potential worsening of hypokalemia by transcellular shift as the patient becomes relatively more alkalotic. Surgical intervention is only needed if there is a specific underlying cause that can be found, such as renal artery stenosis, adrenal adenoma, or intestinal obstruction. Finally, once supplementation has returned the potassium level back to normal, it is important to monitor the potassium levels over the next few days to ensure stable values and to be sure the cause of the hypokalemia was correctly determined and treated. Ultimately, some patients may need to be on a long-term potassium supplementation and/or have long-term monitoring of serum potassium levels.

## REFERENCE

1. Greenlee M, Wingo CS, McDonough AA, et al. Narrative review: evolving concepts in potassium homeostasis and hypokalemia. Ann Intern Med. 2009;150(9):619-25.

## FURTHER READING

1. Frank JD, Robert AB, Jeremy G, et al. The 5-Minute Clinical Consult 2012 20th Edition, Lippincott Williams & Wilkins; 20 edition (March 30, 2012): B005O3HG3M.

## CASE STUDY 95: HYPONATREMIA

## CASE HISTORY

A 50-year-old male long-distance runner was feeling slightly fatigued when he woke up 2 days before he planned to compete in a local marathon. To help himself feel better, he began to hydrate himself by drinking large amounts of water. The following morning, he continued drinking large amounts of water since he felt that it was helping. He decided that he was well enough to compete in the marathon. During the race, he continued to drink water at every opportunity. Although he was struggling at the end, he managed to finish the race. While he was sitting in a recovery tent, he appeared slightly confused and his friends helped him hydrate with more water. This did not seem to

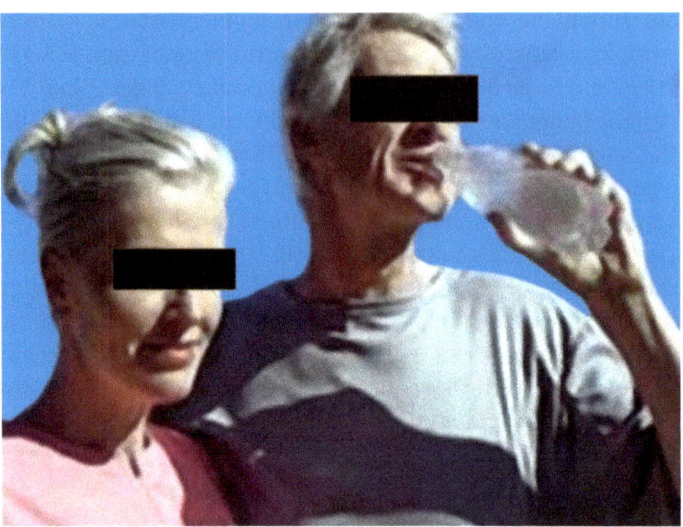

**Fig. 1:** Hyponatremia is a risk for those exercising in excessive heat.
*Source:* Available online at http://www.cdc.gov/meningococcal/index.html.

help, and over the next 15 min, he became increasingly confused and progressively less responsive.

He was immediately transported to the emergency department. Upon arrival, he remained minimally responsive and obviously confused. Laboratory values were rapidly determined and showed a serum sodium (SNa) level of 124 mEq/L and a serum osmolarity of 265 mOsm/kg. On clinical examination, he did not show apparent signs of dehydration. He was immediately put on water restriction and a hypertonic saline infusion was started (Fig. 1). After 2 h, he was no longer exhibiting any neurological deficits and his SNa was 128 mEq/L. The hypertonic saline was discontinued and over the next 48 h he continued with water restriction and replacement of each 1 mL of urine output with 0.5 mL normal saline. He continued to have routine SNa values checked every 6 h. After 48 h, his SNa returned to 138 mEq/L. He was discharged with no residual neurological deficits.

## CASE DISCUSSION

This patient developed an acute hyponatremic episode, which is considered <48 h. The result of the relatively quick decrease in extracellular SNa is a fluid shift to the intracellular space that overwhelms the bodies' compensatory responses. The effects are most pronounced in the central nervous system since the cranium is a rigid structure that does not allow for expansion. The brain cells swell and cause neurological deficits as seen in this patient (e.g., confusion and decreased responsiveness). He was predisposed to hyponatremia due to several factors (Flowchart 1). These included the general stress

**Flowchart 1:** Types of hyponatremia.

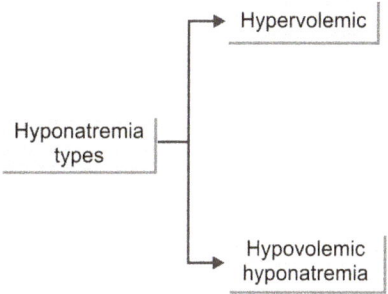

of his illness, excessive hydration with hypotonic fluids (i.e., water), and the large amount of fluid loss (i.e., sweating) associated with his marathon.[1] With the acute and symptomatic nature of his episode, it was important to enact a brief period of relatively rapid increase of SNa concentration of approximately 4–6 mEq/L over the first 1–2 h and then follow that with a slower increase over the following days.

## HYPONATREMIA DISCUSSION

### General

Hyponatremia is defined as a SNa concentration of <135 mEq/L and is considered severe when below 125 mEq/L. This is a common electrolyte disorder in the hospitalized population. People of any gender or age can be affected, but it may be most significant or more frequent in the elderly as they are more likely to have comorbid conditions and/or multiple medications.

### Pathophysiology and Causes

True hyponatremia is associated with low plasma osmolarity, and therefore, this should be assessed as well. A normal or high osmolarity with a low SNa is evidence of either redistributive hyponatremia or pseudohyponatremia. These are related to excessively high levels of glucose, mannitol, triglycerides, or proteins in the serum. True hyponatremia (i.e., with low plasma osmolarity) can then be divided into three subtypes: (1) hypovolemic, (2) euvolemic, and (3) hypervolemic. These are based on physical examination assessment of volume status and may prove beneficial in directing the physician to the cause of the hyponatremia. Since the ultimate treatment may depend on the underlying cause, a hyponatremia algorithm can be used to systematically evaluate the likely cause.[2]

In general, the possible causes can be narrowed down by assessing the volume status; although if there is more than one compounding factor, then this can be more difficult. The most distinctive subtype is likely hypervolemic hyponatremia. Examples include nephrotic syndrome, congestive heart failure, cirrhosis, and chronic renal failure. In general, these disorders lead to a volume overloaded state with much of the volume located within either the venous system or the interstitial space. This causes an apparent volume deficiency in the arterial network (i.e., decreased effective arterial volume) leading to activation of the renin–angiotensin–aldosterone and vasopressin [antidiuretic hormone (ADH)] systems. The abnormal activation of these systems leads to inaccurate regulation of the salt and water balance. On the opposite end of the volume status is hypovolemic hyponatremia. This occurs when there is loss of both water and sodium, but the extent of the sodium loss is greater. This sodium loss can occur via two mechanisms, either renal or extrarenal. These are distinguished by the urine sodium concentration. Renal losses cause the urine sodium concentration to be >30 mmol/L, while extrarenal losses are associated with concentrations of <30 mmol/L. Renal losses may result from cerebral salt wasting (CSW) syndrome, diuretics, or mineralocorticoid deficiency. Extrarenal causes may include vomiting, diarrhea, excessive sweating and heat-related illness, or third-spacing from burns, peritonitis, pancreatitis, or other causes. In general, the low-vascular volume of these disorders leads to fluid retention and thirst, which can lead to dilution of the SNa. Additionally, CSW syndrome may involve various natriuretic peptides that will also decrease SNa. The final subtype is euvolemic hyponatremia, in which the patient does not show sign of either hypervolemia or hypovolemia. This can be due to several mechanisms which can be distinguished to some extent by urine osmolarity or urine sodium concentration. If urine sodium is <20–30 mEq/L or urine osmolarity <100 mOsm/L, this indicates a normal ability for the kidneys to produce dilute urine. This is most often the case with excessive hypotonic fluid intake (i.e., primary polydipsia) or even a reset osmostat. If the urine sodium and osmolarity are more concentrated, this suggests an inability to adequately dilute the urine and therefore predicts a nonosmotic release of ADH. This may be the case in hypothyroidism, hypopituitarism, or adrenal insufficiency leading to glucocorticoid deficiency, or the syndrome of inappropriate ADH secretion (SIADH). Note that SIADH is a diagnosis of exclusion, so you must determine that the hyponatremia is of the euvolemic type with concentrated urine and no evidence of thyroid or adrenal dysfunction. Furthermore, SIADH may be idiopathic or due to a variety of neurologic or pulmonary disorders, so further evaluation for the cause of SIADH should be instituted. One last cause of hyponatremia that should be evaluated in all patients is iatrogenically induced via medications. Due to the different mechanisms of action of the variety of medications, it may occur with any volume status, although euvolemic hyponatremia is the most common. Evaluation of patient medications should occur as part of the workup of all hyponatremia patients.

## Assessment

Since the volume status may be important in determining the cause of the hyponatremia, it is necessary to assess the volume status as part of the physical examination. Examples of hypovolemic evidence may be diminished skin turgor, dry mucous membranes, tachycardia, or orthostasis. Hypervolemia may be suggested by peripheral edema, increased jugular venous distention, ascites, pulmonary rales or an S3 gallop. Lack of any of these physical findings is consistent with euvolemic. Outside of the physical examination findings, a good patient history and some laboratory tests will help to determine the ultimate cause. Much of the time, the hyponatremia is found incidentally upon routine laboratory blood work. This often suggests a chronic nature of the disease and usually has no associated symptoms. In an acute setting, symptoms are more likely to develop, and the severity depends on the extent of the hyponatremia (*Source*: 5MinuteConsult). Initial symptoms may include nausea, vomiting, and malaise which may proceed further to headache, lethargy, confusion, and decreased awareness or responsiveness. If very severe or rapid decreases in sodium occur, then seizure, coma, or respiratory arrest may result. Recall that the underlying physiology of the symptoms is due to the fluid shift from extracellular to intracellular spaces, which primarily affects the brain in the rigid cranium, thus leading to primarily neurologic symptoms.

Besides symptoms of the hyponatremia itself, some patients may exhibit symptoms of the underlying cause of the hyponatremia. For example, a patient with incidental hyponatremia may also have weight gain, fatigue, constipation, and sensitivity to cold which could suggest hypothyroidism as the underlying cause for the hyponatremia. Whether or not symptoms are present, various laboratory analyses may be helpful in determining the diagnosis. As previously mentioned, SNa, plasma osmolarity and volume status must be assessed to determine the specific subtype of hyponatremia (i.e., hypo-, hyper-, or euvolemic). If indicated, additional laboratory tests may include urine sodium and osmolarity, renal function, hepatic function, thyroid function, adrenal function, serum glucose, and lipids. Furthermore, if SIADH is ultimately diagnosed, then a legitimate effort should occur to rule out underlying CNS or respiratory causes, which may require chest X-ray and/or head CT.

## Treatment

The mainstay of treatment for hyponatremia is correction of the SNa abnormality. This must be tailored to the nature of the hyponatremia, whether or not symptoms are present and any underlying pathology. For asymptomatic patients, correction of the sodium deficit should be less aggressive. In hypovolemic patients, isotonic saline should be used to replenish the intravascular volume. This should inhibit the further release of ADH. With hypervolemia, additional fluids are not indicated, and instead the patient should be treated with salt and fluid restriction (<1 L/day) and loop diuretics. A vasopressin-2 (V2) receptor antagonist (i.e., conivaptan or tolvaptan) may be considered to decrease the effect of the inappropriate release of ADH. Furthermore, it is very important to provide treatment for the underlying disease, as this is the ultimate cause for the hyponatremia in the first place. Lastly, in euvolemic patients, fluid restriction is used as well. If fluid restriction of <1 L/day does not improve the hyponatremia, it may be necessary to further restrict fluids or add a V2 receptor antagonist to aid in the correction. In all of these patients, correction of the SNa should not exceed 8–12 mEq/L/day.

Acutely symptomatic patients (i.e., neurologic deficit) should undergo an initial brief period of relatively quick correction of the sodium deficit to reverse the symptoms. This brief (2–3 h) intervention can utilize either hypertonic saline alone or isotonic saline with a loop diuretic. Both of these actions intend to provide relatively more sodium compared to water for a more rapid reversal of symptoms. During this period, correction should be approximately 2 mEq/L/h until the symptoms resolve. Then the previously described treatment for asymptomatic patients can be used. Complications of acute and severe hyponatremia include cerebral edema and neurological symptoms, as the electrolyte balance in the brain adjusts more slowly than in peripheral tissues.[3]

Symptomatic patients with chronic hyponatremia represent the population that is most difficult to treat. Although all patients should be corrected conservatively, these patients are most likely to encounter severe side effects from correction that is too rapid. Sodium correction should be limited to 0.5–1 mEq/L/h and not to exceed approximately 8–10 mEq/L/day. Patients with chronic hyponatremia have had time to compensate for the fluid shifts, and this represents higher risk for neurologic damage by adding more extracellular sodium. This could lead to cell shrinkage from fluid outflow, potentially resulting in central pontine myelinolysis (CPM) and/or extrapontine myelinolysis (EPM). These can lead to irreversible neurological damage. In contrast, acute hyponatremic patients have not had time to compensate for the hyponatremia and therefore are less likely to be harmed by the rapid fluid outflow from the cells and can tolerate a relatively more rapid correction.

## REFERENCES

1. Backer HD, Shlim DR. Problems with heat & cold. Centers for Disease Control and Prevention. [Online]. Available from http://wwwnc.cdc.gov/travel/yellowbook/2012/chapter-2-the-pre-travel-consultation/problems-with-heat-and-cold.htm; 2011 [accessed April 2, 2013].
2. Lien YH, Shapiro JI. Hyponatremia: clinical diagnosis and management. Am J Med. 2007;120(8):653-8.
3. Sterns R., (2018). Osmotic demyelination syndrome (ODS) and overly rapid correction of hyponatremia. In Melin JA (Ed.), UpToDate. Retrieved October 16, 2018 from https://www.uptodate.com/contents/osmotic-demyelination-syndrome-ods-and-overly-rapid-correction-of-hyponatremia.

# CASE STUDY 96: HYPERKALEMIA

## CASE HISTORY

A 60-year-old diabetic patient is presented to the emergency department with the chief complaint of feeling weak, tired, confused for the past 24 h. He also has hypertension for which he is taking lisinopril and spironolactone. On examination, his vitals are stable. He also complains of nausea, vomiting, diarrhea, abdominal pain, paresthesia, such as tingling and numbness, muscle weakness, flaccid paralysis, tachypnea due to respiratory muscle weakness and bradycardia.

## LABORATORY TESTS

Laboratory tests ordered for basic metabolic profile, complete blood count (CBC), and arterial blood gas (ABG) (Fig. 1).

## ELECTROCARDIOGRAM

Electrocardiogram (ECG) shows complete heart block, peaked T-waves, prolonged PR intervals and widened QRS complexes (Fig. 2).

## CAUSES OF HYPERKALEMIA

Hyperkalemia is defined as serum $K^+$ >5.5 mEq/L and can lead to life-threatening consequences.

**Fig. 1:** Toxic levels of hyperkalemia.

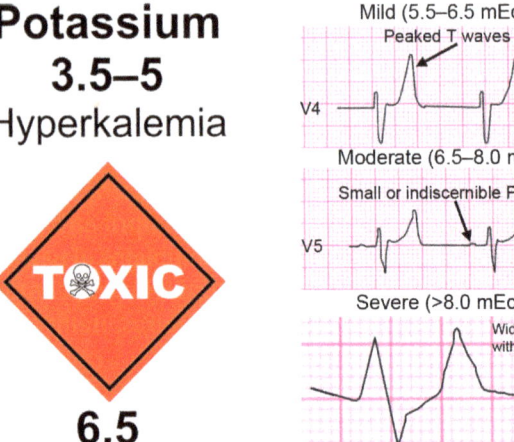

**Fig. 2:** ECG changes.
*Source:* Wikimedia.com.

Pseudohyperkalemia has been reported in as high as 20% of blood samples with elevated potassium levels. Traumatic venipuncture is the most common cause of traumatic hemolysis. Potassium release from muscles usually occurs distal to tourniquet placement. Lastly, when blood clots form in the specimen tube, potassium is released from cells; this usually occurs in the presence of leukocytosis or thrombocytosis. Therefore, if hyperkalemia is present in an asymptomatic patient, it is vital to repeat with a new blood sample.

If repeat testing confirms hyperkalemia, then the source of hyperkalemia needs to be determined. Urine potassium can be helpful to differentiate between potassium released from cells and decreased renal potassium excretion. Urine potassium >30 mEq/L suggests a transcellular shift, and lower urine potassium excretion suggests impaired renal excretion.

Hyperkalemia is often associated with acidosis; however, no evidence demonstrates acidosis as a cause of hyperkalemia. Metabolic acidosis and hyperkalemia are often present together in conditions, such as renal failure and renal tubular acidosis secondary to impaired renal excretion of potassium. Rhabdomyolysis in association with impaired renal clearance can also lead to hyperkalemia, since the kidneys are unable to clear the increased amount of potassium released into the extracellular space by muscle cells.

Drugs can also be a cause for hyperkalemia, therefore it is important to review medication history in patients with hyperkalemia. β-Receptor antagonists and digitalis are most commonly associated with hyperkalemia resulting from a transcellular shift. Digitalis toxicity can result in severely high potassium levels, which can lead to significant cardiac consequences. Several more drugs are associated with hyperkalemia secondary to decreased excretion, such as angiotensin-converting enzyme (ACE) inhibitors, angiotensin receptor blockers (ARBs), potassium sparing diuretics, and nonsteroidal anti-inflammatory drugs (NSAIDs). They impair excretion by inhibiting the renin–angiotensin–aldosterone system.

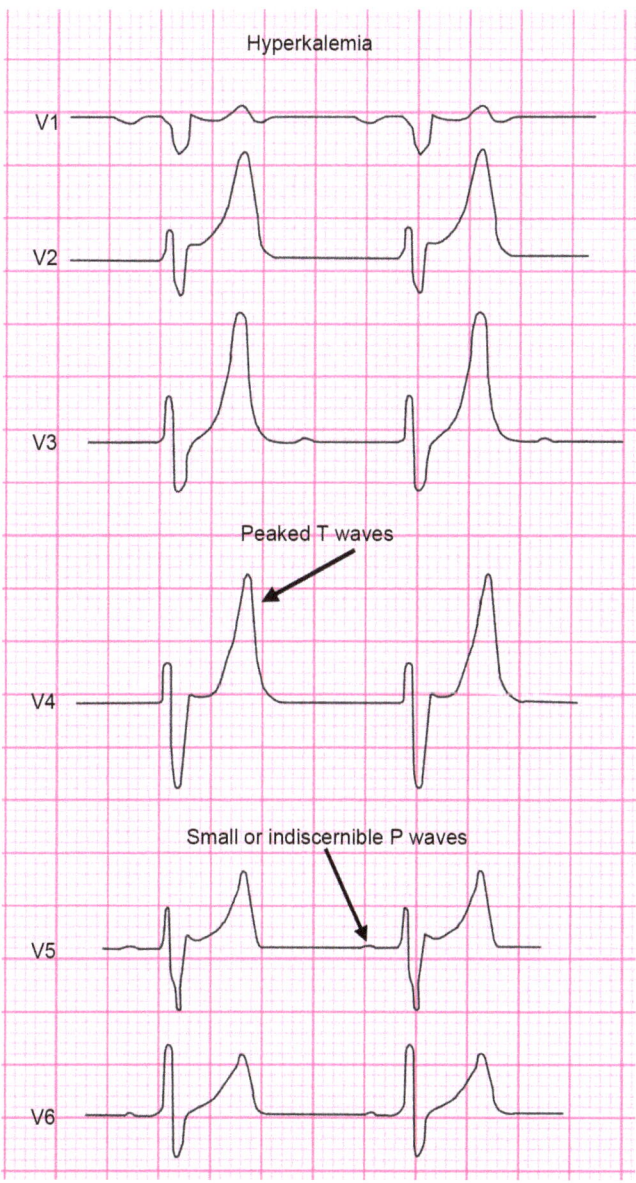

**Fig. 3:** ECG changes associated with hyperkalemia.
*Source:* Wikimedia.org.

Renal and adrenal insufficiency can result in hyperkalemia. This should be suspected if the patient's glomerular filtration rate (GFR) is below 10 mL/min or urine output is lower than 1 L/day.

## CLINICAL MANIFESTATIONS

The most concerning manifestation of hyperkalemia is slowing of electrical conduction in the heart. The effect on the electrical conduction depends on the potassium serum level. Figure 3 shows ECG changes associated with progressive hyperkalemia.

"Peaked T-waves" are usually the first ECG manifestations in hyperkalemia. These are usually appreciated on precordial leads vasopressin-2 (V2) and V3. Progressive hyperkalemia causes decrease in the P-wave amplitude and progressive increase in the PR interval leading to first-degree heart block. Eventually, QRS duration is increased and P-waves disappear resulting in complete heart block seen at serum $K^+$ levels >10 mEq/L. The final event seen at serum $K^+$ levels of 14 mEq/L is ventricular asystole.

"Peaked T-waves" are often observed in patients with metabolic acidosis.

## TREATMENT

The treatment plan of hyperkalemia using cardiac monitor is described in Flowchart 1.

**Flowchart 1:** Treatment of hyperkalemia.

*Courtesy:* Badar M Zaheer, MD, Chicago, USA

Following are the additional treatment options:
- Nebulized albuterol 2.5 mg in 3 mL normal saline (NS) every (q) 20 min
- Sodium bicarbonate one ampule 50 mEq in 5 min
- Furosemide 20–40 mg intravenous pyelogram (IVP).

*Note*: Treat the underlying cause, if it is secondary to Addisonian crisis; give steroids. Antigen-binding fragments (Fab) are given for digoxin toxicity. If digoxin toxicity as well as hyperkalemia coexists, never give calcium gluconate/calcium chloride.

## FURTHER READING

1. National Institute of Health. High potassium levels, http://www.nlm.nih.gov/MedlinePlus/ency/article/001179.htm; 2013.

# CASE STUDY 97: HYPOMAGNESEMIA

## CASE HISTORY

A 45-year-old male is brought to the emergency room for the chief complaint of muscle weakness, confusion, decreased reflexes, jerky movements, high blood pressure, and irregular heart rhythms. He has been drinking heavily but not eating. He is a known hypertensive and takes hydrochlorothiazide (HCTZ) 25 mg daily.

## DISCUSSION

Hypomagnesemia is commonly observed in hospitalized patients and has been reported in as high as 65% of patients in the intensive care unit (ICU). Therefore, it is vital to recognize conditions that predispose a patient to hypomagnesemia (Flowchart 1) and closely monitor their serum magnesium levels.

Aminoglycosides, amphotericin, and pentamidine have been shown to cause hypomagnesemia. Aminoglycosides have been reported to cause hypomagnesemia in approximately 30% of patients by blocking the reabsorption of magnesium in the ascending limb of the loop of Henle.

Diuretic therapy, especially loop diuretics, is most often associated with drug-induced hypomagnesemia. They interfere with magnesium reabsorption while inhibiting sodium reabsorption. Fifty percent of patients on chronic diuretic therapy with furosemide are found to have decreased magnesium levels. Thiazide diuretics, on the other hand, are only associated with hypomagnesemia in elderly patients.

**Flowchart 1:** Causes of hypomagnesemia.

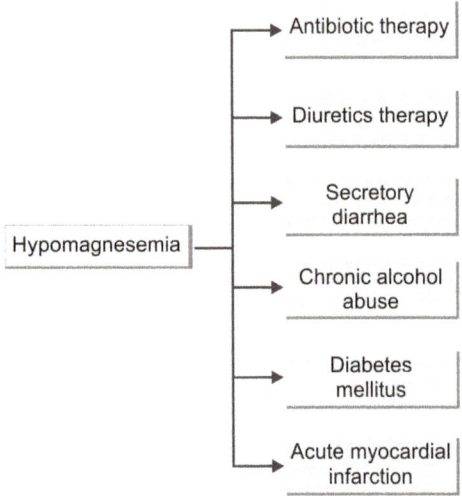

The most common cause of hypomagnesemia in the United States is alcoholism. Patients with chronic alcohol abuse are at an increased risk for hypomagnesemia secondary to poor nutrition and chronic diarrhea. Since magnesium is required in the conversion of thiamine to thiamine pyrophosphate, it is often associated with thiamine deficiency. Magnesium levels should be closely monitored in patients on thiamine supplementation.

Secretory diarrhea predisposes a patient to hypomagnesemia since lower gastrointestinal (GI) excretions consist of high concentrations of magnesium (10–14 mEq/L). Upper GI excretions, on the other hand, are lower in concentration of magnesium.

Hypomagnesemia is also commonly seen in patients with insulin-dependent diabetes secondary to urinary magnesium loss accompanied with glycosuria. Additionally, up to 80% of patients with an acute myocardial infarction have been found to have hypomagnesemia in the first 48 h. This decrease in magnesium serum levels has been hypothesized to be secondary to endogenous catecholamine excess.

## CLINICAL MANIFESTATIONS

Hypomagnesemia is often accompanied with associated electrolyte abnormalities, such as hypokalemia, hypophosphatemia, and hypocalcemia.

## Emergency Room Care and Disposition

- Correct volume deficits and any associated potassium, calcium, or phosphate deficiencies

- In alcoholic patients, who have delirium tremens (DT), or pending DTs, give 2 g of magnesium sulfate in the first hour, and then 6 g in the first 24 h. Check for DTs every 15 min until the serum magnesium levels come back to 3.5 mEq/L or above.

## FURTHER READING

1. National Institute of Health. Hypomagnesia, http://www.nlm.nih.gov/medlineplus/ency/article/000315.htm; 2013.

# CHAPTER 20

# Ocular Emergencies

## CASE STUDY 98: RED EYE

### CASE HISTORY

A 20-year-old male is brought to a rural emergency room by his mother. The man has a bandana wrapped around his eyes. He is placed in an examination room, and his mother quickly turns off the lights until the nurse arrives. Upon arrival to the room, the mother tells the nurse that light hurts her son's eyes. The patient has redness and pain in his right eye that started 2 days ago. There is no drainage and his mother, who has checked his eyes, claims there is nothing inside them. The patient states he has had a loss in focus and clearness of vision in his right eye for the past 2 days. The patient's medical history has nothing notable. Upon examination, the eyelids and lashes are normal. Some ciliary congestion is seen in the sclera on the right eye, but not the left. The patient experiences 8/10 pain when the pupils are examined with light. The right pupil is smaller, irregularly shaped, and less reactive than the left pupil to light. The doctor gives a few drops of tetracaine with no relief. Fluorescein uptake is negative. The anterior-chamber depth is narrow, and the slit-lamp examination is positive for cell and flare. Diagnosis by the emergency department (ED) physician is acute iritis, and long-acting cycloplegic topical medicine is given for the ciliary spasm. Upon consultation with the ophthalmologist, a prescription for a topical steroid is written. A follow-up appointment is arranged with the ophthalmologist within 24 h.

### DISCUSSION

Table 1 discusses symptoms and diagnosis of red eye.

### CAUSES

The possible causes of acute uveitis in patients include infections like tuberculosis, herpes simplex, herpes zoster, toxoplasmosis, cytomegalovirus, or syphilis. Autoimmune, idiopathic diseases, and trauma are other possible causes.

## Ocular Emergencies

**Table 1:** Symptoms and diagnosis of red eye.

| Diseases | Symptoms | Diagnosis |
|---|---|---|
| Conjunctivitis (Fig. 1) 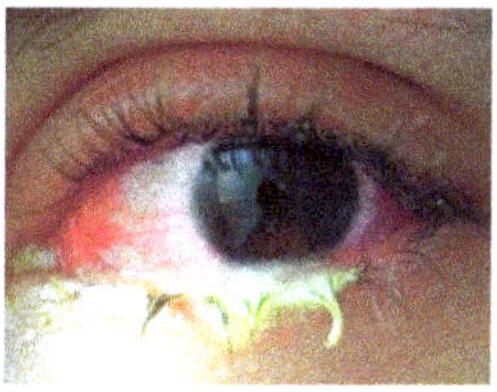 | Red eye + gritty foreign body + discharge | Red eye without change in vision or pain |
| Subconjunctival hemorrhage (Fig. 2) 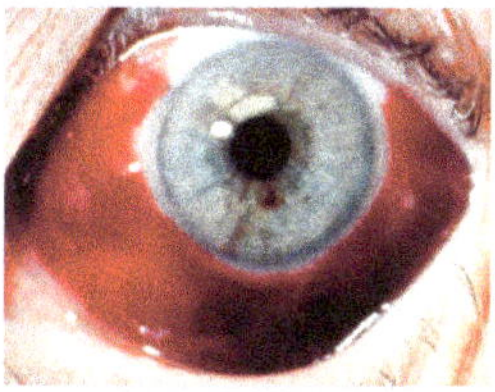 | Blood between the conjunctiva and the sclera | Hemorrhage seen after trauma; may be spontaneous or related to systemic injury |
| Corneal abrasion (Fig. 3) 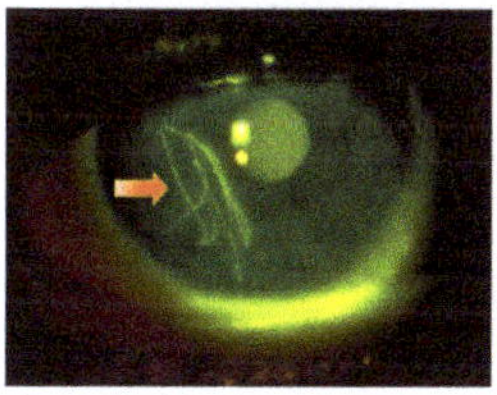 | Pain + foreign body + tearing + photophobia | Abrasions, usually the result of trauma; patient may or may not remember the event. Patient may have blurry vision if abrasion is big enough/covers more of the eye |
| Acute uveitis (Fig. 4) 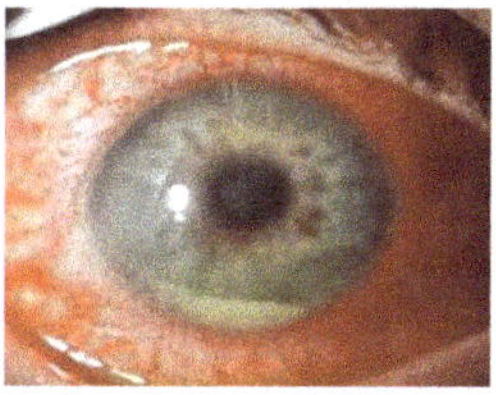 | Severe photophobia + red eye + blurred vision + irregular pupil | Inflammation of the uveal tract. Acute iritis is the most common |

**Fig. 1:** Conjunctivitis.

**Fig. 2:** Subconjunctival hemorrhage.

**Fig. 3:** Corneal abrasion.

**Fig. 4:** Acute uveitis.

Few things you should never miss in the eye:
- Acute glaucoma
- Temporal arteritis
- Anterior uveitis (iritis)
- Central retinal artery occlusion
- Retinal detachment.

## TREATMENT

The treatment of acute uveitis involves topical corticosteroids. This treatment involves risk of development of glaucoma, cataracts, reactivation of herpes, and thus an ophthalmologist must be consulted immediately.

# CASE STUDY 99: ACUTE ANGLE-CLOSURE GLAUCOMA

## CASE HISTORY

A 65-year-old woman presents to emergency room (ER) with right eye pain, redness, severe headache, and blurred vision for the past 4 h after painting picture for several hours. The pain is progressively worse. The left eye feels normal and has no problem with vision. She accidentally injured her head 1 week ago, and she believes this may be the cause. She denies any photophobia, tearing, or discharge. There is no similar eye pain or blurring vision in the past. She only wears glasses and is farsighted. When seen in the ER, she sees halos around her eye.

### Past Medical History

No medical problem was observed, and no use of any medication was found.

### Past Surgical History

Negative.

## PHYSICAL EXAMINATION

On examination the patient has visual acuity of 20/30 in the left eye. Visual acuity is finger counting in the right eye. Visual field is within normal limits. Gentle palpitations of closed right eye reveal that it is harder than left eye. Her left pupil is 5 mm fixed and unreactive. Her left eye appears normal. Size of pupil is 3 mm and brisk reaction is present. Extraocular movements are intact and painless. Right cornea is slightly cloudy and because of the cloudy cornea, fundoscopy is impossible. The left fundus appears normal; temporal arteries are nontender and they are pulsatile. The rest of physical examination is normal.

## DIAGNOSTIC TESTS

Slit-lamp examination measured an intraocular pressure of 52 mm Hg in the right eye and normal pressure in the left eye. The pressure was found using Tono-Pen. Slit-lamp examination also revealed narrow anterior chambers.

## DISCUSSION

Acute close angle glaucoma commonly presents with:
- Headache
- Halo around vision
- Severe eye pain with redness of the eye
- Nausea and vomiting.

## DIFFERENTIAL DIAGNOSIS

- Anterior uveitis
- Conjunctivitis
- Corneal ulcer
- Traumatic endophthalmitis.

## PATHOLOGICAL FINDINGS

- Atrophy and cupping of optic nerve.
- Loss of retinal ganglion cells and their axons produces defects in the retinal nerve fiber layer.
- Funduscopic examination shows optic nerve cupping.

## TREATMENT PLAN

Treatment goal is to lower intraocular pressure with an ophthalmology consult. Carbonic anhydrase inhibitor, acetazolamide (Diamox) 250 mg po qid (four times a day) every 6 h can be given orally or locally. Also, osmotic agents such as mannitol are used to dehydrate the vitreous humor to in turn decrease intraocular pressure.

## PRACTICE PEARL AND LESSON TO LEARN

Never ever in your life miss a case of glaucoma, acute uveitis, temporal arteritis, and other causes of sudden loss of vision. Consider every red eye and headache a potential for these diagnoses. For malpractice law suits, missing diagnosis makes up for about 70% of claims.

## FURTHER READING

1. Bainter PS. (2018). Subconjunctival Hemorrhage (Bleeding in Eye). Retrieved October 16, 2018, from Emedicinehealth website: https://www.emedicinehealth.com/subconjunctival_hemorrhage_bleeding_in_eye/article_em.htm.

2. Eye emergencies. (2018, October 1). Retrieved October 16, 2018, from Medline Plus website: https://medlineplus.gov/ency/article/000054.htm.

## CASE STUDY 100: CENTRAL RETINAL ARTERY OCCLUSION

### CASE HISTORY

A 68-year-old woman is presented to the emergency department (ED) with the chief complaint of sudden loss of vision in the left eye. She was eating dinner with her family after gardening when she experienced the vision loss. She denies nausea, vomiting, or eye pain. She has a history of hypertension and atrial fibrillation. She is not diabetic.

### PHYSICAL EXAMINATION

On examination, she has complete loss of vision in the left eye. Right eye vision is 20/40. Pupils are equal in size and reactive to light. Sclera and intraocular pressure in both eyes are normal. Left eye shows pale fundus with cherry-red spot.

### ASSESSMENT AND PLAN

The diagnosis is central retinal artery occlusion. The differential diagnoses of vision loss can be visualized in Flowchart 1.

**Flowchart 1:** Differential diagnosis of vision loss.

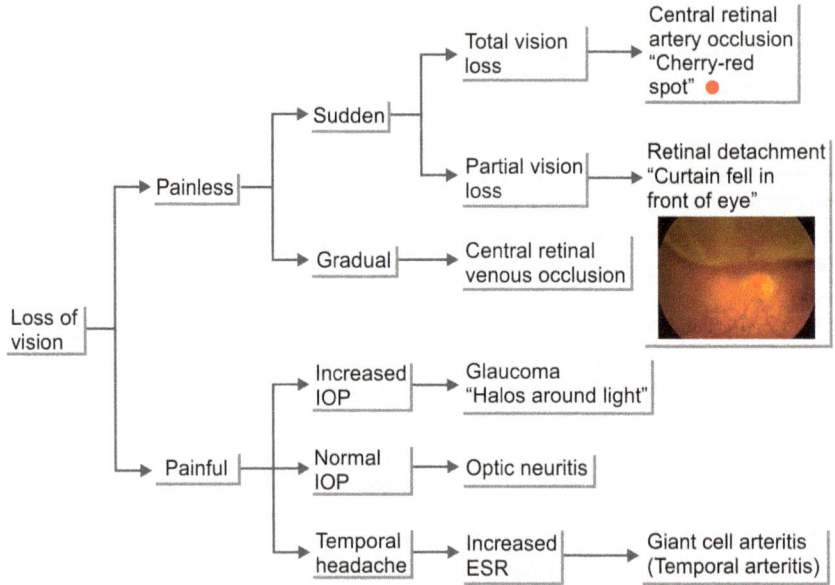

In the ED, the management goal was to dilate the artery to minimize further ischemic injury to the retina and to refer to ophthalmology for advanced treatment.
- Timolol 0.5% eye drops
- Intravenous acetazolamide 5 mg
- Patient was instructed to hyperventilate into a paper bag during the encounter to increase her arterial $CO_2$ in attempt to further dilate the affected artery.
- Intermittent, 5-s digital massage of the entire globe was performed by both physician and patient for 15 min.

## FURTHER READING

1. Graham RH, Lee AG. (2018, September 6). Central Retinal Artery Occlusion (CRAO). Retrieved October 16, 2018, from Medscape website: https://emedicine.medscape.com/article/1223625-overview.
2. Retinal artery occlusion. (2018, October 1). Retrieved October 16, 2018, from MedlinePlus website: https://medlineplus.gov/ency/article/001028.htm.

# CHAPTER 21

# Disaster Management

## CASE STUDY 101: MASS CASUALTY—TRAIN ACCIDENT

### CASE HISTORY

In 1999, a semi-truck driving down the highway pulled in front of an Amtrak train in Kankakee, Illinois, USA. The train was derailed and crashed resulting in 122 persons injured and 11 dead (Fig.1).

For this scenario, let us imagine that a passenger train carrying 110 passengers is travelling down the track on a hot summer night when it collides with a tanker train hauling highly flammable liquids. The commercial train is operated by a small crew of eight members. The collision occurs at night, and when the trains collide, one of the tankers bursts into flames and two more cars simply rupture and their contents go everywhere. After the collision, emergency teams arrive on the scene and do an initial assessment. There are 70 injuries in total with 20 deaths including two firemen who died trying to put out the fire. The paramedics who arrived on the scene start to triage out the victims and come up with 20 Category Red patients (12 with extensive second- and third-degree burns), 19 Category Yellow patients (5 with second-degree burns), 25 Category Green patients (5 with limb deformities), and 6 Category Blue patients (4 with catastrophic third-degree burns). The train crash occurred within 12 miles (mi) of a major hospital with 35 open beds. In 50 mi, there is a hospital with a major trauma center that has a dedicated burn unit.

### DISCUSSION

In disaster situations, there are many factors that need to be taken into consideration in a very short period of time. The first responders will often set up a triage system as illustrated in the case example (Figs. 2A and B). Color coding victims is an easy way to determine which patients need to receive treatment first and which patients can wait till others are done. In this situation,

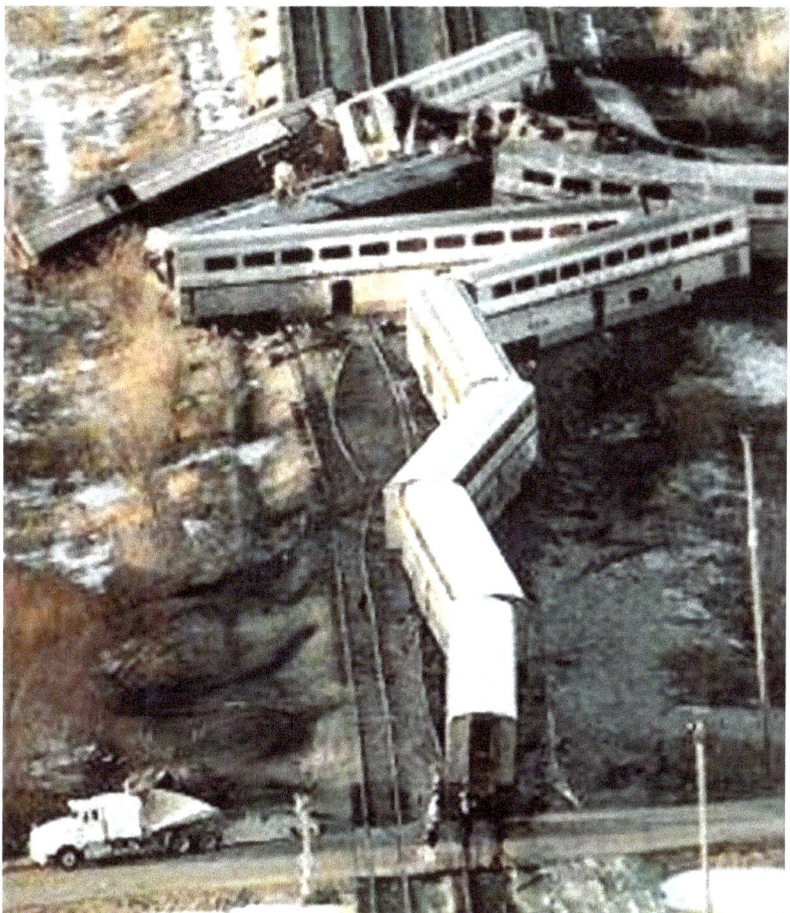

**Fig. 1:** Train accident in Kankakee, Illinois, USA in 1999.
*Source:* Wikimedia.org.

Red injury is for a life-threatening injury that requires immediate attention or operation. Yellow injuries are ones that may become life (or limb) threatening if care is not given within a couple of hours.

Green patients are considered the walking-wounded; these patients have suffered only minor injuries and may be asked to get up and walk away from the disaster area by themselves (note this is also a good way to find Green label patients). Lastly, patients listed as black were dead when the primary triage went through the casualties. Sometimes, triage units list patients as Blue, or severely injured. The prognosis of these patients depends on the current number of casualties to receive care (Red and Yellow patients). Blue patients are often given palliative care hoping they survive until patients with a better probability of surviving make it to the hospital, and then they will be taken.

A situation like this may be considered as mass casualty incident (MCI), a situation where personnel and equipment are overwhelmed. This includes emergency responders to the scene of the accident as well as local hospitals and hospital staff. In this scenario, there is a local hospital within 25 mi of the scene with 35 open beds, but the next hospital is 50 mi away. Emergency medical teams will need to set up alternative areas to stabilize and treat victims until emergency medical vehicles arrive and hospital beds can be found for all injured in the accident. These stabilization areas should be accessible to emergency medical vehicles. Caution should be taken, and these areas should be far enough from the disaster area as not to cause further injury (chemical, mechanical, or otherwise) to the patients within those areas. Typically, as patients are brought into the stabilization area, they are triaged again to assess severity of conditions. They should then be moved to the appropriate area of the stabilization zone to receive treatment and await extraction.

Once all hospital-bound patients have made it on an ambulance, the disaster crew will come in and start the cleanup on the area. Part of this cleanup involves dealing with the casualties from the disaster and getting those bodies to the morgue.

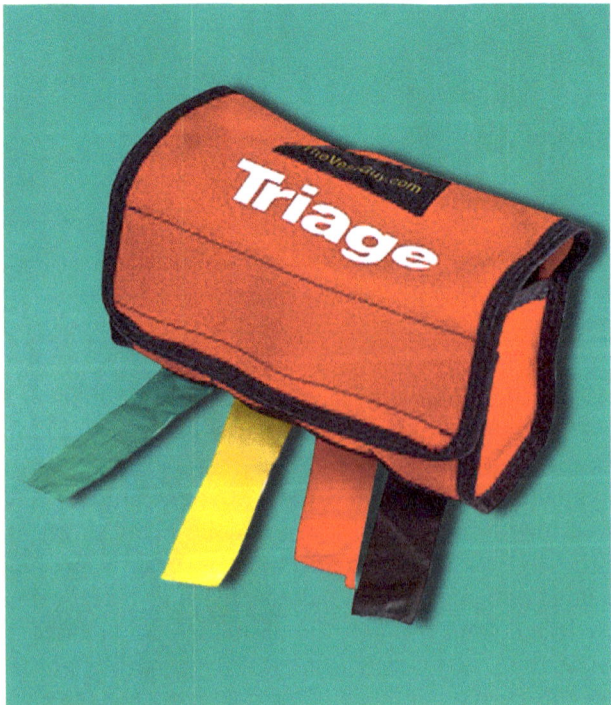

**Fig. 2A:** Triage systems.
*Source:* www.thevestguy.com and wikimedia.org.

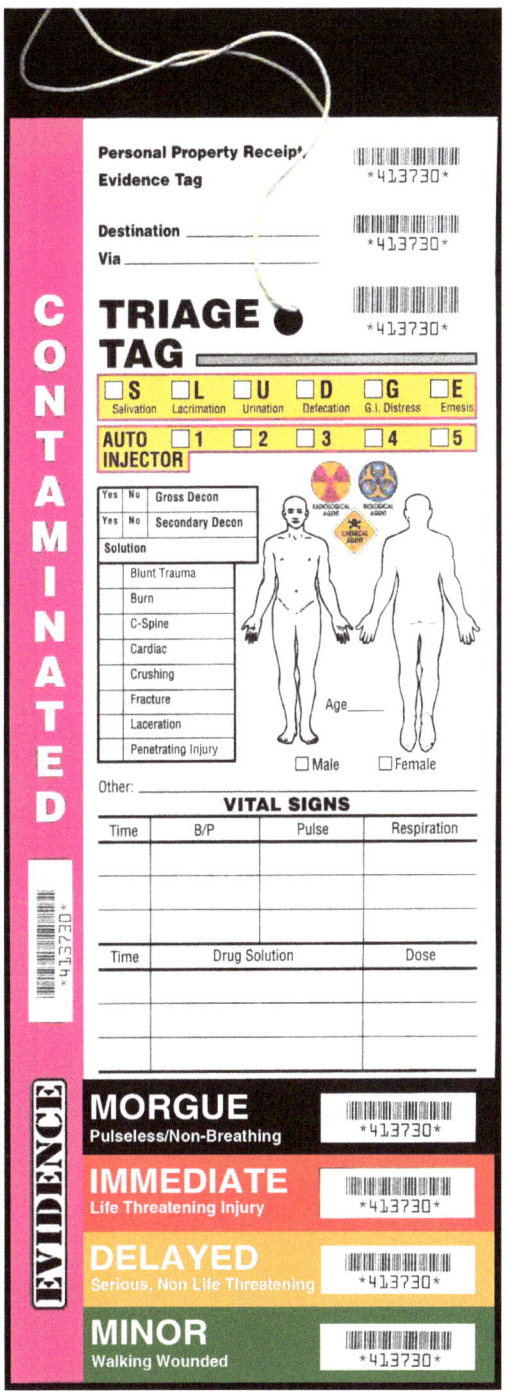

**Fig. 2B:** Triage tag

## PRACTICE PEARL

Remember! In the event of electrical injury, it is never a good idea to put low priority on initial pulseless patients. If a group of persons is struck by lightning, attention should be directed to those with no signs of life (black tagged), because the others will probably recover. Immediate CPR and prevention of anoxic death are essential.

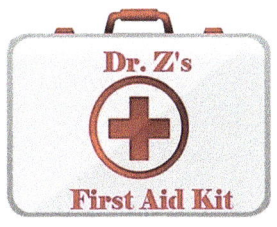

© Property of Badar Zaheer MD

### Dr. Z's First Aid Kit
Pulse oximeter
Airways adult and child size
Ambu bag (Bag valve mask)
Epinephrine
IV NS 1 liter with IV set
Tourniquet/bandages/gauze/alcohol swabs
Thoracostomy Needle (2nd intercostal space mid axillary line) (optional)

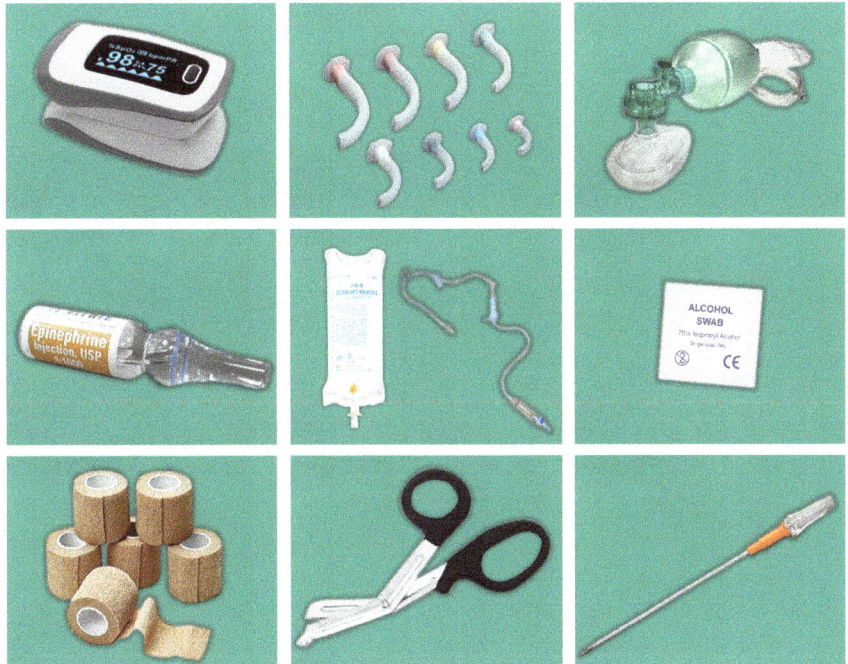

# Index

Page numbers followed by *b* refer to box, *f* refer to figure, *fc* refer to flowchart, and *t* refer to table

## A

Abdomen 31, 119
  examination 202
Abortion, septic 271
Abscess 314
  epidural 155
  peritonsillar 318*f*
  retropharyngeal 317, 319*f*
  tubo-ovarian 270
Absolute neutrophil count 323
Acamprosate 179
Accommodation 202
Acetazolamide 377
Acetycholinesterase 168
Acetylsalicylic acid 67, 74
Aching 78
Acidic urine 325
Acidosis 206
  metabolic 325
Acquired immunodeficiency syndrome 274, 358
Acromioclavicular joint
  anatomy of 148*f*
  injury 148
    features of 148
  separation 148, 149*f*, 149*fc*
Activated partial thromboplastin time 70
Acute coronary syndrome 39, 64, 65, 72, 74, 77
  management of 67
Acute respiratory distress syndrome 39, 61, 63*f*, 134, 252
  Berlin definition of 62*t*
Addison disease 33
Addisonian crisis 211
Adenopathy 34, 273
Adjuvant therapy 70
Adrenal crisis 211
  signs in 214*f*
  symptom in 214*f*
Adrenal function 365
Adrenal insufficiency, acute 91
Advanced trauma life support 92*t*, 195
Aggression 16
Agitation 249, 265
Agoraphobia 216

Air sacs 5
Airway 100, 101, 331
  breathing, circulation 3, 16, 25, 26, 44, 48, 105
  deformity 21
  disability, and exposure 52, 238
  management 227
  obstruction, location of 291*f*
Alanine
  aminotransferase 130
  transaminase 165
Albumin 93
Alcohol 33, 184, 222, 358
  consumption, heavy 120
Alcoholism 1, 175
Aldosterone 212
Alkaline
  burn 265, 267*f*
  phosphatase 165
Allergic alveolitis, extrinsic 39
Allergic reaction 220, 241
Allergy 239
Allopurinol 326
Alprazolam 217
Alteplase 44
Ambisome 354
Amenorrhea 308
American Association for Emergency Psychiatry 218
American College of Emergency Physicians 159
Aminoglycoside 125, 168
Amnesia 16
  post-traumatic 26
  retrograde 26
Amoxicillin 128
Amphetamines 180*f*, 197
  abuse 258
  overdose 258
    adverse effects of 259*f*
Amphocin 354
Ampicillin 318
Amylase 126
Anal sphincter tone, absent 156
Analgesia 134, 278
Anaphylaxis, cutaneous 241
Androgen hormones 212

Anemia 165
Aneurysm
    aortic 89
    ruptures, prevention of 14*f*
Angina 239
Anginal symptoms, severe 79
Angiocath 48*f*
Angioedema 225, 234*f*
Angiogram, selective pulmonary 42*f*
Angiography 72, 86*f*, 95, 338
    pulmonary 41
Angioplasty 67, 187*f*
Angiotensin receptor blockers 369
Angiotensin-converting enzyme 76, 110, 224, 233, 234*f*, 369
    inhibitor 71, 234*f*, 241
Angle-closure glaucoma, acute 376
Animal antiserum 222
Animal bites 220
Anorectic agents 34
Anorexia 128
    nervosa 358
Anterior dislocation, reduction of 152*f*
Antiacetylcholine receptor 166
Antianxiety medications 217
Antibiotics 128, 166, 278
Antibody, antinuclear 32
Anticholinesterase drugs 167
Anticoagulant
    current use of 185
    therapy 1
Antiepileptics 167
Antigen, prostate-specific 162
Antihistamines 227
Anti-PD-1-monoclonal antibodies 168
Antiplatelet therapy 70, 186
Antistreptolysin O titer 95
Antithrombin therapy 70
Anxiety 73, 177, 249, 265
    disorders 39
Aorta
    abdominal 84*f*
    enlarged abdominal 83*f*
    scan 86
Aortic aneurysm
    abdominal 82, 82*f*, 83, 84*f*, 85*f*, 88, 155
    dissecting 71, 75
Aortic arch anomalies 59
Aortic dissection 70, 94
Aortic stenosis 33, 39, 71, 75, 91, 94
Apnea, central 39
Appendicitis 83, 127, 275
Appendix diameter 278
Arachnoid cysts 1
Arrhythmia 177
Arterial occlusions, meningococcemia-induced 343*f*

Arterial oxygen, partial pressure of 62
Arteritis, temporal 376
Artery
    anterior segmental 41*f*
    enlarged central pulmonary 32*f*
    femoral 57*f*
Arthritis 127
Aspartate aminotransferase 130
Aspartate transaminase 165
Aspirin 69, 71, 186, 241
Asthma 53, 59, 60, 239, 240
    exacerbation 33, 240
Astrocytoma 23*f*
Ataxia 209
Atherosclerosis 310
Atrioventricular block 33, 67
Atropine 228, 248*f*
Automated external defibrillator 99, 102*f*
    Universal sign for 99*f*
Automobile accidents 15
Azathioprine 109, 167

**B**

Back pain 39
    assessment of 156
    low 154
    mechanical low 161
Bacteremia 193, 295
Bacteremic origin 144
Bacteriuria 127
Balloon-catheter removal 316
Barbiturates 33
Barium enema study 289*f*
Cough, barking 294
Bartter-Schwartz criteria 210
Basal metabolic
    profile 3
    panel 83, 165, 353
Basilar artery
    occlusion 170
    thrombosis 185
Basilar skull fracture 15
Bath salts 180*f*
Bee sting 238
Bell's palsy 190, 191*f*
Benzodiazepines 33, 178, 196, 217, 260
Benztropine mesylate 219
Beta-blockers 33, 71, 167, 168, 203, 204, 233
Beta-human chorionic gonadotropin 307
Bicarbonate 209
Bile acid sequestrants 204
Bilirubin 165
Biopsy, endomyocardial 95
Bird's beak 289
Biting flies 243
Bladder 251

distended 197
  incontinence 156
Bleeding
  active 70
  control 338*f*
  diathesis 70
  external 91
  gastrointestinal 260
  identifying source of 91
  vaginal 270, 308
Blind spots 10
Blood 5, 189
  cultures 95
  disorders 56
  gases, arterial 36, 45, 62, 254, 367
  glucose 133
    levels 208
  loss of 90
  pressure 82, 107, 196, 211, 233, 266, 302, 333
    control 213
    dropping 239
    high 10
    low 264
    maintain 8
    systolic 10, 11
  tests 198
  transfusion of 93, 122*f*
  type 308
  urea nitrogen 165, 304
Body mass index 135
Body temperature 90
Bone 5
  cysts, aneurysmal 161
*Borrelia burgdorferi* 244*f*
Botulinum toxin 168
Botulism 165, 170
  diagnosis of 172
Bowel 156
  ischemic 83
  obstruction, large 83
Bradyarrhythmia 91
Bradycardia 7, 33, 166, 197, 198, 246
  persistent profound 43
Bradypnea 7
Brain 5, 69, 215
  abscess 258, 324
  astrocytomas 22
    frequency of 23*f*
  injury 197
    chronic traumatic 29
  matter 189
  neoplasms 24
  tumor 23*f*
Brainstem infection 170
Braunwald classification 79*t*
Breathing 100, 101, 331
  shortness of 39, 82, 216, 239

Bronchial lesions 59
Bronchitis 239
Bronchoconstriction 240
Bronchorrhea 246
Bronchospasm 246
Brugada syndrome 111
  types of 112*fc*
Bundle branch block 69
Bunny ear 36
Burns 90, 282, 331

**C**

Calcium 100, 372
  channel blocker 36, 167
  containing stones 349
  levels 325
  phosphate stones 349
  stones 351
Calf swelling 58
*Campylobacter jejuni* 174
Canabanoid hyperemesis syndrome 262
Canadian C-spine rule 20*f*
Cancer, active 58
Cannabis abuse 260
Carbamazepine 209
Carbon monoxide 253
  poisoning 253, 254*t*
Carbonic anhydrase inhibitor 377
Carboxyhemoglobin 253
Carcinoid syndrome 197
Carcinoma, esophageal 320
Cardiac arrest 99, 100*f*, 101*f*, 103*b*
  acute 102*f*
  outside hospital 104
Cardiac biomarkers 69, 75
  elevated 76
Cardiac death, sudden 39, 111
Cardiac enzymes, elevated 94
Cardiac monitoring 69, 227
Cardiomyopathy 39, 91, 260
Cardiovascular system 94, 126, 177
Catecholamine surge 259
Catheter
  directed therapy 43
  insertion 49*f*
C-collar 50
Ceftriaxone 278
Celebrex 354
Cement burns 267*f*
Centers for Disease Control and Prevention 243, 248, 281
Central nervous system 31, 249, 304, 324
  tumors 11
Central pulmonary veins, extrinsic compression of 34

Central retinal artery occlusion 376, 378
Central venous catheter site 324
Cephalosporin, third-generation 125
Cerebral
    abscess 184
    angiography 10
    contusion 29
    edema, reduce 8
    salt wasting 364
    spinal fluid 158
    vascular disease 165
    venous thrombosis 158, 159
Cerebrospinal fluid 12$f$, 172, 304, 332
Cerebrovascular accident 158
Cerebyx 354
Cervical
    arthritis 331
    motion tenderness 306
    spine
        anatomy of 19$f$
        injury 17, 20$f$
Cervix 144
Chest 31
    computed tomography 45
    discomfort 216
    imaging 62
    pain 65, 82, 216, 223
        causes of 66$fc$
        symptom of 259
    radiograph 95, 177, 210
    tube 49$f$
    wall 294
    X-ray 32, 34, 39, 44, 52, 53, 60, 61, 66, 77, 83, 95, 323, 330
*Chlamydia* 308
    *trachomatis* 270
Chlordiazepoxide 178
Chloroquine 168
Cholangiopancreatography, endoscopic retrograde 131
Cholangitis 136
    primary sclerosing 127
Cholecystectomy 136
    laparoscopic 136, 137$f$
Cholecystitis 271
    acute 135, 136, 136$f$
Cholecystostomy 136
Cholelithisasis 83
Cholinesterase enzyme permitting 247
Chronic obstructive pulmonary disease 33, 39, 45, 67, 85
Ciprofloxacin 278
Circulation 331
Citrus fruits 326
Clammy sweat 90
Clavulanic acid 128
Clindamycin 168
Clonazepam 217
Clonidine 354
C-loop, widening of 131
Clopidogrel 70, 71, 186
Coagulation 223
    abnormalities 146
Coagulopathy 1, 310
Cocaine 197
Codeine 241
Coffee
    bean sign 289$f$
    ground emesis 120
Cold 90
    agglutinin titer 95
    stimulus 158
Collagen vascular disease 34
Colloid 93
Colon cut-off sign 131
Colonoscopy 120
Colovaginal fistulae 129
Coma 16, 249, 254, 264
Compartment syndrome 339, 340$f$
Complete blood count 1, 45, 55, 83, 91, 94, 100, 114, 126, 130, 135, 162, 165, 192, 218, 233, 256, 275, 288, 308, 341, 353, 367
Comprehensive metabolic panel 126, 233, 256, 353
Compression 100
    external 158
    fracture, contralateral anteroposterior 335$f$
    lateral 335$f$
    ultrasound 40
Computed tomography 1, 6, 9, 13, 16, 21, 22, 26, 41$f$, 53, 61, 63$f$, 66, 83, 84$f$, 92$f$, 96, 114, 123, 124$f$, 127, 129, 130, 156, 158, 165, 166, 170, 177, 182, 192, 195, 210, 235, 275, 277, 314, 317, 330, 333, 346
    severity index 133$t$
Concussion 25, 27, 29
    symptom of 29
    syndrome 29
Condylomata acuminata 273$f$
Condylomata lata 273
Confusion 249, 254, 325
Conjunctivitis 375$f$, 377
Connective tissue disorders 10
Consciousness 294
    level of 182
    loss of 26, 157
Conservative method 8
Constipation 264
Constriction 91
Continuous positive airway pressure 62, 107
Contusion, pulmonary 44, 46$f$

Index

Convulsions 325
Cor pulmonale 39
Corneal abrasion 375*f*
Coronary angioplasty, percutaneous transluminal 75*f*, 76
Coronary artery
 bypass
  graft 67, 75*f*, 76
  surgery 71
 disease 74, 78, 82, 95, 108, 177
 vasospasm 94
Corticosteroids 109, 227, 228
Corticotropin-releasing hormone 213
Costochondritis 71, 75
Cough 240
Coumadin 354
Cramping, abdominal 246, 265
Cranial nerves 181
Craniofacial disorder 158
Craniotomy 4*f*
Cranium 158
C-reactive protein, elevated 94
Creatine kinase 215, 360
 muscle 69, 75, 215
 and brain 75, 94, 165
Creatine phosphokinase 304
Creutzfeldt-Jakob disease 184
Crisis, hypertensive 114*fc*, 203
Croup
 acute 291
 mild 294
Crystalloids, infusion of 308
Cullen sign 307*f*
Cyanosis 294
Cyclobenzaprine 352
Cyclophosphamide 167, 209
Cyclosporine 109, 167
Cystic fibrosis 59, 286
Cystine stones 351
Cytokines 287
Cytomegalovirus 374

## D

D-dimer 32, 39, 55, 58
 positive 39
 test 40
Deep tendon reflexes 55, 90, 165, 182
Deep venous thrombosis 38, 40, 55, 58
 Doppler ultrasound of 57*f*
 venograms of 57*f*
Degenerative disk disease 85*f*
Dehydration 205
Delirium 209, 249, 264
 tremens 174, 175, 373
Delusions 218
Dentition 331

Depression 16, 177
Dermatitis, exfoliative 90
Dexamethasone 204
Dextran 93, 222
Dextrose, intravenous 203
Diabetes 1, 74, 78
 mellitus 73
  non-insulin-dependent 82
Diaphoresis 73, 79, 177
Diarrhea 166, 251, 260, 346, 367
 symptom of 259
Diastolic dysfunction 331
Diazepam 178
Diazoxide 198
Dichlorodiphenyltrichloroethane 249
Diethylstilbestrol 308
Diphtheria 172, 238
Diplopia 168
Dipyridamole 186
Dirty fat 131
Disaster management 380
Disseminated intravascular coagulation 213, 259, 297, 341
Distal ureter 346
Distention, jugular venous 365
Distress
 abdominal 216
 gastrointestinal 246
Disulfiram 179
Diuretics 107, 328
Diverticular disease 83
Diverticulitis 123, 127, 128, 271
 acute 129
 complicated 129
 severe 124*f*
Diverticulum, true 128
Dizziness 26, 33, 223, 234, 249
Dobutamine 228
Dopamine 259
Dopaminergic neuron 260
Doppler flow 139
Doppler ultrasound 40
Dorsiflexion 39
Drawing blood 100
Drowsiness 26, 197, 234, 264
Drug abuse 216
Dry drowning 296
Dry mouth 264
Dry oral mucus 202
Dual energy radiographic absorptiometry 162
Dying, fear of 216
Dysarthria 182, 209
Dyspareunia 270
Dysphagia 317, 320
Dyspnea 39, 79, 239, 240, 317
Dysreflexia, autonomic 196

Dysrhythmia 91, 296
  cardiac 230, 325
  re-entry 331
  ventricular 118
Dystrophy, muscular 165
Dysuria 127

# E

Ear, nose and throat 126
  emergencies 310
Echocardiogram 95
  transesophageal 109
Echocardiography 32, 111
Ectopic pregnancy 271, 306, 307*f*
Eczema, venous 56*f*
Edema 5, 94
  acute pulmonary 203
  interstitial 64*f*
  laryngeal 239, 240
  origin of 62
  peripheral 239
  pitting 58
  pulmonary 39
  submucosal 347
Edrophonium 166
Ejection fraction 71
Electrical injury 229, 232*f*, 237*t*
Electrocardiogram 32, 35, 42*f*, 64, 69, 74, 77*f*, 82, 94, 96*f*, 100, 111, 183, 235, 356, 367
Electrocardiography 35, 53, 60, 62, 65*f*, 198, 215, 353
Electroencephalogram 192
Electroencephalography 193
Electrolyte 100, 165
  abnormalities 179
  balance 213
Electromyography 166, 172
Emergency eye wash tool 268*f*
Emergency medical services 22, 61, 208, 262, 333
Emergency room 9, 59, 64, 99, 106, 164, 174, 192, 215, 302, 304, 376
  care and disposition 212, 324, 372
  management 174
  treatment 278
Emesis 120
Emotional liability 26
Emphysema 39, 239
Encephalitis 184, 193, 258, 295, 324
Encephalopathy
  hepatic 184
  hypertensive 184
Endarterectomy, carotid 186
Endocarditis, bacterial 341
Endocrine 33, 201

Endometriosis 127
Endophthalmitis, traumatic 377
Endothelin receptor antagonists 37
Endotoxin 287
Endovascular therapies 186
Enzymes, cardiac 215, 233
Epididymo-orchitis 138
Epidural compression syndrome 155
Epidural hematoma 3, 3*f*, 4*f*, 6, 7*f*, 8, 29, 188*f*, 193, 295
  neurosurgical exposure of 7*f*
Epigastric discomfort 120
Epiglottitis 291
Epilepsy 1, 295
  type 193
Epinephrine
  administration 228
  autoinjector 242*f*
Episode, acute 217
Epistaxis 239, 310
  management of 311*fc*
Erythema migrans 243*f*
Erythrocyte sedimentation rate 94, 162, 271
Esophageal button battery 321*f*
Esophageal rupture 94
Esophageal spasm 94
Esophagitis 94
*European honey bee* 241*f*
Exercise 59
Extracorporeal membrane oxygenators 109
Extracorporeal shock wave lithotripsy 351
Extremities 31, 126, 170
Eye
  contact 249
  severe eye pain with redness of 377
Eyelid drooping 10

# F

Facet arthropathy, lumbar 161
Facial 29
Fasciculation 166
Fasciotomy procedure 340*f*
Fat embolism 39
Fatigue 26, 205
  generalized 79, 165
Febrile 201
  seizures 294
    complex 295*t*
Female reproductive system, anatomy of 271*f*
Femur fracture 280*f*
Fever 124*f*, 127, 145*f*, 273, 295, 317
  high 197
  history of 155
  neutropenic 323
Fibrillation, atrial 39, 185
Fibrinolysis 70

Fistula formation 129
Fitz-Hugh-Curtis syndrome 271
Flail chest, Computed tomography of 46*f*
Flank pain 127
Fleas 243
Flesh burns 232*f*
Fluid 179, 206
  and electrolytes, loss of 90
  loss 93
  restriction 210, 328
Flu-like symptoms 79
Fluoroquinolones 168
Focal neurologic signs 159
Forced expiratory volume 36
Fosphenytoin 196
Foul 127
  rhinorrhea 316
Fracture 282
  long-bone 91
  lumbar compression 160
Free ventricular wall 91
Fresh frozen plasma 330
Fungizone 354

## G

Gait 177
Gallbladder disease 71, 75
Gastric
  dilatation, acute 51
  ulcer, deep 121*f*
Gastritis 83, 94
Gastroesophageal reflux disease 59, 65, 75, 93, 130
Gastrointestinal
  abnormalities 273
  bleeding management, lower 122*fc*
  system 94
Glasgow Coma
  Scale 1, 6, 8, 14, 52
  Score 296
Glaucoma, acute 376
Glenohumeral joint dislocation 150
Glenoid rim fractures, anterior 151
Glioblastoma 22, 23*f*
  multiforme 22
Glomerular filtration rate 113, 370
Glucocorticoids 167, 173, 204, 212, 213
  intravenous 203
Glucose 100, 165
  serum 365
Glyceryl trinitrate 107
  intravenous 108
Glycoprotein 68, 70
Gonococcemia 341
Gonorrhea 308
Graves' disease 203

Greater tuberosity avulsion fracture 151
Guillain-Barré syndrome 169, 170, 173, 173*f*, 197
  clinical stages of 171*f*
  phases of 171*f*

## H

Hallucinations 179, 218
Halo sign, positive 313*f*
Haloperidol 219
Hantavirus pulmonary syndrome 64*f*
Head
  and neck 1, 202
  elevation 328
  eyes, ears, nose and throat 126, 158
  injury 184, 280*f*
  trauma 158, 197
Headache 5, 26, 52, 67, 90, 145, 157, 158, 197, 249, 273, 377
  atypical 22
  cluster 158
  different types of 24*f*
  frontal 254
  miscellaneous 158
  tension-type 158
  throbbing 254
  thunderclap 10
  types of 24*fc*
Heart
  disease
    atrial 34
    valvular 34, 109
    ventricular 34
  failure
    acute right 109
    congestive 39, 56, 59, 67, 75, 78, 85, 90, 97, 106, 110*fc*, 117, 177
  pounding 216
  rate, accelerated 216
  rhythm 103
  sounds 202
Heat
  emergency 256
  stroke 203
*Helicobacter pylori* 120, 121
Hemangiomas 161
Hemangiomatosis, pulmonary capillary 34
Hematemesis 120, 251
Hematochezia 120
Hematocrit 120, 207, 323
Hematoma 90
  postictal subdural 184
  septal 314
  subdural 1, 3, 3*f*, 4*f*, 8, 29, 188*f*
Hematuria 127
Hemicrania, chronic paroxysmal 158
Hemodialysis 325

Hemodynamics 107
Hemoglobin 120, 121
Hemoperitoneum 89, 90
Hemopneumothorax 50
    blood, chest X-ray for 51*f*
Hemoptysis 40, 239
Hemorrhage 92*f*, 93
    external 90
    internal 90
    intracranial 3*t*, 70
    ocular 198
    subarachnoid 3, 3*f*, 9, 11*f*, 15, 158, 159, 184, 188*f*, 197
    subconjunctival 375*f*
Hemothorax 90, 91
Heparin 185
    unfractionated 42, 70
Hepatic necrosis 260
Hepatitis 179, 273
Heroin abuse 262
Herpes simplex 374
Herpes zoster 374
Hiatal hernia 71, 75
High-tension pneumothorax needle 49*f*
Hinchey classification system 129
Hippocratic technique, modified 152, 152*f*
Histamine 226
    administration 228
Hoarse cry 294
Hoarseness 239
Homan's sign 39
Hormone 56
    adrenocorticotropic 211
    antidiuretic 208, 364
Human immunodeficiency virus 160, 272, 273, 344
    infection 34
Human papilomavirus 273*f*
Hydration 325
Hydrocarbon, chlorinated 249
Hydrocephalus 5
Hydrochlorothiazide 113, 157, 201, 356, 371
Hydrocortisone 212
Hydromorphone 354
Hydrostatic pressure, minimizing 328
Hydroxychloroquine 168
Hydroxyindoleacetic acid levels 226
Hyperaggression 179
Hyperbaric therapy, indications for 254
Hyperbilirubinemia 146
Hypercholesterolemia 79
Hyperemia, conjunctival 304
Hyperglycemia 72, 145, 184, 206
Hyperkalemia 325, 367, 369*f*
    causes of 367
    toxic levels of 367*f*
    treatment of 370*fc*

Hyperosmolar hyperglycemic nonketotic state 208*t*
Hyperphosphatemia 325
Hyperplasia
    benign prostatic 347
    thymic 166
Hyperpyrexia, severe 259
Hypersensitivity reaction 240
Hypertension 7, 64, 78, 79, 113, 177, 352
    arterial 33
    history of 74
    paroxysmal 197
    persistent pulmonary 34
    portal 34
    primary pulmonary 34
    pulmonary venous 34
    questionable 310
Hypertensive emergency 108, 113, 115*f*, 203
    causes of 115*fc*
    treatment of 115*fc*
Hyperthermia
    malignant 203, 258
    severe 179
Hyperthyroidism 216
Hypertrophy, ventricular 35, 35*f*
Hyperuricemia 325
Hyperventilation 8
Hypervolemia 364
Hypocalcemia 133, 184, 325
    symptomatic 326
Hypoglycemia 33, 184, 296
Hypokalemia 171, 356, 357
    symptom of 357*f*
Hypomagnesemia 371
    causes of 372*fc*
Hyponatremia 184, 208-210, 259, 361, 362*f*, 363
    causes of 210
    correction of 210
    degree of 210
    types of 363*fc*
Hypoperfusion 107
Hypophosphatemia 171
Hyporeflexia 209
Hyposmolality 208
Hypotension 107, 145*f*, 240, 254, 303
    arterial 145
    orthostatic 33
Hypothalamus-anterior-pituitary-ACTH pathway 213
Hypothermia 145
Hypothyroidism 210
Hypovolemia 331, 364
Hypoxemia 133
    arterial 146

# Index

## I

Idiopathic diseases 374
Iliopsoas compartment 92*f*
Immunoglobulin 222
   serum 172
Immunosuppression 272
Immunosuppressive therapy 167
Impression 127, 166, 170, 203, 240
In vitro fertilization 308
Indinavir stones 351
Infantile spasms 193
Infarction 5, 72
   inferior 73
Infections 5, 97, 347
   epidural 193, 295
   subdural 193, 295
Infectious diseases 341
Infectious Diseases Society of America 243
Inferior vena cava 58, 89
   filter 43
Inflammatory bowel syndrome 127
Inguinal hernia 138
Injury
   environmental 220
   heat related 256*t*
   levels of 18*f*
   mechanism of 8
   mild 15
   types of 237
Inotropes 107
Inotropic support 43
Inspired oxygen, fraction of 61, 62
Insulin 206
Integrase strand transfer inhibitors 274
Intensive care unit 371
International normalized ratio 58, 121
Intestinal spasms 264
Intra-aortic balloon pump 110
Intracranial disorder, nonvascular 158
Intracranial mass lesion 165
Intracranial pressure 3, 5, 9, 15, 160, 195
Intraosseous line 104
   placement 104
Intrauterine device 308
Intravenous Keppra levetiracetam 194
Intussusception 278, 283
   computed tomography scan of 285*f*
   management plan of 286*fc*
   operative management of 287*f*
Iodine 204
Iritis 376
Iron
   poisoning 250
   tablets 252*f*
   toxicity, stages of 251
Ischemia
   accurate test for 182
   myocardial 39
   recurrent 67
Itching 239
   symptoms 240

## J

Jelly stools 283
Jolt test, positive 159

## K

Kallikrein-kinin systems 223
Kerley B lines 64*f*
Ketoacidosis
   alcoholic 179
   diabetic 90, 205, 208*t*
Ketolides 168
Ketosis 206, 208
Kidney 251
   disease, chronic 113
   injury 238, 331
   stones 348, 349
Kiesselbach's plexus 310
Klonopin 354

## L

Lacrimation 246
Lactate dehydrogenase 95, 207
Lactic acidosis 325
Ladd's procedure 290
Lambert-Eaton syndrome 165, 168
Large infarction, large 73
Laryngomalacia 291
Laryngoscopy 320
Laryngotracheitis, acute 291
Laryngotracheobronchitis, acute 292
Left ventricular
   assist device 109, 116
   ejection fraction 76, 78
Leg pain 85*f*
   unilateral 39
Lethargy 249
Leukemia 325
   chronic myelogenous 324
Leukocytosis 128, 145, 165
Leukopenia 145
Lichtenberg figure 236*f*
Light aerobic exercise 30
Light bulb 154
Lightning injury 235, 237*t*
Limb paresis, asymmetric 170
Lip, edema of 233
Lipase 126, 130
Lipids 365
Lisinopril 157

Liver
   disease 177
   enzymes 207
   function test 165, 218
Lorazepam 178, 217, 219, 259
Lumbar puncture 158, 170, 177, 198
   locations 12$f$
Lung 39
   arteriovenous malformation 39
   contusion, right 51
   injury, acute 62
Lyme disease 190, 243, 244$f$, 245
   antibody titer 95

## M

Macroglossia 331
Maculopapular rash 273
Magnesium 100, 167
Magnetic resonance
   angiogram 10
   cholangiopancreatography 131
   imaging 10, 25, 85, 85$f$, 96, 156, 158, 162, 182, 198, 210, 332
Malaise 273
Malformation, arteriovenous 158
Malignancy 40, 56, 155
Mallory-Weiss syndrome 120
Mania 177
Marijuana
   abuse 260
   preparation 261$f$
Massive pulmonary embolism 43, 43$f$
Mastoid air cells fractures 5
Maxillary sinus nontender 240
Mean arterial pressure 10, 195
Mecamylamine 198
Meckel's diverticulitis 278
Mediastinitis, fibrosing 34
Medical expulsion therapy 351
Medical gallstone dissolution 136
Melanocyte stimulating hormone 213
Melena 89, 120
Memory 16, 177
Meningeal signs 159
Meningitis 193, 258, 295, 324
Meningococcal disease 343
   peripheral complications of 344$f$
Meningococcemia 341, 342$f$
Mental disorders
   diagnostic manual of 216
   statistical manual of 216
Mental status 5, 10, 145, 177, 202, 218, 246
Metabolic disorders 158
Metallic taste 224
Metaphyseal corner fractures 282
Metformin 157, 354

Methicillin-resistant *Staphylococcus aureus* 303
Methylprednisolone 240
Metronidazole 278, 354
Microstomia 331
Midazolam 259
Midgut volvulus 289
Migraine 158
   pulmonary 59
Mild sensory
   signs 172
   symptoms 172
Mineralocorticoids 212
Miosis 246
Missing sepsis 147
Mitochondrial myopathy 165
Mitral regurgitation 73
   murmur 94
Mitral stenosis 39, 91
Mitral valve prolapse 71, 75
Monobactam 125
Morphine 69, 107, 241, 354
Mosquito bites 243
Motor vehicle accident 14, 161, 331, 333
Motor weakness, major 156
Mucosa swollen 240
Mucous membranes 90, 304
Muffled voice 317
Muscle
   cramps 325
   spasticity 264
   weakness, generalized 209
Muscular dystrophy, oculopharyngeal 165
Myalgia 10, 265
Myasthenia 172
   gravis 166, 166$f$, 168$b$, 172
Myasthenic crisis, acute 167
Mycophenolate 167
Mycoplasma 132
Myelin sheath, destruction of 173$f$
Myelinolysis, extrapontine 366
Myelitis, transverse 170
Myocardial infarction 39, 53, 65, 78, 83, 88, 94, 108, 215, 296
   acute 80$f$, 113
   new classification of 73$f$
Myocardial perfusion imaging 72
Myocardial stiffness 331
Myocarditis 71, 75, 109
Myoclonus 209
Myopathy 171
Myxoma, atrial 91

## N

Naltrexone 179
Nasal
   cautery 313$f$

congestion 197
foreign body 316
    removal hook 317*f*
fracture 314, 315*f*
vascular anatomy 312*f*
Nasopharyngeal fragility 331
National Electronic Injury Surveillance
    System 300
National Institute of Allergy and Infectious
    Diseases 226
National Institute of Neurological Disorders
    and Stroke 193
National Stroke Association 189*f*
Nausea 5, 10, 166, 197, 216, 251, 346, 367, 377
    symptom of 259
Near drowning 296
Neck 158
    pain 11
    stiffness 10, 317
    veins 94
*Neisseria gonorrhoeae* 143, 270, 341, 342
*Neisseria meningitidis* 343*f*
    diplococcal bacteria, gram-negative 342*f*
Neoplasm 33, 97, 310
Neostigmine 167
Nephrolithiasis 83, 346
Nephrolithotomy, percutaneous 351
Nesiritide 107
Neuralgias 158
Neuroleptic malignant syndrome 197, 258
Neuromas, acoustic 190
Neuromuscular blocking agents 168
Neuropathy 177
    toxic 171, 172
Neuropsychiatric abnormalities 260
Neuropsychiatric testing, abnormal 254
Neuropsychologic testing 30
Nicotinic effects 246
Nifedipine 198
Nitrates 33, 71
Nitroglycerin 69, 198
    paste 68
Nitroprusside 107
Nitrous oxide 36
N-methyl-D-aspartate 175
Noncritical coronary stenosis 72
Non-Hodgkin's lymphoma 323
    high-grade 325
Noninvasive positive pressure ventilation 107
Non-nucleoside reverse transcriptase
    inhibitors 274
Nonsteroidal anti-inflammatory drugs 119,
    155, 222, 241, 332, 369
Non-ST-segment elevation myocardial
    infarction 74
    clinical management of 75*f*
Norepinephrine 108, 259

Novolin 354
Novolog 354
Nutrient artery 128
Nystagmus 177

## O

Obesity 56
Obstipation 128
Obstruction
    atherosclerotic 72
    coronary 72
    small-bowel 83
Ohm's law 231*f*
Oliguria, acute 146
Opioids 167, 222
Oral antibiotics 128
Oral calcium channel blockers 36
Oral injuries 282
Organ dysfunction 146
Organochlorine pesticides 249
Organophosphate 249
    poisoning 246
Orthopnea 239
Osmolality, serum 209
Osteoporosis 161
Ovarian cyst 127, 271
    ruptured 278
Oxcarbazepine 209
Oxygen 76, 130
    saturation 45
        maintenance of 107
    support 328

## P

Packed red blood cells 308
Pain 347
    abdominal 79, 124*f*, 127, 171, 251, 278,
        308, 367
    chronic 270
    control 69
    misdiagnosing lower-back 157
    musculoskeletal 83
    patterns 24*f*
Pallor 294
Palpitations 216, 239
    symptom of 259
Panbronchiolitis, diffuse 59
Pancolonic diverticula 128
Pancreas, normal 133
Pancreatic necrosis 133
Pancreatitis 83, 136, 177, 179
    acute 96*f*, 130
Panic attack 215, 240
Papillary muscle malfunction 73
Paralysis 58
    descending 170

extent of 18*f*
periodic 171
Paralytic ileus 131
Paraneoplastic disease 172
Paranoia 179
Paresis 58
Paresthesia 216, 367
Parkland formula 232*f*
Paroxysmal nocturnal dyspnea 239
Pelvic fractures 91, 333
    classification of 333
    lateral compression 333
    treatment of 337
Pelvic girdle 91
Pelvic hemorrhage, controlling 337
Pelvic inflammatory disease 127, 270, 278, 307
    pyrosalpinx in 272*f*
Penicillamine 168
Penicillins 239, 241
Peptic ulcer
    active 70
    disease 71, 75, 83, 94
Percutaneous coronary intervention 68, 69, 76, 109
Perfusion 40
    lung scan 32
Periappendiceal fat changes 277*f*
Pericardial disease 91
Pericardial friction rub 94
Pericardial tamponade 88
Pericardiocentesis 96, 97*f*
Pericarditis 39, 53, 71, 75, 93
    constrictive 96
    neoplastic 96
    restrictive 96
    staging 96
Pericardium 98*f*
Peripheral nervous system 197
Peritoneal cavity 91
Peritoneal lavage, diagnostic 332
Peritonitis, generalized 128
Pertussis 238
Phencyclidine 179
Phenothiazines 33, 167
Phenoxybenzamine hydrochloride 198
Phenytoin 241
Pheochromocytoma 203
Phlegmon, ill-defined fluid collection of 133
Phonophobia 26
Phosphate 207, 325
    deficiencies 372
Photophobia 10
Pinpoint pupils 264
Piperacillin 278
Placenta
    previa 304
    types of 305*f*

Plasma
    C-reactive protein 145
    glucose 145
    loss of 90
    osmolarity 365
Plasmapheresis 167
Plasminogen activator 183, 187
Platelets 126
Pleural cavity 91
Pleurisy 53
Pleuritis 71, 75
Pneumonia 39, 53, 97, 179, 239
Pneumothorax 33, 39, 47, 48, 50, 53, 71, 75
Poliomyelitis 170, 172
Polycystic kidney disease, history of 10
Polycythemia 56
Polydipsia 205
Polymerase chain reaction 144
Polymorphonuclear neutrophil 275
Polymyositis 170
Polyphagia 205
Polysomnography 36
Polyuria, classical symptoms of 205
Pontine myelinolysis, central 366
Porphyria 171
Porphyrin metabolism, abnormal 172
Positive end-expiratory pressure 47, 62, 63
Positron emission tomography 162
Posterior epistaxis, management of 311*fc*
Potassium 206, 372
    chloride 353
    iodide 204
    levels 234
    serum 212
    sparing diuretics 369
Pralidoxime chloride injections 248*f*
Prednisone 204
Pregnancy 272
Pressure
    central venous 257
    compression fracture, anterior 334
    jugular venous 31
Procainamide 167, 168
Profunda femoris vein 57*f*
Prominent systolic flow murmur 202
Propranolol 204
Propylthiouracil 204
Prostacyclin
    analogs 37
    intravenous 36
Protamine 222
Protease inhibitors 274
Pseudodiverticulum 128
Pseudohyperkalemia 368
Pseudohyponatremia 363
*Pseudomonas aeruginosa* 324
Psychiatric emergencies 215
Psychiatric issues 177

Psychosis 171, 217
Psychotropic drugs 33
Ptosis 168
   senile 165
Pubic rami 335*f*
Pubic ramus fracture 336*f*
Pulmonary arterial hypertension 34
   treatment of 37*fc*
Pulmonary embolism 33, 38-40, 53, 58, 59, 71, 75, 88, 94, 215
   colored computed tomography 42*f*
   computed tomography 41
Pulmonary function test 32, 36
Pulmonary hypertension 31, 33, 39, 91
   diagnosis of 33
Pulmonary veno-occlusive disease 34
Pulse
   rate 73
   symmetry of 21
Pump failure 91
Pupillary size 126, 170, 202
Pure calcium phosphate stones 349
Pure matrix stones 351
Pyelogram, intravenous 371
Pyelonephritis 83, 127, 271
Pyoderma gangrenosum 127
Pyridostigmine 167
Pyuria 127

## Q

Quinidine 168
Quinine 168
Quinolones 241
Q-wave 76

## R

Radioactive albumin 41
Ramsay Hunt syndrome 190
Randomized controlled trials 160, 346
Range of motion 126, 157
Ranson's criteria 133*b*
Ranson's CT severity index 132
Rapid bolus injection 69
Rectum 144, 197
Red blood cell 91, 158, 246
Red eye 374
   diagnosis of 375*t*
   symptom of 375*t*
Renal dysfunction, preexisting 325
Renal emergencies 346
Renal failure 260
   acute 325
   post-treatment 325
Renal function 365
Renin angiotensin-aldosterone system 369
Repetitive nerve stimulation 165

Respiration 31, 51, 126, 209
Respiratory 33, 223, 237, 239
   equipment 100
   failure 254
      impending 294
   findings 224
   rate 90
   system 94
Resuscitation, cardiopulmonary 38, 99, 102, 104, 116, 235, 300
Reteplase 69
Retinal detachment 376
Rhabdomyolysis 171, 260
   nephrology for 238
Rhesus 308
Rheumatoid arthritis 143
Rh-immunoglobulin 5
Rhinitis 265
Rhino rocket applicator and packing 312*f*
Rhinorrhea 239
Rib fractures 45, 46*f*
Richmond agitation-sedation scale 61
Right bundle branch block 35
Right ventricular assistive device 116
Ringer's lactate 227
Road traffic accidents 56
Rocky mountain spotted fever 341
Rotator cuff tears 151
Rule of nine 232*f*

## S

Sacral fracture 336*f*
Sacroiliac complex 336*f*
Sacroiliac ligaments, complete disruption of 336*f*
Saddle anesthesia 156
Saline, normal 61, 174, 302, 303, 371
Salivation 246
Salpingitis 308
Sarcoidosis 34, 172
Schistosomiasis 34
Schizophrenia 218
Sclera icterus 126
Sclerosis, multiple 184
Segmental wall motion abnormalities 95
Seizures 10, 254
   complex 33
   differential diagnosis of 193, 295
   disorders 192, 194
   epileptic 184
   generalized 209
   symptom of 259
Selective serotonin reuptake inhibitor 209
Sensation, loss of 10
Sensory loss, perianal 156
Sensory syndrome 172
Sentinel loop 131

Sepsis  127, 193, 203, 258, 295
    diagnostic management of  146*f*
Septal hypertrophy, asymmetric  33
Septic arthritis  143
    X-ray of  144*f*
Serial electrocardiograms  45
Serotonergic neuron  260
Serotonin
    release  259
    syndrome  197
Serum glutamic
    oxaloacetic transaminase  304
    pyruvic transaminase  304
Serum lactate  145
Sexually transmitted
    diseases  306
    infections  138, 270, 273
Sheehan syndrome  213
Shock  91
    anaphylactic  91
    cardiogenic  39, 91
    distributive  90, 91
    hemorrhagic  88, 92*t*
    hypovolemic  90, 92*t*
    neurogenic  90, 91
    obstructive  90, 91
    septic  91, 203
Shockwave lithotripsy  351
Shoulder
    dislocation, types of  151*fc*
    X-ray of  149*f*, 151*f*
Sigmoid colon  128
Sigmoid malignancy  127
Simple febrile seizure  295*t*
Sinus  5, 158
    disease  59
    node disorders  33
Sinusitis  59, 314
Skeletal injury  237
Skin  90, 126, 249
    color changes  197
    examination  170
    turgor  205
Skull fracture  29, 165
Sleep
    apnea, obstructive  36
    disturbance  26
    study  36
Sodium
    bicarbonate  207
    continued renal exertion of  210
    hydroxide  267
    serum  212, 362
Soft-tissue compartments  91
Solitary toxic adenoma  203
Sore throat  239
Spasmodic croup  292

Speech
    incoherent  26
    slurred  26
Sphincterotomy, endoscopic  136
Spinal cord
    compression  170
    injuries  197, 296, 332
Spinal stenosis  155
Spiral computed tomography  39, 40
Splenectomy  56
Spondylolisthesis  161
Spondylolysis, lumbar  161
Spontaneous pneumothorax  53, 54
    pathophysiology of  54*t*
    presentation of  54*t*
    progression diagnosis of  54*t*
    treatment of  54*t*
Spontaneous ureteral stone expulsion  348*f*
Sporadic disorder  34
Sputum  239
Squeezing  65
*Staphylococcus aureus*  143, 304, 324
Steeple sign  293*f*
Stiffness  11, 197
Stigmata  177
Stimson's technique  152, 153, 153*f*
Stones, types of  349, 350*fc*
Streptokinase  44
    contraindications of  70
Stridor  317
Stroke  10, 33, 180
    golden hour of acute ischemic  184
    ischemic  70
    types of  183*fc*
    warning signs of  189*f*
ST-segment elevation myocardial infarction
        64, 67, 77
Stupor  249
Subarachnoid space  13*f*
Substance abuse  258
Sudden infant death syndrome  111
Sulbactam  318
Superficial veins, collateral  58
Superior iliac spine, anterior  276
Superior vena cava  326
    syndrome  39, 326, 327*f*
Sweating  58, 197, 216, 265
    excessive  90
Swelling
    cloudy  250
    periorbital  242*f*
Symphysis, slight widening of  335*f*
Syncope  31, 33, 76, 166, 223, 240, 254, 296
    neurogenic  314
Syndrome of inappropriate secretion of
        antidiuretic hormone  208
Synovial fluid analysis  147*f*

Syphilis 273, 374
Systemic inflammatory response syndrome 130, 147
Systemic lupus erythematosus 143

## T

Tachyarrhythmia 91, 203
Tachycardia 90, 177, 179, 198, 240, 294
   supraventricular 33
   ventricular 33, 76, 230
Tachydysrhythmia 67
Tachypnea 145, 177
Tamponade 91
Tazobactam 278
Tenecteplase 69
Tension pneumothorax 47, 54, 91
   left 51
   pathophysiology of 54$t$
   presentation of 54$t$
   progression diagnosis of 54
   treatment of 54
Test tubes 12$f$
Testicle, torsion of 139$f$
Testicular torsion 138, 140$f$
   treatment of 140$fc$
   types of 139$fc$
Tetanus 238
Tetany 325
Thoracic-lumbar-sacral orthosis 162
Thoracoscopy, video-assisted 53
Throat, inflammation of 318$f$
Thrombectomy 43
   mechanical 186, 186$f$
Thrombocytopenia 1, 146, 165
Thrombolysis 43, 79
Thrombolytics 44
   benefits 44
   therapy 184$f$
Thrombosis 56, 239
Thymoma 166
Thyroid 202
   function 365
   stimulating hormone 202
      level 218
   storm 201, 203
Tick bites 243
Tidal volume 61
Tissue
   perfusion variables 146
   plasminogen activator 43, 68, 90
Tongue
   angioedema affecting 234$f$
   discoloration 264
   edema of 233
Tonsillar enlargement 240
Topiramate 179
Toradol 354

Total iron binding capacity 251
Total parenteral nutrition 133, 358
Toxic multinodular goiter 203
Toxic shock syndrome 302, 303$b$, 304, 304$b$, 314, 341
   typical rash of 303$f$
Toxicology 220
Toxoplasmosis 374
Traction-counter-traction technique 152, 152$f$
Tramadol 354
Transcatheter aortic valve implantation 109
Transcranial Doppler ultrasounds 10
Transient ischemic attack 165
Transthoracic echo 96
Trauma 56, 177, 179
   focused abdominal sonography for 332
Traumatic brain injury 14, 15, 27$f$
   conta sports-related 16
   major causes of 15$f$
Trazodone 354
Tremors 177, 209
*Treponema pallidum* 273
Tricyclic antidepressant 33
Troponin 45, 69, 165, 233
Tuberculosis 97, 213, 239, 374
Tubular necrosis, acute 132
Tumor 34, 184
   cardiac 91
   lysis syndrome 324
   testicular 138
T-wave 183, 356
   normalization of 96
Tympanic membrane rupture 237

## U

Ulcer
   corneal 377
   perforated 83
Ultrasound 131
Unstable angina 68, 72, 75, 77
   Braunwald classification of 79$t$
Upper airway
   anteroposterior radiograph of 293$f$
   normal anteroposterior radiograph of 292$f$
Upper extremity, right 181
Upper gastrointestinal bleed 119
Upper quadrant, right 130, 284
Uremia 171
Ureteral muscle spasm 347
Ureteral stones, tamsulosin for 346
Ureterolithiasis 346
Ureters 251
Urethra 144
Uretoscopy 351
Uric acid 325

blood levels 350*f*
crystals 350*f*
  formation of 350*f*
levels, reduce 326
stones 351
Urinalysis 126, 130, 165, 177, 218, 275
Urinary 5-hydroxyindoleacetic acid 226
Urinary frequency 127
Urinary tract infection 83, 127
Urine
  cloudy 127
  culture 192
  osmolality 209
  sodium 365
  tests 198
Urokinase 44
Urticaria, acute 241
Uveitis
  acute 375*f*
  anterior 376, 377
U-wave 356

## V

Vaginal discharge 270
Vague abdominal pain 39
Valproic acid, intravenous 194
Valvular disease 95
  obstructive 91
Valvular dysfunction, acute 91
Vancomycin 168, 222
Varicose veins 239
Vascular disorders 158
Vasculitic neuropathies 172
Vasculitis 341
  risk of 260
Vasoactive systems 223
Vasodilator 33, 107
  challenge, acute 37*fc*
  drugs 91
Vasodilatory test, acute 36
Vasopressin 209, 366, 370
Vasovagal reflex 33
Vein, femoral 57*f*
Ventilation 32, 40, 101, 331
Ventricles 5, 189
Ventricular assistive device 116
Ventricular septum, rupture of 91
Vertebroplasty, transcutaneous 162*f*

Vesicle fistulae 129
Vienna Concussion Conference 29
Vinblastine 354
Vincristine 354
Viral infection 286
Vision 16
  blurred 197
  double 10
  halo around 377
  loss 10
    differential diagnosis of 378*fc*
Visual disturbances 26
Vital signs 90, 177, 202, 331
Vitamin $B_{12}$ level 218
Vocal cord dysfunction 59, 291
Volume depletion, absence of clinical
    evidence of 210
Vomiting 5, 10, 79, 127, 225, 251, 346, 367, 377
  symptom of 259
von Willebrand disease 328, 329*f*

## W

Water and electrolyte imbalance 356
Water ice therapy 258
Waterhouse-Friderichsen syndrome 213, 342
Weak pulses 264
Weakness
  abdominal 171
  extreme 16
Weight
  heparin, low-molecular 43, 58
  loss 127
  low-molecular 223
Well's criteria 40*t*, 58*b*
Well's score 58*b*
Wernicke-Korsakoff syndrome 179, 184
Wheezing 239, 240, 296
White blood cell 123, 126, 135, 143, 271, 275
  count 271
White cell casts 127
Willis tower 235*f*
World Health Organization's Diagnostic
    Classification of Pulmonary
    Hypertension 34*b*

## X

Xanthochromia 12*f*

EU GSPR Authorised Reprsentative
Logos Europe, 9 rue Nicolas Poussin
1700, La Rochelle, France
Phone: +33 (0) 6 67 93 73 78
E-mail: contact@logoseurope.eu

www.ingramcontent.com/pod-product-compliance
Ingram Content Group UK Ltd.
Pitfield, Milton Keynes, MK11 3LW, UK
UKHW051922060825
461530UK00006B/76